Drug Therapy in Infants and Children with Cardiovascular Diseases

Drug Therapy in Infants and Children with Cardiovascular Diseases

Adam Schneeweiss, M.D.
Heart Institute
The Chaim Sheba Medical Center
Tel Hashomer, Israel

Lea & Febiger 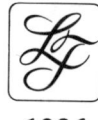 Philadelphia

1986

Lea & Febiger
600 Washington Square
Philadelphia, PA 19106-4198
U.S.A.
(215) 922-1330

Library of Congress Cataloging in Publication Data

Schneeweiss, Adam.
　Drug therapy in infants and children with cardiovascular diseases.

　Includes bibliographies and index.
　1. Cardiovascular agents.　2. Cardiovascular system—
Diseases—Chemotherapy.　3. Pediatric cardiology.
I. Title.　[DNLM: 1. Cardiovascular Agents—therapeutic
use.　2. Cardiovascular Diseases—drug therapy.
3. Cardiovascular diseases—in infancy & childhood.
QV 150 S358db]
RJ424.5.C47S36　1985　　618.92'12061　　85-10384
ISBN 0-8121-1001-3

Copyright © 1986 by Lea & Febiger. Copyright under the International Copyright Union. All rights reserved. This book is protected by copyright. *No part of it may be reproduced in any manner or by any means without written permission from the publishers.*

PRINTED IN THE UNITED STATES OF AMERICA

Print No.　4　3　2　1

PREFACE

Twenty-five years ago, when extensive research into pediatric cardiovascular drug therapy had begun, few agents were available to the cardiologist and even fewer to the pediatric cardiologist. Pediatric cardiovascular therapy consisted almost exclusively of digitalis glycosides and diuretic agents. Quinidine and procainamide were the only antiarrhythmic drugs available. Adult cardiologists used also nitrates, hydralazine, and beta-blockers, which had just been introduced into clinical use. Some centrally acting antihypertensive drugs were also available. The alpha-adrenoreceptor blockers known at that time were not suitable for clinical use.

Since then, cardiovascular drug therapy has progressed. New positive inotropic drugs, including sympathomimetic amines, bipyridine derivatives, and other agents, are used clinically and investigationally. Class I antiarrhythmic agents now include, in addition to quinidine and procainamide, about ten other drugs that are routinely used. Moreover, a new class of antiarrhythmic agents, Class III, was developed, including some effective agents such as amiodarone, and these are widely used in adults as well as in children. In the group of beta-adrenoreceptor blockers, propranolol is still widely used; however, modern agents with ancillary properties that partially overcome the disadvantages of beta-blockers are available. The short and sad episode of practolol, a selective beta-blocker that caused severe side effects diagnosed late after initiation of therapy, left some bad feelings, but safe and effective beta-1-selective adrenoreceptor blockers, such as atenolol, are now available. Beta-adrenoreceptor blockers with intrinsic sympathomimetic activity, such as pindolol, are considered to be safer than beta-blockers devoid of this property in patients with pulmonary or peripheral vascular diseases.

Several direct-acting vasodilators are now used in treatment of cardiovascular diseases in infants and children. For example, nitroprusside and hydralazine are used for hypertension or congestive heart failure. Modern alpha-adrenoreceptor blockers such as prazosin are also used. Perhaps the most important achievement of cardiovascular drug therapy in the past 25 years has been the development of calcium antagonists. These agents have changed the treatment of hypertension, ischemic heart disease, and certain cardiomyopathies and arrhythmias. One of these agents, verapamil, is widely used in infants and children for treatment of supraventricular arrhythmias.

Angiotensin-converting-enzyme inhibitors were developed and introduced for treatment of systemic hypertension and congestive heart failure. One of these agents, captopril, has been used in children, primarily for treatment of hypertension. In children, there is perhaps an optimal indication for captopril—coarctation of the aorta with high-renin hypertension and congestive heart failure. Several new centrally acting antihypertensive agents have been developed, and some of these have also been tried in children.

Thus, cardiovascular drug therapy has undergone revolutionary changes in the past 25 years. It appears that most of this progress is applicable to pediatric cardiovascular therapy because most indications for treatment in adults may be found also in children. Nonetheless, the introduction of new achievements to cardiovascular drug therapy in infants and children has been slow and this has been attributed to the conservative approach of pediatric cardiologists as well as to the known difficulties of introduction of any new drug into pediatric practice.

It is the purpose of this book to summarize the experience gained in the use of modern cardiovascular drugs in infants and children. Unlike in adults, only part of the pediatric knowledge in the field is based on well-controlled studies. The remaining is based on isolated case reports and on open studies. In many cases, the experience in adults has been used and interpolated for children. In addition to summarizing the experience in children, I have tried also to discuss new achievements in adult cardiovascular therapy and some new drugs that have not yet been used in children. This discussion is important in presenting pediatric cardiologists with new possibilities and in stimulating research and clinical use of these drugs.

Tel Hashomer, Israel   Adam Schneeweiss

CONTENTS

Section I. **Positive Inotropic Agents** 1
  Chapter 1. *Digitalis Glycosides* 3
          2. *Dopamine* 35
          3. *Dobutamine* 43
          4. *(Isoproterenol) Isoprenaline* 51
          5. *Bipyridine Derivatives* 55
Section II. **Calcium Antagonists** 61
  Chapter 6. *Verapamil* 63
          7. *Nifedipine* 85
          8. *Diltiazem* 95
Section III. **Vasodilators** 105
  Direct-Acting Vasodilators 107
  Chapter 9. *Hydralazine* 107
          10. *Nitroprusside* 121
          11. *Nitroglycerin* 133
          12. *Minoxidil* 137
          13. *Diazoxide* 145
  Alpha-Adrenoreceptor Blocking Agents 149
  Chapter 14. *Prazosin* 149
          15. *Tolazoline* 157
  Agents Affecting the Renin-Angiotensin System 159
  Chapter 16. *Captopril* 161
          17. *Saralasin* 179
Section IV. **Beta-Adrenoreceptor Blocking Agents** 181
  Chapter 18. *Propranolol* 189
          19. *Other Beta-Adrenoreceptor Blocking Agents* 219
Section V. **Antiarrhythmic Agents** 233
  Chapter 20. *Quinidine* 237
          21. *Procainamide* 245
          22. *Disopyramide* 255
          23. *Lidocaine* 261
          24. *Phenytoin* 265
          25. *Mexiletine* 275
          26. *Flecainide* 285
          27. *Propafenone* 287
          28. *Ethmozin* 301
          29. *Amiodarone* 305

30. *Bretylium Tosylate* 327
31. *Adenosine and Adenosine Triphosphate* 331

Section VI. **Prostaglandins and Prostaglandin-Synthesis Inhibitors** 337
  Chapter 32. *Prostaglandin E* 341
  33. *Prostacyclin* 359
  34. *Indomethacin* 365

Section VII. **Centrally Acting Antihypertensive Agents** 377
  Chapter 35. *Clonidine* 379
  36. *Methyldopa* 385

Index 389

Section I
POSITIVE INOTROPIC AGENTS

Positive inotropic agents are used in patients with congestive heart failure or those in shock, to improve hemodynamics by enhancement of myocardial contractility. The concept of enhancing myocardial contractility in patients with hemodynamic deterioration appears logical, but it has several drawbacks: (1) the failing heart is already stimulated by compensatory mechanisms such as sympathetic activation, and further stimulation often does not enhance contractility; (2) if a considerable portion of the myocardium is damaged, then stimulation of the remaining may extend the damage, up to mechanical complications such as perforation; (3) an increase in contractility not associated with a decrease in other determinants of oxygen consumption increases the myocardial oxygen demand, and in patients with coronary artery disease, myocardial ischemia may be enhanced by this mechanism; and (4) most positive inotropic agents available for clinical use have an arrhythmogenic potential.

Despite all these disadvantages, under some conditions no alternative exists to the administration of positive inotropic agents. The positive inotropic agents available for clinical use may be classified as follows: (1) digitalis glycosides, acting by the sodium-potassium adenosine triphosphatase (Na-K ATPase) system; (2) sympathomimetic amines, including isoproterenol, dopamine, and dobutamine, acting by stimulation of adrenoreceptors and possibly also other specific receptors; (3) bipyridine derivatives such as amrinone and milrinone, acting possibly by inhibition of phosphodiesterase; and (4) glucagon. The first three groups are used in infants and children and are discussed in the following chapters.

Several problems may complicate the use of positive inotropic agents in infants and children. Some infants and children, such as those with primary endomyocardial diseases, may require continuous treatment for longer than 10 years. The immature heart of low-birth-weight neonates and even small infants may respond to these agents differently from the mature myocardium of older patients. Such is the case with amrinone. A high proportion of infants and children with congestive heart failure have congenital cardiac anomalies with mechanical disturbances. Most of the studies of positive inotropic agents were performed in adults without such disturbances. It is not clear whether data obtained in these studies may be extrapolated to infants and children with congenital heart diseases. These problems are further discussed in the following chapters.

Chapter 1

Digitalis Glycosides

Digitalis glycosides have been used for treatment of heart diseases for about 200 years. They are effective mainly in patients with congestive heart failure and certain arrhythmias. Digitalis glycosides are the most widely used positive inotropic agents and the only such agents used for long-term treatment of congestive heart failure in infants and children. In treatment of arrhythmias, digitalis glycosides are effective mainly in controlling the ventricular rate in cases of atrial fibrillation or flutter and in terminating supraventricular tachycardia. The digitalis glycosides most widely used in children are digoxin and digitoxin. In this chapter, the features of these drugs are described together, except for the section on clinical pharmacology, in which they are discussed separately.

Several problems are unique to the use of digitalis glycosides in the pediatric population. For example, the resting level of myocardial function in the neonate is higher than in the adult,[1] and it is not clear whether digitalis glycosides can further enhance contractility. The pharmacokinetic profile of digoxin in premature neonates differs from that in older children and in adults. Accidental ingestion of high doses of digitalis glycosides is common in young children. On the other hand, under certain conditions, digitalis glycosides are the drug of choice in infancy but not at older ages. For example, in adults with Wolff-Parkinson-White syndrome and reentrant arrhythmias, digitalis glycosides are contraindicated, whereas in neonates and small infants with this disease, they are the drugs of choice.

Mechanism of Action

The positive inotropic effect of digitalis glycosides is exerted by inhibition of the membrane sodium-potassium adenosine triphosphatase, which supplies energy for maintenance of cation balance across the cell membrane. This process causes an increase in intracellular concentration of sodium and, as a result, of calcium as well. The increase in intracellular calcium concentration enhances myocardial contractility.[2] The validity of this theory has been questioned, but other suggested mechanisms have not been confirmed.

Hemodynamic Effects

The primary hemodynamic effect of digitalis glycosides is the positive inotropic effect. This phenomenon has been directly demonstrated by application of digitalis glycosides to isolated myocardial strips, both ventricular and atrial. The increase in cardiac output resulting from the positive inotropic effect may have various secondary effects. For example, an increase in cardiac output from enhanced contractility can result in sympathetic withdrawal and a decrease in peripheral vascular resistance. This process is, at least partially, opposed by a direct peripheral vasoconstricting effect of the drug. It is still controversial whether digitalis glycoside can enhance the contractility of the normal heart as well as that of the failing heart. In patients with congestive heart failure, the increase in cardiac output results in a decrease in the elevated left ventricular filling pressure and the increased cardiac volumes.

Digitalis elevates the systemic arterial pressure because of increases in cardiac output and systemic vascular resistance. Digitalis has also a direct venoconstricting effect.[3] Almost all studies show acute hemodynamic improvement in patients with congestive heart failure after short-term administration of digitalis. The effect of long-term digitalis therapy is controversial. It has been evaluated mainly by withdrawal studies, in which hemodynamic measurements are performed during and after discontinuance of long-term treatment with digitalis glycosides.

The most widely quoted study that shows a sustained beneficial effect of long-term digoxin treatment in patients with congestive heart failure was reported by Arnold and associates in 1980.[4] These workers studied 9 patients with congestive heart failure and sinus rhythm. After discontinuance of prolonged digoxin treatment, the patients' hemodynamic status deteriorated, as noted by decreases in cardiac index (from 2.4 ± 0.7 to 2.1 ± 0.6 L/min/m^2), ejection fraction, stroke volume index, and stroke work index, as well as by an increase in pulmonary capillary wedge pressure from 21 ± 8 to $29 \pm$ mm Hg. After readministration of digoxin, sudden hemodynamic improvement was observed. In most patients, symptomatic worsening accompanied the hemodynamic deterioration.

Opposing data were reported by Gheorghiade and Beller,[5] who studied 24 patients with congestive heart failure and sinus rhythm. Discontinuance of long-term treatment with digoxin resulted in no hemodynamic or clinical deterioration. Contrasting data were obtained in several other studies. Withdrawal studies were not performed in children.

My colleagues and I have encountered six episodes of abrupt discontinuance of digitalis in five children with primary endocardial fibroelastosis and congestive heart failure. In five of these episodes, congestive heart failure was worsened, or, if it had disappeared during treatment, it developed again on discontinuance of digitalis. In patients with atrial fibrillation and congestive heart failure, digitalis is definitely effective, in part because of regulation of the ventricular response. This finding is of little relevance in children with congestive heart failure, however, because they are usually in sinus rhythm.

From my experience and that of my colleagues and from a review of the literature, I conclude that the beneficial effect of digitalis glycosides is usually sustained throughout long periods of treatment in patients of all ages with congestive heart failure.

Renal Function

Digitalis increases cardiac output and reduces the sympathetic tone in patients with congestive heart failure. Both these effects can contribute to improvement of renal function. Withdrawal studies in patients with congestive heart failure showed that renal function deteriorates when long-term treatment with digitalis is discontinued.[4]

Effect of Age on Inotropic Response

Age is an important determinant of the response to digitalis glycosides. It has a significant implication on the use of digitalis in the pediatric age group. In most mammalian species, the sensitivity to the inotropic and toxic effects of digitalis glycosides in the neonatal period is different from that in young adulthood.[6-9] These differences have been attributed to variations in the effects of these agents at the cellular level,[10-12] as well as to maturational changes in the volume of distribution.[13,14] The differences are not attributable to different plasma concentrations because these concentrations are similar in animal neonates and in adults treated with digoxin.[12] The metabolism of digoxin and its protein binding do not vary with age, and the differences in effect cannot be thus explained.[15,16]

Because of the reduced effect of these drugs in newborn infants, these patients are treated routinely with higher doses of digoxin per kilogram of body weight than adults. These higher doses are controversial because they raise problems of tolerance.

Endocardial Fibroelastosis

My colleagues and I have reviewed a series of 49 infants and children with the dilated form of primary endocardial fibroelastosis. All were under 2 years of age when first diagnosed. Because endomyocardial biopsies were not performed, it may be questioned whether some of these patients had congestive cardiomyopathy rather than endocardial fibroelastosis. It was not considered justified to perform a biopsy that would have no therapeutic implications, however. Diagnosis was based on the following criteria: (1) congestive heart failure in the first 2 years of life; (2) electrocardiographic signs of left ventricular hypertrophy with inversion or flattening of T-waves in leads V_5 to V_6; (3) a dilated, poorly contracting left ventricle visible angiocardiographically (ejection fraction less than 0.4); (4) the absence of shunts; and (5) the absence of pressure gradients across the aortic and pulmonary valves.

The patients were followed for 4 months to 12 years. Ten patients were lost from follow-up. The remaining 39 were treated with digitalis from the time of diagnosis and for several years thereafter; the longest period of treatment was 9 years. Eleven of the 39 patients died; 2 of them, siblings, died suddenly, 7 died of severe congestive heart failure, and 2 died at home of unknown causes. Twenty-eight patients are alive after 1 to 9 years of treatment with digitalis and show clinical improvement. Several of these patients who were treated for at least 5 years stopped taking digitalis and were apparently cured, at least clinically. These findings suggest that continued treatment with digitalis for several years may change the natural course of primary endocardial fibroelastosis.

To evaluate the late consequences in these clinically "cured" patients, I studied, by serial cardiac catheterization, 8 patients with the dilated form of primary endocardial fibroelastosis in whom congestive heart failure disappeared with treatment.[17] All patients had been asymptomatic for at least 3 years before the second cardiac catheterization. No patients were receiving digoxin at the time of repeated catheterization. Four patients showed regression of the abnormal electrocardiographic findings, 3 showed persistence, and 1 showed progression of left ventricular hypertrophy. In 6 of the patients, repeated cardiac catheterization showed left ventricular dilatation with poor contraction (mean ejection fraction 0.32). Left ventricular end-diastolic pressure was elevated, up to 28 mm Hg. Only 2 of these patients, with regression of the abnormal electrocardiographic findings, had no abnormal findings at repeated catheterization. The highest left ventricular end-diastolic pressure was found in a patient in whom the abnormal electrocardiogram almost reverted to normal.

These findings indicate that treatment with digitalis can cause clinical improvement in patients with the dilated form of primary endocardial fibroelastosis. The "cure" is incomplete, however. The abnormal findings may explain some of the cases of sudden death or late clinical deterioration in patients with "cured" primary endocardial fibroelastosis. The electrocardiogram is of little value in assessing these processes. Echocardiography may be useful for follow-up of the children throughout the period of treatment.

Left-to-Right Shunt and Congestive Heart Failure

In infants and children, symptoms of heart failure may follow circulatory congestion. This condition results from hemodynamic consequences of anatomic defects, usually ventricular septal defect or patent ductus arteriosus. In this condition, volume overload of the heart causes symptoms and signs of congestive heart failure, in the presence of normal myocardial contractility.

Traditional medical management of infants and children with circulatory congestion consists of the administration of diuretic agents and digitalis glycosides.[18, 19] Stimulation of myocardial contractility may improve the hemodynamic condition, although the myocardium is basically normal. The distinction between congestive heart failure and circulatory congestion is rarely made by pediatric cardiologists, and the usual treatment of infants and children with both conditions includes digitalis glycosides.

Several studies have demonstrated that infants with circulatory congestion do not show hemodynamic improvement after inotropic stimulation, however.[17, 20, 21] This finding suggests that digitalis glycosides may not be useful in infants with circulatory congestion due to a large left-to-right shunt. Because some infants show hemodynamic improvement and others show clinical improvement even in the absence of hemodynamic improvement, however, the question whether or not to use digitalis glycosides in infants with this condition is not settled. For example, Berman and colleagues studied the effect of digoxin in 21 infants (mean age 2.7 months, mean weight 3.8 kg) with ventricular septal defect.[22] The dose of digoxin was individually adjusted, and therapeutic plasma concentrations were achieved in all cases. Only 6 of the 21 infants had an inotropic response, as reflected by echocardiographic indices of contractility. In these 6 infants, as well as in 6 others without such response, the drug was of clinical benefit. These results show that only a minority of infants with circulatory congestion and symptoms of heart failure benefit hemodynamically from digoxin therapy. Those who do improve hemodynamically, as well as several others, show clinical improvement, however.

Selection of infants for treatment with digoxin may be improved if the distinction between heart failure and circulatory congestion is made. For example, White and Lietman stated that myocardial contractility is normal in most infants with left-to-right shunt, the symptoms reflect circulatory congestion, and digitalis is of little value in the management of these infants.[23] Also important are the studies of O'Rourke and associates, who evaluated the effect of digitalis in dogs with chronic volume overload caused by a surgically created aortocaval fistula.[24] These investigators did not observe any hemodynamic alteration produced by digoxin, whereas nitroprusside produced hemodynamic improvement.

In my opinion, it is still controversial whether myocardial contractility is normal or even supernormal in infants with left-to-right shunt or whether it is depressed. Several studies have shown that ejection fraction, systolic time intervals, velocity of circumferential fiber shortening, and other indices of cardiac performance suggest normal or improved contractility.[21, 25, 26] Because afterload is reduced in these infants, however, the improved myocardial performance cannot be attributed directly to enhanced contractility.

If it is accepted that contractility is normal, then the role of digitalis is questionable. Digitalis may, to a limited extent, enhance the contractility of normal myocardium and may have various other effects on conduction and vascular tone, but it is difficult to suggest a therapeutic role of digitalis in the presence of normal contractility. Despite these theoretic considerations, in my experience digitalis is beneficial, as part of combined therapy. This experience is based on treatment of hundreds of infants and children with left-to-right shunting and symptoms and signs of congestive heart failure. Controlled clinical trials of a large number of patients are required to confirm the role of digitalis in these patients, however.

Obstructive Cardiac Lesions

Most of the discussion in the previous section of this chapter is relevant also for infants and children with obstructive cardiac lesions. Many of them, and especially those with aortic stenosis, are treated with digitalis glycosides, even at early stages of the diseases when myocardial function is not impaired. This subject has not been systematically studied, and no conclusions can be drawn. In patients with disorders with a dynamic obstructive component, such as hypertrophic subaortic stenosis or infundibular pulmonic stenosis, however, digitalis glycosides should not be used.

Electrophysiologic Effects

The electrophysiologic effects of digitalis result from its direct action on the conduction system and the myocardium, as well as from its actions on the autonomic nervous system.

Action Potential

Digitalis shortens the action potential's duration, primarily by shortening its plateau phase. It increases the slope of phase 4 depolarization, and at high concentrations, it may also decrease the resting membrane potential and the rate of rise and amplitude of phase 0 depolarization.[27, 28] The increase in slope of phase 4 depolarization is especially evident in the presence of hypokalemia.

Sinoatrial Node

Many reports have been published on the electrophysiologic effects of digitalis on the sinoatrial node in adult animals and human subjects. Kugler and co-workers have reported results of intracardiac electrophysiologic studies in children.[29] The effect of digitalis on the sinoatrial node appears to be the net result of the direct action of the drug and its vagotonic effect.

Usually, digitalis either does not alter or prolongs the sinoatrial conduction time in adults.[30–32] This action results from the drug's direct effect on the sinoatrial node,[33] as well as from its vagotonic effect.[33–35] In a group of 10 children (mean age 10.5 years) with various arrhythmias, ouabain, 0.01 mg/kg, increased the sinoatrial conduction time in all subjects.[29] The increase in sinoatrial conduction time for the whole group increased from 149 ± 11 msec to 182 ± 13 msec. In adults, digitalis, at therapeutic doses, depressed the sinus node automaticity and increased the sinus cycle length.[30] This phenomenon was observed in patients with normally functioning sinoatrial node, as well as in patients with sick sinus syndrome.[30, 36, 37] In a group of 10 children, ouabain increased the sinus cycle length in 6 and decreased it in 4 children.[29] For the whole group, no statistically significant difference was observed.

Variable effects of digitalis on the sinus node recovery time have been reported. In patients with normal sinus node function, digitalis usually prolonged the sinus node recovery time,[32, 37, 38] but changes or shortenings were not always observed. In 7 of 10 children, ouabain prolonged the sinus node recovery time, but for the whole group, no statisically significant difference was noted.[29] In a study of adults with sick sinus syndrome, digitalis shortened the sinus node recovery time.[37] This change could be attributed to prolongation of sinoatrial conduction.

In summary, the effect of digitalis on the sinoatrial node in children appears to be similar to that in adults. Digitalis prolongs the sinoatrial conduction time. This effect may artificially shorten the sinus node recovery time.

Karpawich and colleagues studied the effect of digoxin on the sinus node of beagle puppies.[39] At doses of 0.04 mg/kg/day, the drug decreased the sinus rate from 176 ± 9 to 136 ± 15 beats/min and prolonged the corrected sinus node recovery time from 69 ± 4 to 198 ± 66 msec. Lower doses of digoxin did not alter the sinus node recovery time. The high does of digoxin (0.04 mg/kg/day) prolonged the sinoatrial conduction time from 53 ± 5 to 110 ± 36 msec. Lower doses had only minimal effects on sinoatrial conduction. These findings in puppies are similar to those observed in children and adults. Atropine abolished the effect of digoxin on the corrected sinus node recovery time.

Atria

Digitalis decreases the duration of the action potential of atrial myocardial fibers and shortens or does not alter the atrial effective refractory period. In puppies, digoxin did not alter the mean atrial effective refractory period.[39] At high concentrations of digitalis, changes in amplitude and configuration of P wave may be observed. In a group of 10 children, digitalis did not alter the atrial effective refractory period.[29]

Atrioventricular Node

Digitalis slows conduction and prolongs refractoriness in the atrioventricular node.[40-42] In this node, the direct effect of digitalis and the indirect vagal effect act in the same direction. Digitalis may produce advanced atrioventricular block, which can be partially reverted by atropine administration.

In puppies, digoxin prolonged the P-R interval from 82 ± 4 to 134 ± 21 msec. In 5 of 6 puppies who received 0.04 mg/kg digoxin, second-degree atrioventricular block was observed.[39] Puppies treated with digoxin developed Wenckebach periodicity at slower pacing rates than before digoxin (170 versus 364 beats/min). The functional refractory period of the atrioventricular conduction system was increased in these puppies. The administration of atropine partially prevented the effect of digoxin.

Accessory Atrioventricular Pathways

The effect of digitalis on accessory atrioventricular pathways was found by several investigators to be unpredictable,[43] but most investigators have stated that digitalis usually decreases the antegrade effective refractory period of accessory atrioventricular pathways. For example, Wellens and Durrer reported that, in adults with Wolff-Parkinson-White syndrome, digitalis decreased the antegrade effective refractory period of the accessory pathway by 40 msec.[44] Jedeikin and co-workers found a 43% decrease in this parameter in children and young adults.[45] The decrease in the effective refractory period of the accessory pathway by digitalis may result in a rapid ventricular rate in patients with Wolff-Parkinson-White syndrome who develop atrial fibrillation. Therefore, digitalis is contraindicated in such patients unless electrophysiologic studies have confirmed its safety. Such is not the case, however, in neonates with Wolff-Parkinson-White syndrome and supraventricular arrhythmias. In these neonates, digitalis is effective and safe and is considered to be the drug of choice.

Ventricles

Digoxin shortens the duration of action potential in His-Purkinje and ventricular myocardial fibers. This change shortens refractoriness. In puppies, digoxin did not alter the ventricular effective refractory period.[39] In adults, digoxin usually decreased the QTc interval.[46,47] This effect was found to be related to the plasma concentration of digitalis glycosides at any age.[48] Digoxin shortened the QTc interval in puppies.[39] In intact adult dogs and human patients, digoxin may increase or may not alter the refractoriness of the His-Purkinje system.[46,47]

In isolated myocardial fibers, digoxin and other digitalis glycosides increase the slope of the plateau phase and decreases the slope of phase 3 action potential. These effects result in electrocardiographic ST segment depression and T-wave inversion in human patients. This electrocardiographic effect of digitalis resembles the strain pattern.

Myocardial Infarction

Acute myocardial infarction is rare in infancy and childhood. Infants with certain congenital anomalies of the coronary arteries may, however, develop acute myocardial infarction and congestive heart failure. Because these infants are candidates for treatment with digitalis, it is important to review the experience with digitalis in acute myocardial infarction.

The risk of digitalis toxicity is not increased in patients with acute myocardial infarction. The drug improves global left ventricular function and enhances contractility in the normal and ischemic zones, but not in the infarcted zone.[49] Potentially, however, digitalis may increase the risk of mortality in patients with acute myocardial infarction by several mechanisms. The enhanced myocardial contractility increases the myocardial oxygen demand, and this change enlarges the ischemic and necrotic zone. The combined arrhythmogenic effect of digitalis and ischemia may result in the development of lethal arrhythmias. In adults with acute myocardial infarction, digitalis therapy is associated with a higher mortality rate.[50, 51] In patients with coronary artery disease but without acute myocardial infarction, digitalis is not associated with increased mortality rates. I have treated with digitalis several infants with anomalous origin of the left coronary artery from the pulmonary artery, myocardial infarction, and congestive heart failure. In no case was death attributable to digitalis treatment. Two patients died in progressive heart failure. One infant had impaired left ventricular contractility visible by radionuclide ventriculography; after a few months of treatment with digitalis, left ventricular contractility improved.

Arrhythmias

The main use of digitalis glycosides in arrhythmias is to control the ventricular rate in patients with atrial tachyarrhythmias and to terminate such arrhythmias. Digitalis is rarely used for treatment of ventricular arrhythmias.

Supraventricular Tachycardia

In adults, digitalis glycosides are used for termination of supraventricular tachycardia or, if the drug fails to terminate the arrhythmia, for control of the ventricular response. This indication is limited in adults because the use of digitalis in adults with Wolff-Parkinson-White syndrome and supraventricular tachycardia is controversial. In these patients, digitalis may enhance anterograde conduction over the accessory pathway and may accelerate the ventricular response.[43, 52] Such is not the case in children.

Garson and associates reported the largest series of children with supraventricular tachycardia treated with digoxin.[53] Short-term treatment with digoxin was effective in 57 of 84 children (68%). Electrical cardioversion was effective in 60% of the children, and vagal maneuvers were effective in 63%. After initial treatment, 113 of 191 patients (72%) received long-term treatment. Digoxin, at a dose of 0.01 mg/kg/day, was the most common drug used in the first month of treatment, either alone or in combination with propranolol or quinidine. In 116 patients, tachycardia recurred at least once. Digoxin reduced the rate of recurrences in these patients.

Garson and associates recommend treatment for at least a year in all children with supraventricular tachycardia, whether or not the first episode terminates spontaneously.[53] The success of digoxin was unrelated to age, the presence of congestive heart failure, heart rate, or other electrocardiographic features, including the presence of Wolff-Parkinson-White syndrome.

Atrioventricular junctional tachycardia, a form of supraventricular tachycardia that is most often seen in infants and children during the immediate postoperative period after correction of congenital cardiac anomalies, is resistant to treatment. Digoxin may be used to reduce the abnormal junctional rate or to induce a second-degree atrioventricular block in children with this arrhythmia, however. If hemodynamic deterioration occurs, electrocardioversion will be required.[54]

In contrast to the favorable results obtained by many investigators, Dick and associates recently suggested that digitalis is of little value for the prophylaxis of supraventricular tachycardia.[54a] These workers studied 5 infants, aged 29 to 111 days, with supraventricular tachycardia. In all infants, digoxin therapy was started. Clinical supraventricular tachycardia disappeared in 3 of 5 patients and decreased in the remaining 2 patients. The arrhythmia could have been induced by programmed stimulation in 4 of 5 patients, however, despite therapeutic levels of digoxin. These researchers speculated, based on electrophysiologic studies, that the spontaneous decrease in clinical supraventricular tachycardia occurred independently of digoxin administration, and thus digoxin is of little value in preventing this arrhythmia.

Fetal Supraventricular Tachycardia Treated with Maternal Digoxin. Sustained supraventricular tachycardia may occur in fetuses in utero. It is an established cause of fetal congestive heart failure and of nonimmune hydrops fetalis. For example, in 3 of 13 fetuses with nonimmune hydrops fetalis before birth, reported by Kleinman and colleagues, supraventricular tachycardia was the sole cause of this condition.[55]

Various forms of transplacental pharmacologic treatment attempting to terminate this arrhythmia have been reported. The first attempt to terminate the arrhythmia with digoxin failed;[56] the first attempt to terminate it by maternal treatment with the combination of digoxin and propranolol also failed.[57] Several cases of successful termination of supraventricular tachycardia in the fetus by maternal digoxin therapy have been reported since 1980, however. In these patients, digoxin was used either alone or in combination with drugs known to terminate supraventricular tachycardia at older ages, such as verapamil and propranolol.[58-62]

The first case of successful treatment of fetal supraventricular tachycardia by maternal administration of digoxin was reported by Lingman and co-workers in 1980.[58] The arrhythmia was terminated in a 29-week-old fetus within 24 hours of administration of digoxin. The neonate was healthy, with normal sinus rhythm. Six other cases have been reported in the literature.[55, 58, 59, 63-65] In all of them, the arrhythmia was terminated within a week of initiation of treatment. In most, signs of congestive heart failure disappeared after termination of the arrhythmia. Only one case was exceptional.

King and associates reported a case of a 26-week-old fetus with supraventricular tachycardia and congestive heart failure diagnosed by demonstration of ascites and scalp edema by ultrasound.[63] Normal sinus rhythm was restored within 60 hours of initiation of oral digoxin, 0.125 mg daily. Scalp edema decreased, but ascites persisted. Treatment with digoxin was continued until birth. After birth, echocardiography revealed normal cardiac features. Digoxin maintenance treatment was begun, and the infant was well throughout 11 months of follow-up. That this fetus had only partial resolution of signs of congestive heart failure after termination of the arrhythmia may have resulted from the early onset of the arrhythmia (20 weeks' gestation) and its long duration prior to initiation of treatment (6 weeks).[63]

Wolff and colleagues reported that, in a fetus with supraventricular tachycardia, the combination of digoxin and verapamil restored normal sinus rhythm within 5 days of treatment.[61]

Digoxin can be used safely during pregnancy because fetuses are resistant to the arrhythmogenic effect of digitalis glycosides.[10, 60] In 5 of the 7 cases reported, normal sinus rhythm was observed after birth; 1 neonate had Wolff-Parkinson-White syndrome with short bursts of supraventricular tachycardia,[65] and the other had chaotic atrial rhythm requiring treatment with digoxin and propranolol.[55]

In summary, maternal administration of digoxin is an effective and safe treatment for fetal supraventricular tachycardia. It has not been accurately determined whether digoxin should be given to the neonate, and for what period.

Atrial Flutter

Digitalis can prevent a rapid ventricular response in patients with atrial flutter. This effect results from impairment of atrioventricular conduction by the drug. Occasionally, digitalis converts atrial flutter to normal sinus rhythm.

Rowland and co-workers reviewed the experience of 3 institutions in the management of atrial flutter in infants under 2 years of age.[66] Eight infants with atrial flutter but otherwise normal cardiac findings were included in the study. Five patients had congenital atrial flutter, diagnosed electrocardiographically at the age of 2 days to 7 weeks. Three patients had paroxysmal flutter, diagnosed at the age of 6 weeks to 17 months. A 2-day course of digoxin was given to each infant. In the 5 infants with congenital atrial flutter, this course resulted in uncomplicated resolution of the arrhythmia, although one of these infants continued to suffer episodes of paroxysmal supraventricular tachycardia for 6 years. The longest period of therapy until conversion of the arrhythmia was 14 days. Digoxin was less effective in the 3 infants with paroxysmal atrial flutter. In 2 of them, quinidine was subsequently added. One of them developed ventricular fibrillation, and the other developed 1:1 atrioventricular conduction of atrial flutter with a rapid ventricular response. Both required emergency electrocardioversion, which was successful. These authors concluded that digoxin is the preferred initial therapy for nonacutely ill patients with atrial flutter in infancy. Patients showing signs of cardiac decompensation should be treated with D.C. countershock.[66]

Dunnigan and colleagues reported 6 infants with congenital atrial flutter, diagnosed before 8 weeks of age. Three of them had congestive heart failure,[67] 3 of them had anatomically normal hearts, 1 had Ebstein's anomaly, 1 had simple transposition of the great arteries, and the remaining patient had an atrial septal defect. Normal sinus rhythm was achieved within 24 hours of administration of digoxin in one infant. In all other 5 infants, various forms of electrocardioversion were used. It was not mentioned whether digoxin had been given and had failed in these 5 patients. A short course of digoxin treatment should be attempted in all infants with atrial flutter who are not critically ill and who do not require immediate conversion of the arrhythmia. The question whether the drug should be discontinued before electrical conversion is still controversial.

Atrial Fibrillation

In adults with cardiac arrhythmias, the most important indication for digitalis glycosides is atrial fibrillation. Digitalis glycosides are used for control of the ventricular rate. The ability of digitalis glycosides to convert atrial fibrillation to sinus rhythms is controversial. Digitalis glycosides probably do not directly convert atrial fibrillation to normal sinus rhythm. They may exert an indirect effect mediated by control of ventricular rate and overall hemodynamic improvement, however.[68, 69, 70] One study demonstrated a direct converting effect of digoxin in cases of atrial fibrillation.[71]

Atrial fibrillation is rare in pediatric patients, except for those undergoing cardiac operations involving the atria. Most of these patients also have damage to the sinoatrial node. Therefore, treatment of atrial fibrillation with digitalis glycosides in these patients may cause severe bradycardia. Some of these patients may require insertion of a cardiac pacemaker for treatment of sick sinus syndrome.

Ventricular Arrhythmias

Digitalis glycosides are not usually used for treatment of ventricular arrhythmias. Several studies have shown, however, that these agents may be effective for suppression of chronic ventricular premature beats.[72, 73] The antiarrhythmic efficacy of digoxin for this indication is moderate. The mechanism of action is probably sympathetic withdrawal, owing to the overall hemodynamic improvement.

Clinical Pharmacology

The clinical pharmacologic features of digoxin and digitoxin are discussed separately.

Digoxin

Digoxin is the most widely used digitalis glycoside, because of its favorable pharmacokinetic profile. In adults, up to 85% of a dose of digoxin is absorbed from the gastrointestinal tract. Maximal plasma concentration is achieved within an hour of oral administration. Coadministration with food may change the rate of absorption, but not its magnitude.[74-76] These findings are also valid for children and full-term infants. For example, Hernandez and associates reported that in a group of 20 infants with congenital heart disease, digoxin could be detected in the plasma within 5 to 10 min of oral administration, and peak plasma concentrations were evident within 60 to 180 min.[77] The validity of these data for preterm infants has not been confirmed. The peak hemodynamic effect is evident within 6 hours of oral administration.

Digoxin can also be given intravenously, for rapid effect. The peak hemodynamic effect is evident within 3 hours of intravenous administration. Intramuscular injections are rarely used because they may cause pain.

The half-life of distribution of digoxin is 30 min after intravenous administration of digoxin.[78] Wettrell has suggested that the tissue distribution of digoxin is more extensive in infants than in adults.[79] Protein binding of digoxin is low.

Digoxin reaches its highest concentrations in the myocardium and kidneys, but most of the drug present in the body concentrates in skeletal muscles.[80] The concentration of digoxin in adipose tissues is low. Therapeutic serum concentrations of digoxin range between 1 and 2 ng/ml. In a group of 12 infants aged 1 to 12 months who were receiving long-term digoxin therapy, the serum digoxin concentration was 1.48 ± 0.77 ng/ml.[63] Pinsky and colleagues reported that, in premature neonates, the serum digoxin concentration after a digitalizing dose of 30 µg/kg ranged between 1.4 and 7.5 ng/ml (mean + S.D. 3.5 ± 0.39 ng/ml).[81] After a digitalizing dose of 20 µg/kg, the serum concentration ranged between 1.2 and 3.0 ng/ml (mean + S.D. 1.73 ± 0.15 ng/ml). Lang and Von Bernuth reported that the serum digoxin concentration ranged between 1.2 and 3.5 ng/ml in mature newborns and between 1.5 and 4.5 ng/ml in premature newborns.[82]

The concentration of digoxin is much higher in the myocardium than in the plasma, in adults as well as in children. For example, Krasula and co-workers studied 42 children, 18 of whom were treated with digoxin for at least a month, and found a mean digoxin concentration of 62 ng/g in the right atrial appendage and 12 ng/ml in the plasma.[83] Wagner and associates used a specific assay and found that the concentration of digoxin in right atrial tissue was 100 times higher than that in the serum.[84]

Tissue concentrations of digoxin have been reported in a few infants and children.[77, 83, 85, 86] These concentrations are affected by age, dosage, period of treatment, and route of administration. Recently, Hastreiter and Van der Horst studied the concentration of digoxin in tissues and the content of the drug in various organs in 36 infants and children evaluated post mortem.[87] Upper therapeutic concentration thresholds for digoxin were established in various tissues. They were different for preterm and full-term neonates than for older children and adults. In adults and neonates, postmortem digoxin blood values were 8 and 15 ng/ml, respectively, and concentrations for ventricular myocardium were 250 and 450 ng/ml, respectively. Premature infants receiving long-term digoxin treatment had larger fraction of digoxin in most tissues than older infants and children.[87] This finding is in accord with the findings of Pinsky and colleagues, who noted higher serum concentrations of digoxin in premature infants than in full-term infants.[81] In another study of tissue concentrations of digoxin obtained during surgical procedures, neonates had higher concentrations in the right and left ventricular myocardium than older children and adults.[83] Renal concentrations of digoxin in premature infants receiving long-term digoxin therapy were 71 ± 66 ng/g; in full-term infants, concentrations were 231 ± 153 ng/g, and in children, they were 122 ± 98 ng/g.[87]

Reported digoxin concentrations in the liver and gastrointestinal tract were also higher in neonates than in older children.[87] Lang and co-workers studied tissue and plasma digoxin concentrations in 13 premature and 6 full-term neonates and in 5 older infants.[85] Concentrations of digoxin in tissues, and especially in the myocardium and skeletal muscles, were higher in the neonates than in the older infants. The renal concentrations of digoxin were lower in preterm than in mature newborns, although differences in digoxin concentrations were noted among infants of various gestational ages.

Several theories have been suggested to explain the higher plasma levels and slower elimination of digoxin in premature infants. In my opinion, these phenomena are probably attributable to the impaired ability of premature infants to excrete digoxin. Digoxin is eliminated primarily by renal excretion of the unchanged drug. Up to 40% of the absorbed amount may be metabolized in the liver to dihydrodigoxin and other derivatives, which are pharmacologically inactive. About 90% of these metabolites are excreted in the urine. That the remaining 10% are excreted in the feces indicates the presence of an enterohepatic cycle. Some of the unchanged drug, which is not absorbed, is also found in the feces.[88,89] In about 10% of patients, active metabolites may be formed.[90]

In adults with normal renal function, and mainly a normal glomerular filtration rate, the elimination half-life of digoxin is about 35 hours. In the neonate, digoxin is excreted unchanged, by glomerular filtration.[82] Premature infants have a glomerular filtration rate lower than that of full-term infants.[91] This feature may account for the prolonged elimination half-life of digoxin in neonates. Pinsky and associates reported that the elimination half-life of digoxin in 7 premature infants ranged from 56 to 88 hours, with a mean of 72 ± S.E. 5.2 hours.[81] These data are close to those noted by Lang and Von Bermuth in low-birth-weight infants.[82] These investigators found the elimination half-life of digoxin to range between 17 and 52 hours in mature newborns and between 38 and 88 hours in premature newborns. In patients with impaired renal function, the elimination half-life of the drug is prolonged, and digoxin and its metabolites may accumulate.

Digitoxin

Digitoxin may be given intravenously or orally. It is rapidly and almost completely absorbed from the gastrointestinal tract after oral administration.[92] The onset of action is evident within 3 hours of oral administration. About 90% of the drug in the plasma is protein-bound.[93] About two-thirds of a dose of digitoxin is eliminated by hepatic metabolism, and about one-third is excreted unchanged in the urine and feces. The elimination half-life of digitoxin is several days,[92,94] and it is prolonged in patients with hepatic dysfunction.

The pharmacokinetic profile of digitoxin in infants and children has been evaluated by several investigators. Larsen and Storstein reported that children had larger volumes of distribution of digitoxin (1.0 L/kg) than adults (0.57 L/kg).[95] The mean serum elimination half-life was shorter in children (6.4 days) than in adults (8.2 days). Total body clearance was much greater in children than in adults, mainly because of a greater metabolic clearance. In this study, the bioavailability of digitoxin in children was complete. Peak plasma levels of 23 to 50 ng/ml developed within 90 to 120 minutes of administration of an oral dose.

Treatment During Pregnancy

Digoxin readily crosses the placenta and reaches high concentrations in the fetal myocardium. The fetus may be exposed to digoxin on two occasions: (1) during treatment of heart disease in the mother; and (2) during administration of digoxin to the mother to treat a heart disease, such as supraventricular tachycardia, in the fetus.

Fetal digoxin concentrations, estimated by analysis of umbilical cord blood, are usually high. Rogers and co-workers[96] and Lingman and colleagues[58] found equal digoxin concentrations in umbilical cord blood and in maternal blood. Kerenyi and associates[65] and Chan and colleagues[60] reported lower digoxin concentrations in umbilical cord blood than in maternal blood, however. King and co-workers reported a case in which the digoxin concentration of umbilical cord blood was 0.4 ng/ml, whereas the maternal digoxin blood level was 3.6 ng/ml.[63]

The fetal myocardium is resistant to the arrhythmogenic effect of digitalis. Because the safety of digitalis during pregnancy has not been accurately determined, the drug should be used only if the potential risk is lower than the expected benefit.

Digitalis Toxicity

Toxicity is an important problem associated with therapeutic and accidental ingestion of digitalis glycosides. In recent years, the incidence of digitalis toxicity has declined, but because of the widespread use of the drug, digitalis toxicity still remains a major public-health problem. In large-scale studies performed more than 10 years ago, the incidence of digitalis toxicity was reported to be 8 to 20% among hospitalized adults.[97] The incidence is higher in infants and children, as well as in elderly patients, than in young and middle-aged adults. Digitalis toxicity, an important problem in children and adolescents, is encountered under the following circumstances: (1) accumulation of the drug during use of therapeutic doses in infants and children with heart diseases; (2) accidental ingestion of high doses of digitalis; (3) suicide attempts. For example, 98 of 145 cases of accidental ingestion of digitalis glycosides reported by the National Clearinghouse of Poison Control Centers in the United States occurred in children under 5 years of age.

Rarely, digitalis toxicity is due to ingestion of poisonous plants. For example, McNamara and colleagues reported a case of serious toxicity in a child who ingested the leaves of a day lily plant.[98]

In recent years, digitalis toxicity attributed to therapeutic doses has become uncommon in infants and children. This change is due to the use of digoxin rather than other digitalis glycosides and to reduction in dosage. Most cases of digitalis toxicity associated with therapeutic doses are mild, occur mainly in premature infants, and respond within several days to discontinuance of the drug. The most severe cases are observed after accidental ingestion of high doses of digitalis. Mortality rates in these patients are high, especially in infancy.

Controversy exists concerning the incidence of digitalis intoxication in premature infants. Several investigators have emphasized the lack of digitalis toxicity in premature infants,[81] whereas others have stated that the risk of digitalis toxicity in children is highest in premature infants.[82] I believe that digitalis toxicity is uncommon in premature infants. The controversy may be explained by the finding of high serum digoxin concentrations in premature infants without toxicity. In my experience, digitalis-induced cardiac toxicity is uncommon in premature infants, despite serum concentrations higher than those found in children and adults. In a comparative study of neonatal and adult dogs, neonatal dogs developed toxicity at a higher serum concentration of digoxin than did adult dogs, in contrast to the finding of no difference in the inotropic effect of equal levels of digoxin serum concentrations in the two groups of dogs.[99] In neonates and in infants under 3 months of age, poor renal clearance of digoxin may result in high plasma levels of the drug, which may overcome the natural myocardial resistance in these age groups.

Clinical Manifestations

Digitalis toxicity may have serious clinical manifestations soon after ingestion of a high dose of the drug, or it may be mild, such as during long-term minimal toxicity. These manifestations include cardiac effects, which are the most serious, and extracardiac effects.

Cardiac Effects. The cardiac effects of digitalis toxicity include arrhythmias and conduction disturbances. Almost all reported types of arrhythmias and conduction disturbances have been observed in association with digitalis toxicity.

The arrhythmias associated with digitalis toxicity vary with the patient's age. Supraventricular arrhythmias and conduction disturbances are more common in infants and children, whereas ventricular arrhythmias are more common in elderly patients. In adults, the most frequently observed arrhythmias and conduction disturbances in digitalis toxicity are ventricular premature beats, junctional tachycardia, atrial tachycardia with block, and various degrees of atrioventricular block. These arrhythmias and conduction disturbances also predominate in children. For example, Nadas and co-workers reported that, in their series of infants and children with cardiac manifestations of digitalis toxicity, 27% of the patients had first-degree atrioventricular block, 27% had premature ventricular beats, 9% had sinus arrest or sinoatrial block, and another 9% had atrioventricular junctional rhythms.[100] In other series of infants and children, the incidence of atrioventricular junctional tachycardia or atrioventricular dissociation was high.[101-103] Greenwood and colleagues reported that 22% of infants and children with cardiac manifestations of digitalis toxicity had sinus bradycardia.[101] The reported incidence of sinus bradycardia was especially high in premature infants with digitalis toxicity.[104, 105] The incidence of ventricular arrhythmias was reported to be higher in children with severe myocardial damage, severe electrolytic disturbances, or acute ingestion of high doses of digitalis glycosides than in other children.[106]

Atrial fibrillation, atrial flutter, multifocal atrial tachycardia, polymorphous ventricular tachycardia, and ventricular parasystole are rarely associated with digitalis toxicity, especially in children.

Extracardiac Effects. The predominant extracardiac manifestations of digitalis toxicity in all age groups are related to the central nervous and gastrointestinal systems. Symptoms related to the central nervous system include drowsiness, lethargy, weakness, and many visual disturbances, such as impairment in color vision, especially yellow or green.[107] Rarely, seizures or psychotic manifestations are observed. Drowsiness is the most important central-nervous-system manifestation in infants and small children. The gastrointestinal manifestations of digitalis toxicity are nausea, vomiting, anorexia, failure to thrive, weight loss, and abdominal pain.[97, 100, 108]

Determination of Plasma Levels in Digoxin Toxicity

Measurement of digoxin plasma levels is an important tool in the diagnosis of digoxin toxicity. The therapeutic concentration range of digoxin is 0.8 to 2.0 ng/ml. In almost all children and in about 90% of adults with digoxin toxicity, the digoxin plasma concentration exceeds 2.0 ng/ml.[97] Most of these patients, and especially those who develop toxicity during treatment with therapeutic doses, have plasma concentrations lower than 6.0 ng/ml. Neonates and small infants require high levels of digoxin to develop signs of toxicity, however. They rarely develop toxic manifestations at plasma concentrations lower than 3.5 ng/ml and often have levels of 20 ng/ml or more.[109] A significant overlap exists between plasma digoxin concentrations in infants and children who do not have digoxin toxicity and plasma drug concentrations in those who do have such toxicity.

Serum potassium levels should be determined whenever digoxin levels are measured. Determination of plasma concentrations of digitalis is also prognostic. Hastreiter and associates, who recently reviewed the subject, stated that patients with plasma concentrations below 20 ng/ml who were appropriately treated usually survive,[106] whereas patients with plasma levels higher than 20 ng/ml rarely survive.[110-112] The introduction of digoxin-specific Fab antibody fragments can improve survival rates in children with plasma concentrations higher than 20 ng/ml.

Most of the criteria for monitoring digoxin plasma concentrations were developed in adults. In children, especially in those less than a year old, the condition is complicated both by the altered sensitivity of these patients to digoxin and by the altered pharmacokinetic profile of the drug.

In a recent review of the subject, Aronson stated that for children over a year old, one may use the criteria for the monitoring of digoxin plasma levels in adults.[90] No formal studies supporting this view are cited, however. In infants under 12 months of age, it is generally accepted that higher concentrations of digoxin are associated with a higher incidence of toxicity. In these small infants, however, and especially in those under 3 months of age, toxicity occurs at higher plasma concentrations than in adults.[90, 113]

Treatment

Treatment of digitalis toxicity includes prevention of further elevation of plasma concentrations of digitalis glycosides, reduction of the toxic concentrations already present, treatment of the potentially deleterious effects of toxicity, and supportive management.

Prevention of Further Elevation of Plasma Concentrations. If digitalis toxicity is suspected, further administration of the drug should be avoided, even in patients who depend on the drug for regulation of heart rate and hemodynamic support. Gastric lavage and induced emesis are of value if performed less than 4 hours after ingestion of a high dose of digitalis glycosides. If these procedures are performed within an hour of drug ingestion, absorption of the drug may be reduced by up to 40%.[114] In children over a year old, administration of ipecac syrup is recommended for induction of emesis. Gastric emptying may be complicated by a vagal reflex resulting in cardiac standstill. Activated charcoal may be used for binding and inactivation of the drug in the bowel. Magnesium sulfate may decrease the absorption of the drug by increasing bowel movement. Cholestyramine may interfere with absorption of digitoxin from the gastrointestinal tract.

Digoxin-Specific Antibody. In the last decade, digoxin-specific antibodies were evaluated for treatment of digitalis toxicity. Both heterologous antibodies and Fab fragments were evaluated and were found to be effective in lowering the plasma digoxin concentration. Animal experiments shows that the Fab fragment is superior in its effect on mortality and arrhythmias, however.[115] The Fab fragment also has a more favorable pharmacokinetic profile than the antibody.

Unlike the original 150,000-dalton antibody, the new 50,000-dalton Fab fragment is excreted by glomerular filtration. Reduction of the plasma digoxin concentration by this antibody results in dissociation of the reversible binding between digoxin and its receptors in the tissues. Soon after administration of the antibody, a higher level of the complex digoxin-specific antibody is found in the plasma. This level declines gradually over several days.

The use of Fab fragments of digoxin-specific antibodies for treatment of severe manifestations of digitalis toxicity in children was first reported in 1982 by two different groups, in the same issue of *Pediatrics*. Murphy and co-workers reported a 20-month-old child who ingested 30 to 50 tablets of digoxin.[116] When admitted to hospital, he was irritable and lethargic. His blood pressure was 90/60 mm Hg, and his heart rate was 80 beats/pmin. The electrocardiogram showed a second-degree sinoatrial block and first- and second-degree atrioventricular block. The patient's serum digoxin concentration was 16.7 ng/ml. Because it was thought that the child was still absorbing the drug, it was decided to treat him with digoxin-specific antibodies. After a skin test with the antibodies, a dose of 1 mg was given as an intravenous bolus. No acute sensitivity reaction was noted. The antibody was than infused intravenously at a dose of 960 mg, equimolar to the estimated amount of digoxin ingested, over 20 minutes. The patient reverted to sinus rhythm within about 4 hours, although the ventricular pacing required because of the condition disturbances masked the exact moment. The patient made an uneventful recovery.

Zucker and colleagues reported a case of massive overdosage of digoxin, in a 2.5-year-old boy, that produced sustained ventricular fibrillation refractory to conventional therapy.[117] The child received digoxin-specific Fab fragments of antibody. A few minutes later, and after a dose of propranolol and D.C. cardioversion, sinus rhythm was restored and sustained. The serum free digoxin level before treatment was over 100 ng/ml, and it rapidly fell to undetectable levels after the antibody was given. The elimination half-life of digoxin bound to antibody in this child was 48 hours.[117] A test for sensitivity is recommended before administration of the full dose of antibody; 60 mg Fab fragment is considered to be equimolar to 1 mg digoxin, and the dose of the antibody is calculated to match the estimated amount of digoxin ingested.

Smith and associates summarized the experience with Fab fragment and stated that up to 1982, 21 of 26 patients with digitalis intoxication who received this new treatment had survived.[118] Hastreiter and co-workers suggested that this form of therapy offers the best therapeutic promise for severe digitalis toxicity.[106]

Other Methods of Reducing Elevated Plasma Concentrations. Hemodialysis and peritoneal dialysis may reduce plasma levels of digitalis glycosides.[119] These techniques are not used clinically. Hemoperfusion with activated charcoal is a promising investigational procedure. Forced diuresis and exchange transfusions are ineffective in reducing the elevated plasma levels of digitalis glycosides.

Conduction Disturbances. Severe digitalis toxicity may be associated with the development of high-degree atrioventricular block. Insertion of a temporary transvenous pacemaker is indicated in patients who suddenly develop such conduction disturbances, in those who ingest high doses of digitalis, or in those with plasma levels higher than 6.0 ng/ml. Hastreiter and associates suggested that acute ingestion of 10 or more times the daily maintenance dose may warrant prophylactic insertion of a temporary pacemaker.[106] A temporary pacemaker may be used also for treatment of refractory arrhythmias in patients with digitalis intoxication.

Disturbances of the sinoatrial and atrioventricular nodes in digitalis intoxication partially respond to atropine.

Arrhythmias. Treatment of arrhythmias associated with digitalis toxicity includes administration of antiarrhythmic agents, D.C. electroshock, and cardiac pacing. Arrhythmias such as ventricular tachycardia, multiple ventricular premature beats, bidirectional tachycardia, and atrioventricular junctional tachycardia with an exit block or a rapid ventricular response respond to most available antiarrhythmic agents, but selection of the appropriate drug depends both on efficacy and safety. Digitalis toxicity is often associated with atrioventricular conduction disturbances. Therefore, antiarrhythmic drugs such as quinidine, procainamide, and verapamil, which may aggravate these conduction disturbances, should not be used. Another important aspect of drug selection when treating arrhythmias associated with digitalis toxicity is drug interactions. Antiarrhythmic drugs that interact with digitalis glycosides to increase their plasma levels, such as quinidine, verapamil, and amiodarone, should not be used. Traditionally, phenytoin is considered to be the drug of choice for arrhythmias associated with digitalis toxicity. It does not interact with digitalis, and it enhances conduction in the atrioventricular node.[120, 121]

I believe that lidocaine is at least as effective as phenytoin in suppression of ventricular arrhythmias associated with digitalis intoxication. Like phenytoin, lidocaine does not interact with digitalis and enhances rather than impairs atrioventricular nodal conduction. Moreover, the pharmacokinetic profile of lidocaine is more favorable than that of phenytoin (rapid onset of action after initiation of infusion and rapid disappearance of effect after discontinuance of infusion), and most cardiologists are more familiar with lidocaine than with phenytoin. Therefore, I recommend that lidocaine be used first for suppression of ventricular arrhythmias associated with digitalis intoxication. The main disadvantage of lidocaine in this setting is that it is not effective when given orally. If lidocaine does not suppress the arrhythmias, phenytoin should be tried. If phenytoin fails, procainamide may be given, although with caution. Bretylium may be used in patients with resistant ventricular fibrillation or tachycardia.

In the near future, new lidocaine-like antiarrhythmic agents and other orally effective class 1 antiarrhythmic agents, such as encainide, tocainide, and flecainide, will probably be tried in the treatment of ventricular arrhythmias associated with digitalis intoxication. For supraventricular arrhythmias, phenytoin, propranolol, or a combination of both drugs may be tried.

In resistant cases of ventricular fibrillation, D.C. cardioversion may be used. Occasionally, multiple D.C. electric countershocks are required to control the arrhythmia. In patients with arrhythmias associated with digitalis intoxication, electrocardioversion should be a last resort; cardioversion in these patients may cause serious ventricular arrhythmias unresponsive to further D.C. cardioversion. If cardioversion is absolutely required, the D.C. electric countershock should be initially attempted at a low energy level and then gradually increased, if indicated. Prophylactic administration of lidocaine or phenytoin before D.C. cardioversion may be effective.

Electrolytic disturbances. Digitalis intoxication is often associated with electrolytic disturbances. Rapid correction of these disturbances may be essential for treatment of the manifestations of intoxication.

HYPOKALEMIA. This disorder is the most common electrolytic disturbance in digitalis intoxication. It is especially frequent when diuretic agents are concomitantly administered. Hypokalemia increases myocardial sensitivity to digitalis intoxication. Rapid correction of hypokalemia, by intravenous or oral administration of potassium salts, can suppress arrhythmias even without administration of antiarrhythmic drugs.[40, 122] Some clinicians administer potassium salts to patients with digitalis intoxication even if their serum potassium level is normal; this practice is controversial and, in my opinion, ineffective. Potassium should not be given to patients with atrioventricular conduction disturbances or renal failure.

HYPERKALEMIA. Massive ingestion of digitalis may be associated with hyperkalemia, which is a sign of poor prognosis in these patients.[106] For example, one report states that serum potassium levels above 5.5

mEq/L are usually associated with early death in patients with acute digitalis toxicity.[123] In cases of severe hyperkalemia, measures to reduce the serum potassium level, such as the use of glucose-insulin solutions, exchange resins, or dialysis, may be justified. In less severe cases, the hyperkalemia usually corrects itself.

Drug Interactions

Several cardiovascular and other therapeutic agents interact with digitalis glycosides and alter their pharmacokinetic profile. These interactions may result in elevation of plasma levels of digitalis glycosides and may cause digitalis toxicity. Study of such interactions is especially important because some of these drugs were used to treat cardiac manifestations of digitalis toxicity before the adverse interactions were recognized. Other drugs may reduce the plasma concentrations of digitalis glycosides.

Quinidine

Co-administration of digoxin and quinidine results in elevation of plasma levels of digoxin. This interaction is described in detail in Chapter 20.

Verapamil

Recently, it was reported that co-administration of verapamil and digoxin prolongs the elimination and elevates the plasma concentration of digoxin. This interaction is described in detail in Chapter 6.

Amiodarone

Two recent studies revealed that co-administration of amiodarone and digoxin may elevate the plasma concentrations of digoxin. This interaction is described in detail in Chapter 29.

Koren studied the amiodarone-digoxin interaction in children.[124] Amiodarone decreased the renal clearance of digoxin without altering the glomerular filtration rate. This change caused a rise in serum concentrations of digoxin. Amiodarone also decreased the volume of distribution of digoxin in children. The effect of amiodarone on the clearance of digoxin resembles the effects of quinidine and verapamil on digoxin clearance. The increase in serum digoxin level with amiodarone was greater in children than in adults. This phenomenon may be attributed to the higher rate of tubular secretion of amiodarone in children than in adults.

Because of the long half-life of amiodarone, the interaction with digoxin may persist long after amiodarone is discontinued. On the other hand, such an interaction may take a long period to develop. In one child reported by Koren, digoxin toxicity appeared more than a month after the addition of amiodarone to the digoxin regimen.[124]

Vasodilators

Co-administration of hydralazine or nitroprusside and digoxin may increase the renal clearance of digoxin by about 50% in patients with congestive heart failure.[125] Children with severe congestive heart failure are often given both digoxin and nitroprusside. This interaction may cause a synergistic effect. When nitroprusside or hydralazine is discontinued, the plasma concentration of digoxin may rise, resulting in digitalis toxicity. The interaction between nitroprusside or hydralazine and digoxin results from an effect of these vasodilators on the tubular secretion of digoxin.

Aspirin

Aspirin may increase the serum concentration of digoxin,[126] but this subject is still controversial.[127]

Indomethacin

Indomethacin, used for closure of patent ductus arteriosus, is commonly given concomitantly with digoxin in infants with patent ductus arteriosus and congestive heart failure. Indomethacin impairs renal function in the majority of preterm infants. Because 90% of a dose of digoxin is excreted by the kidneys, indomethacin may impair the elimination of digoxin.

Schimmel and co-workers reported a neonate who developed severe digitalis toxicity associated with indomethacin-induced renal insufficiency during concomitant administration of digoxin and indomethacin.[128] Koren and associates studied 11 preterm infants treated with digoxin and indomethacin. Administration of indomethacin caused a mean elevation of 50% in digoxin serum concentration, which paralleled a mean reduction of 50% in urine output. The volume of distribution of digoxin was decreased, as often occurs in patients with renal insufficiency. The mechanism of this interaction is a reduction in the filtration rate of digoxin.[130] When indomethacin and digoxin are administered together to preterm infants, the dose of digoxin should be reduced by 50%, and digoxin serum levels and urinary output should be determined.

Antibiotic Agents

Certain antibiotic agents may increase the plasma concentration of digoxin as a result of alteration of intestinal flora. Neomycin, on the other hand, may decrease the absorption of digoxin.[131]

Antacids

Oral administration of high doses of antacids may decrease the absorption of digitalis glycosides from the gastrointestinal tract.

Dosage and Administration

Digitalis glycosides are given at a high loading dose, usually divided into several doses on the first day of treatment, followed by a lower maintenance dose.

Digoxin

Intravenous Administration. The loading dose of digoxin in adults is 1 mg, divided into 2 to 4 doses. Doses of 50 to 80 µg/kg are used in infants and children. The digitalizing dose of digoxin recommended for full-term newborn infants ranges from 25 to 50 µg/kg. Lang and von Bernuth used a digitalizing dose of 26 µg/kg in premature and mature newborns.[82] Pinsky and co-workers suggested that the digitalizing dose in premature infants be 20 µg/kg. The maintenance dose is usually 25% of the digitalizing dose.[81]

Oral Administration. The oral digitalizing dose in adults is 1 mg, whereas the oral digitalizing dose in infants ranges between 25 and 50 µg/kg. A dose of 35 µg/kg is usually considered optimal. The maintenance dose is usually 25% of the digitalizing dose. In infants, an acceptable dose is 10 µg/kg daily.

Maternal Treatment. Fetal supraventricular tachycardia was successfully treated by oral administration of digoxin, 0.125 mg daily, to the mother.[63]

Digitoxin

A loading dose of 20 µg/kg, intravenously or orally, has been recommended for children.[95]

References

1. Berman. W. Jr., and Musselman, J: Myocardial performance in the newborn lamb. Am. J. Physiol., *237*:H66, 1979.
2. Kim, D., et al.: Ouabain binding and changes in ^{42}K uptake, sodium content and contractile state in cultured heart cells. AHA 1983.
3. Hoffman, B.F. and Bigger, J.T., Jr.: Digitalis and allied cardiac glycosides. *In* Goodman and Gilman's: The Pharmacological Basis of Therapeutics, 6th ed. Edited by Gilman, A.G., Goodman, L.S., and Gilman, A. New York, MacMillan, 1980, p. 729.
4. Arnold, S.B., et al.: Long-term digitalis therapy improves left ventricular function in heart failure. N. Engl. J. Med., *303*:1443, 1980.
5. Gheorghiade, M., and Beller, G.A.: Effects of discontinuing maintenance digoxin therapy in patients with ischemic heart disease and congestive heart failure in sinus rhythm. Am. J. Cardiol., *51*:1243, 1983.
6. Keiliher, G.J., and Roberts, J.: Effect of age on the cardiotoxicity of digitalis. J. Pharmacol. Exp. Ther., *197*:10, 1976.

7. Wollenberger, A., et al.: Influence of age on the sensitivity of the guinea pig and its myocardium to ouabain. J. Pharmacol. Exp. Ther., *108*:52, 1953.
8. Rosen, M.R., et al.: Ouabain-induced changes in electrophysiologic properties of neonatal, young and adult canine cardiac Purkinje fibers. J. Pharmacol. Exp. Ther., *194*:255, 1975.
9. Halloran, K.H., et al.: Digitalis tolerance in young puppies. Pediatrics, *46*:730, 1970.
10. Berman, W., Jr., et al.: Differential effects of digoxin at comparable concentrations in tissue of fetal and adult sheep. Circ. Res., *41*:635, 1977.
11. Inturrisi, C.E., and Papaconstantinou, M.C.: Ouabain sensitivity of the Na^+, K^+-ATPase from rat neonatal and human fetal and adult heart. Ann. N.Y. Acad. Sci., *242*:710, 1974.
12. Berman, W., Jr., et al.: The physiologic effects of digoxin under steady-state drug conditions in newborn and adult sheep. Circulation, *62*:1165, 1980.
13. Klaassen, C.D.: Immaturity of the newborn rat's hepatic excretory function for ouabain. J. Pharmacol. Exp. Ther., *183*:520, 1972.
14. Glantz, S.A., et al.: Age-related changes in ouabain pharmacology. Circ. Res., *39*:407, 1976.
15. Berman, W., Jr., and Musselman, J.: The relationship of age to the metabolism and protein binding of digoxin in sheep. J. Pharmacol. Exp. Ther., *208*:263, 1979.
16. Lukas, D.S., and De Martino, A.G.: Binding of digitoxin and some related cardenolides to human plasma proteins. J. Clin. Invest., *48*:1041, 1969.
17. Schneeweiss, A., et al.: Persistent left ventricular disease in clinically "cured" primary endocardial fibroelastosis. Br. Heart J., *50*:252,1983.
18. Artman, M., and Graham, T.P., Jr.: Congestive heart failure in infancy: recognition and management. Am. Heart J., *203*:1040, 1982.
19. Rudolph, A.M. (Ed.): Pediatrics, 16th ed. New York, Appleton-Century-Crofts, 1977.
20. Park, S.C., et al.: Systolic time intervals in infants with congestive heart failure. Circulation, *47*:1281, 1973.
21. Baylen, B., et al.: Left ventricular performance in the critically ill premature infant with patent ductus arteriosus and pulmonary disease. Circulation, *55*:182, 1977.
22. Berman, W., Jr., et al.: Effects of digoxin in infants with a congested circulatory state due to a ventricular septal defect. N. Engl. J. Med., *308*:363, 1983.
23. White, R.D., and Lietman, P.S.: Commentary: a reappraisal of digitalis for infants with left-to-right shunts and "heart failure." J. Pediatr., *92*:867, 1978.
24. O'Rourke, R.A., et al.: Comparative hemodynamic effects of digoxin vs nitroprusside in conscious dogs with aortocaval fistula-induced chronic left ventricular volume overload and normal systolic performance. Am. Heart J., *103*:489, 1982.
25. Shan, D.J., et al.: Echocardiographic detection of large left-to-right shunts and cardiomyopathies in infants and children. Am. J. Cardiol., *38*:73, 1976.
26. Levy, A.M., et al.: Effects of digoxin on systolic time intervals of neonates and infants. Circulation, *46*:816, 1972.
27. Rosen, M.R., et al.: Correlation between effects of ouabain on the canine electrocardiogram and transmembrane potentials of isolated Purkinje fibers. Circ. Res., *47*:65, 1973.
28. Vassalle, M., et al.: Toxic effects of ouabain on Purkinje fibers and ventricular muscle fibers. Am. J. Physiol., *203*:433, 1962.
29. Kugler, J.D., et al.: Electrophysiologic effect of digitalis on sinoatrial nodal function in children. Am. J. Cardiol., *44*:1344, 1979.
30. Comes, J.A.C., et al.: Effects of digitalis on the human sick sinus node after pharmacologic autonomic blockade. Am. J. Cardiol., *48*:783, 1981.
31. Bond, R.C., et al.: The effect of digitalis on sinoatrial conduction in man. (abstract.) Am. J. Cardiol., *33*:128, 1974.
32. Dhingra, R.C., et al.: The electrophysiological effects of ouabain on sinus node and atrium in man. J. Clin. Invest., *56*:555, 1975.
33. Ten Eick, R.E., and Hoffman, B.F.: The effect of digitalis on the excitability of autonomic nerves. J. Pharmacol. Exp. Ther., *169*:95, 1969.

34. Toda, N., and West, T.C.: The influence of ouabain on cholinergic responses in the sinoatrial node. J. Pharmacol. Exp. Ther., *153*:104, 1966.
35. Scherlag, B.J., et al.: The differential effects of ouabain on sinus, A-V nodal, His bundle, and idioventricular rhythms. Am. Heart J., *81*:227, 1971.
36. Rubenstein, J.S., et al.: Clinical spectrum of the sick sinus syndrome. Circulation, *46*:5, 1972.
37. Engel, T.R., and Schal, S.F.: Digitalis in the sick sinus syndrome: the effects on sinoatrial automaticity and atrioventricular conduction. Circulation, *48*:1201, 1973.
38. Reiffel, J.A., et al.: The effect of digoxin on sinus node automaticity and sinoatrial conduction (SAC) in man. (abstract.) J. Clin. Invest., *53*:64a, 1974.
39. Karpawich, P.P., et al.: Comparative electrophysiologic effects of digoxin in the nonsedated chronically instrumented puppy. Am. Heart J., *103*:1001, 1982.
40. Fisch, C., et al.: Effect of digitalis on conduction of the heart. Prog. Cardiovasc. Dis., *6*:343, 1964.
41. Kosowsky, B.D., et al.: The effects of digitalis on atrioventricular conduction in man. Am. Heart J., *75*:736, 1968.
42. Mendez, R., and Mendez, C.: The action of cardiac glycosides on the refractory period of heart tissue. J. Pharmacol. Exp. Ther., *107*:24, 1953.
43. Sellers, T.D., et al.: Digitalis in the preexcitation syndrome. Circulation, *56*:260, 1977.
44. Wellens, H.J., and Durrer, D.: Wolff-Parkinson-White syndrome and atrial fibrillation. Am. J. Cardiol., *34*:777, 1974.
45. Jedeikin, R., et al.: Effect of ouabain on the anterograde effective refractory period of accessory atrioventricular connections in children. J. Am. Coll. Cardiol., *1*:869, 1983.
46. Gomes, J.A.C., et al.: The effect of digitalis on refractoriness of the intact canine His-Purkinje system. Circulation, *58*:284, 1978.
47. Gomes, J.A.C., et al.: Effects of digitalis on ventricular myocardial and His-Purkinje refractoriness and reentry in man. Am. J. Cardiol., *42*:931, 1978.
48. Erbel, R., et al.: Suizidale Digitalisintoxikation—Beziehung zwischen der Digitalis-Serum Konzentration und den elektrokardiographischen Befunden. Z. Kardiol., *68*:590, 1979.
49. Vatner, S.F., and Baig, H.: Comparison of the effects of ouabain and isoproterenol on ischemic myocardium of conscious dogs. Circulation, *58*:654, 1978.
50. Muller, J., et al.: Does digoxin therapy increase mortality following myocardial infarction? AHA 1983.
51. Moss, A.J., et al.: Digitalis-associated mortality in postinfarction patients. AHA 1983.
52. Dreifus, L.S., et al.: Ventricular fibrillation: a possible mechanism of sudden death in patients with Wolff-Parkinson-White syndrome. Circulation, *43*:520, 1971.
53. Garson, A., Jr., et al.: Supraventricular tachycardia in children: clinical features, response to treatment, and long-term follow-up in 217 patients. J. Pediatr., *98*:875, 1981.
54. Krongrad, E.: Postoperative arrhythmias in patients with congenital heart disease. Chest, *85*:107, 1984.
54a. Dick, M., et al.: A new look at digoxin in supraventricular tachycardia in infants. AHA 1984.
55. Kleinman, G.S., et al: Fetal echocardiography for evaluation of in utero congestive heart failure. N. Engl. J. Med., *306*:568, 1982.
56. Newburger, J. W., and Keane, J.F.: Intrauterine supraventricular tachycardia. J. Pediatr., *95*:780, 1979.
57. Klein, A. M., et al.: Fetal tachycardia prior to the development of hydrops—attempted pharmacologic cardioversion: case report. Am. J. Obstet. Gynecol., *134*:347, 1979.
58. Lingman, G., et al.: Intrauterine digoxin treatment of fetal paroxysmal tachycardia. Br. J. Obstet. Gynaecol., *87*:340, 1980.
59. Wiggins, W., et al.: Successful diagnosis and therapy of arrhythmias, congestive heart failure in the fetus with digoxin. (Abstract.) Pediatr. Cardiol., *2*:175, 1982.

60. Chan, V., et al.: Transfer of digoxin across the placenta and into breast milk. Br. J. Obstet. Gynaecol., 85:6059, 1978.
61. Wolff, F., et al.: Prenatal diagnosis and therapy of fetal heart rate anomalies; with a contribution of the placental transfer of verapamil. J. Perinat. Med., 2:203, 1980.
62. Teuscher, A., et al.: Effect of propranolol on fetal tachycadia in diabetic pregnancy. Am. J. Cardiol., 42:304, 1978.
63. King, C.R., et al.: Successful treatment of fetal supraventricular tachycardia with maternal digoxin therapy. Chest, 85:573, 1984.
64. Harrigan, J.T., et al.: Successful treatment of fetal congestive heart failure secondary to tachycardia. N. Engl. J. Med., 304:1527, 1981.
65. Kerenyi, T.D., et al.: Transplacental cardioversion of intrauterine supraventricular tachycardia with digitalis. Lancet, 2:393, 1980.
66. Rowland, T.W., et al.: Idiopathic atrial flutter in infancy: a review of eight cases. Pediatrics, 61:52, 1978.
67. Dunnigan, A., et al.: Atrial flutter in infancy.: clinical features and modes of termination. Pediatr. Cardiol., 4:308, 1983.
68. Sobel, B.E., and Braunwald, E.: Cardiac dysrhythmias. In Harrison's Principles of Internal Medicine. Edited by K.J. Isselbacher et al. New York, McGraw-Hill, 1980, p. 1056.
69. Bellet, S.: Essentials of Cardiac Arrhythmias. Philadelphia, W.B. Saunders, 1972, p. 78.
70. Hurst, J.W.: The Heart. New York, McGraw-Hill, 1978, p. 665.
71. Pick, A.: Digitalis and the electrocardiogram. Circulation, 15:603, 1957.
72. Lown, B., et al.: Effect of a digitalis drug on ventricular premature beats. N. Engl. J. Med., 296:301, 1977.
73. Gradman, A.H., et al.: Effects of oral digoxin on ventricular ectopy and its relation to left ventricular function. Am. J. Cardiol., 51:765, 1983.
74. White, R.J., et al.: Plasma concentrations of digoxin after oral administration in the fasting and post prandial state. Br. Med. J., 1:380, 1971.
75. Marcus, F.I., et al.: The metabolism of digoxin in normal subjects. J. Pharmacol. Exp. Ther., 145:203, 1964.
76. Iisalo, E.: The clinical pharmacokinetics of digoxin. Clin. Pharmacol., 2:1, 1977.
77. Hernandez, A., et al.: Pharmacodynamics of ^{3}H-digoxin in infants. Pediatrics, 44:418, 1969.
78. Doherty, J. E., et al.: Clinical pharmacokinetics of digitalis glycosides. Prog. Cardiovasc. Dis., 21:141, 1978.
79. Wettrell, G.: Distribution and elimination of digoxin in infants. Eur. J. Clin. Pharmacol., 11:327, 1977.
80. Doherty, J.E., et al.: The distribution and concentration of tritiated digoxin in human tissues. Ann. Intern. Med., 66:116, 1967.
81. Pinsky, W.W., et al.: Dosage of digoxin in premature infants. J. Pediatr., 94:639, 1979.
82. Lang, D., and von Bernuth, G.: Serum concentrations and serum half-life of digoxin in premature and mature newborns. Pediatrics, 59:902, 1977.
83. Krasula, R. W., et al.: Serum, atrial, and urinary digoxin levels during cardiopulmonary bypass in children. Circulation, 49:1047, 1974.
84. Wagner, J.G., et al.: Determination of myocardial and serum digoxin concentrations in children by specific and nonspecific assay methods. Clin. Pharmacol. Ther., 33:577, 1983.
85. Lang, D., et al.: Postmortem tissue and plasma concentrations of digoxin in newborns and infants. Eur. J. Pediatr., 128:151, 1978.
86. Gorodischer, R., et al.: Tissue and erythrocyte distribution of digoxin in infants. Clin. Pharmacol. Ther., 19:256, 1976.
87. Hastreiter, A.R., and Van der Horst, R.L.: Postmortem digoxin tissue concentration and organ content in infancy and childhood. Am. J. Cardiol., 52:330, 1983.
88. Peters, U., et al.: Digoxin metabolism in patients. Arch. Intern. Med., 138:1074, 1978.

89. Watson, E., et al.: Identification by gas chromatography mass spectroscopy of dihydrodigoxin as a metabolite of digoxin in man. J. Pharmacol. Exp. Ther., *184*:424, 1973.
90. Aronson, J.K.: Interactions for the measurement of plasma digoxin concentrations. Drugs, *26*:230, 1983.
91. Fenner, A., et al.: Creatine levels in first urines of male preterm and term infants. J. Perinat. Med., *2*:185, 1974.
92. Lukas, D.S.: Some aspects of the distribution and disposition of digoxin in man. Ann. N.Y. Acad. Sci., *179*:338, 1971.
93. Lukas, D.S., and de Martino, A.G.: Binding of digitoxin and some related cardenolides to human plasma proteins. J. Clin. Invest., *48*:1041, 1969.
94. Vohringer, H.F., et al.: Disposition of digitoxin in renal failure. Clin. Pharmacol. Ther., *19*:387, 1976.
95. Larsen, A., and Storstein, L.: Digitoxin kinetics and renal excretion in children. Clin. Pharmacol. Ther., *33*:717, 1983.
96. Rogers, M.C., et al.: Serum digoxin concentrations in the human fetus, neonate and infant. N. Engl. J. Med., *287*:1010, 1971.
97. Beller, G.A., et al.: Digitalis intoxication: prospective clinical study with serum level concentrations. N. Engl. J. Med., *284*:989, 1971.
98. McNamara, D.G., et al.: Accidental poisoning of children with digitalis. N. Engl. J. Med., *271*:1106, 1964.
99. Vargo, T.A., et al.: Comparison between puppies and adult dogs following infusion of digoxin. Pediatr. Res., *9*:335, 1974.
100. Nadas, A.S., et al.: The use of digitalis in infants and children. N. Engl. J. Med., *248*:9, 1953.
101. Greenwood, H., et al.: Development of a highly sensitive radioimmunoassay for digoxin and its application in pediatric practice. Eur. J. Cardiol., *515*:413, 1977.
102. Halkin, H., et al.: Steady state serum digoxin concentration in relation to digitalis toxicity in neonates and infants. Pediatrics, *61*:184, 1978.
103. Loes, M.W.: Relation between plasma and red cell electrolyte concentrations and digoxin levels in children. N. Engl. J. Med., *299*:501, 1978.
104. Johnson, G.L., et al.: Complications associated with digoxin therapy in low-birth-weight infants. Pediatrics, *69*:463, 1982.
105. Levine, O.R., and Somlyo, A.P.: Digitalis intoxication in premature infants. J. Pediatr., *61*:70, 1962.
106. Hastreiter, A.R., et al.: Digitalis toxicity in infants and children. Pediatr. Cardiol., *5*:131, 1984.
107. Rietbrock, N., and Alken, R.G.: Color vision difficiencies: a common sign of intoxication in chronically digoxin-treated patients. J. Cardiovasc. Pharmacol., *2*:93, 1980.
108. Hauck, A.J., et al.: The use of digoxin in infants and children. Am. Heart J., *56*:443, 1958.
109. Hastreiter, A.R., et al.: Accidental digoxin overdose in an infant: postmortem tissue concentrations. J. Forensic Sci., *28*:482, 1983.
110. Harris, M.M., et al.: Asymptomatic digoxin toxicity. (Letter.) N. Engl. J. Med., *305*:643, 1981.
111. Hobson, J.D., and Zettner, A.: Digoxin serum half-life following suicidal digoxin poisoning. JAMA, *223*:147, 1973.
112. Smith, T.W., and Willerson, T.J.: Suicidal and accidental digoxin ingestion: report of five cases with serum digoxin level correlations. Circulation, *44*:29, 1971.
113. Wettrell, G., and Andersson, K.E.: Clinical pharmacokinetics of digoxin in infants. Clin. Pharmacokinet., *2*:17, 1977.
114. Gellis, S.S., and Kagan, B.M.: Current Pediatric Therapy. Philadelphia, W.B. Saunders, 1982, pp. 136 and 654.
115. Lloyd, B.L., and Smith, T.W.: Contrasting rates of reversal of digoxin toxicity by digoxin-specific IgG and Fab fragments. Circulation, *58*:280, 1978.
116. Murphy, D.J., Jr., et al.: Massive digoxin poisoning treated with Fab fragments of digoxin-specific antibodies. Pediatrics, *70*:472, 1982.

117. Zucker, A.R., et al.: Fab fragments of digoxin-specific antibodies used to reverse ventricular fibrillation induced by digoxin ingestion in a child. Pediatrics, *70*:468, 1982.
118. Smith, T.W., et al.: Treatment of life-threatening digitalis intoxication with digoxin-specific Fab antibody fragments: experience in 26 cases. N. Engl. J. Med., *307*:1357, 1982.
119. Holt, D.W., and Benstead, J.G.: Postmortem assay of digoxin by radiommunoassay. J. Clin. Pathol., *28*:483, 1975.
120. Karliner, J.: Intravenous diphenylhydantoin sodium (Dilantin) in cardiac arrhythmias. Dis. Chest, *51*:256, 1967.
121. Halfant, R.H., et al.: Protection from digitalis toxicity with the prophylactic use of diphenylhydantoin sodium. Circulation, *36*:119, 1967.
122. Fisch, C., et al.: Transient effect of intravenous potassium on AV conduction and ectopic beats. Am. Heart J., *60*:220, 1960.
123. Bismuth, C., et al.: Hyperkalemia in acute digitalis poisoning: prognostic significance and therapeutic implication. Clin. Toxicol., *6*:153, 1973.
124. Koren, G.: Digoxin toxicity associated with amiodarone in children. J. Pediatr., *104*:467, 1984.
125. Cogan, J.J., et al.: Acute vasodilator therapy increases renal clearance of digoxin in patients with congestive heart failure. Circulation, *64*:973, 1981.
126. Fenster, P.E., et al.: Kinetics of the digoxin-aspirin combination. Clin. Pharmacol. Ther. *32*:428, 1982.
127. Wilkerson, R.D., et al.: Effects of selected drugs on serum digoxin concentration in dogs. Am. J. Cardiol., *45*:1201, 1980.
128. Schimmel, M.S., et al.: Toxic digitalis levels associated with indomethacin therapy in a neonate. Clin. Pediatr., *19*:768, 1980.
129. Koren, G., et al.: Effects of indomethacin on digoxin pharmacokinetics in preterm infants. Pediatr. Pharmacol., *4*:25, 1984.
130. Koren, G.: Interaction between digoxin and commonly coadministered drugs in children. Pediatrics. In press.
131. Vohringer, H.F., et al.: Der Einfluss von Antacide auf die Plasmakonzentration von Digoxin beim Menschen. Dtsch. Med. Wochenschr., *101*:106, 1976.

Chapter 2
Dopamine

Dopamine is an endogenous precursor of norepinephrine with sympathomimetic properties. It has become useful in the treatment of low cardiac output and hypertension in adults and children with various cardiac and noncardiac disease. In children, this agent has been successfully used to treat cardiogenic and septic shock, as well as low cardiac output following surgical treatment of congenital heart disease.[1-4] The drug also increases cardiac performance and raises systolic blood pressure in the severely asphyxiated neonate.[5] The primary effects of dopamine, and those that make the drug useful under these conditions, are positive inotropic, peripheral vasoconstricting, and renal vasodilatory effects.

Dopamine is the first-line sympathomimetic amine in adult therapy. It is preferred to isoproterenol because it has fewer tachycardiac and arrhythmogenic effects. In children, these effects are less of a problem, and both agents are used.

Structure

Dopamine is 3,4-dihydroxyphenylethylamine.

Pharmacologic Properties

At low concentrations, dopamine has a selective dilatory effect in several vascular beds, the most important of which is the renal arterial bed.[6, 7] This effect may result from stimulation of specific dopaminergic receptors. At high concentrations of dopamine, this effect is overcome by the generalized vasoconstricting action of the drug.

Dopamine has also a sympathomimetic action, resulting in its positive inotropic and peripheral vasoconstricting effects. It stimulates both beta-1- and beta-2-adrenoreceptors. Dopamine also releases norepinephrine from sympathetic nerve terminals. and thereby stimulates the usual effects of norepinephrine.[8] Dopamine also stimulates alpha-adrenoreceptors, but to a lesser extent than epinephrine or norepinephrine.

Hemodynamic Effects

The most important hemodynamic effects of dopamine are its positive inotropic effect, accompanied by various degree of positive chronotropic effect, its peripheral vasoconstricting effect, and at low doses, its direct renal vasodilatory effect. The positive inotropic effect results from both release of norepinephrine and direct stimulation by dopamine of cardiac beta-1-adrenoreceptors.[9] This process is accompanied by various degrees of acceleration of heart rate, which is usually less than that produced by isoproterenol. Occasionally, the heart rate may be slowed because of overall hemodynamic improvement. Increases of heart rate by about 30 to 65% were observed in infants treated with dopamine after corrective heart operations.[1] In a group of 14 severely asphyxiated neonates, dopamine produced no significant change in heart rate.[5] In my experience, dopamine may produce up to a 20% decrease in heart rate in children with low cardiac output, but this response is uncommon and is not seen with high doses of dopamine. Holzer and colleagues found no significant increase in heart rate during dopamine infusions of up to 30 µg/kg/min.[10] During the peak response to dopamine, the heart rate decreased.

The increased contractility and heart rate result in an increase in cardiac output. Dopamine produces peripheral vasoconstriction. This effect and the increase in cardiac output result in elevation of systemic arterial blood pressure, mainly systolic pressure. This action of dopamine is useful in conditions of shock. In conditions of low cardiac output associated with normal or high blood pressure, the effect may be deleterious because the elevation of peripheral vascular resistance increases afterload and prevents the full expression of the positive inotropic and chronotropic effects of dopamine as an increase in cardiac output. At low concentrations, dopamine selectively dilates the renal arterial bed. This process may cause diuresis when diuretic agents have failed. The mesenteric arterial bed is also dilated, although to a lesser extent.

The foregoing effects of dopamine result in the usual hemodynamic profile of the drug: (1) an increase in cardiac output by 20 to 30%,[9,11] although occasionally as high as 87%,[12] with an increase in stroke volume of 5 to 50%; (2) a varying increase in heart rate; (3) a significant increase in systolic systemic arterial pressure, with only a slight increase, if any, in diastolic pressure; (4) a decrease in the pulmonary capillary wedge pressure because of the increase in cardiac output, or no change, or even an increase because of systemic arterial and venous construction.

The effect on the pulmonary circulation is much less than on the systemic circulation. This differential vascular responsiveness may be especially prominent in infants. Durmmond and co-workers reported a full-term infant with persistent pulmonary hypertension who received an accidental bolus of 675 µg/kg dopamine.[13] The drug increased mean aortic pressure from 41 to 78 mm Hg (47%), whereas pulmonary arterial pressure changed from 76 to 78 mm Hg (3% only).

The hemodynamic effect of dopamine may be attenuated during continued therapy. In dogs, a substantial attenuation was observed after 24 hours.[14] This attenuation may result from depletion of catecholamine stores, on which the effect of dopamine partially depends, or from changes in the density of adrenoreceptors. In children, development of tolerance is of little clinical relevance because dopamine is usually used only for short periods.

In addition to the renal arteries, dopamine dilates the mesenteric, coronary, and cerebral arteries. This effect can be inhibited by phenothiazines and haloperidol, but not by beta- or alpha-adrenoreceptor blocking agents.

Pediatric Use

Review of the hemodynamic effects of dopamine indicates that the drug is especially suitable for treatment of low cardiac output associated with hypotension. Many studies in adults confirm the efficacy of dopamine in patients with this condition. In children, the most important use of dopamine is to treat low cardiac output following repair of congenital heart defects.

Lang and associates studied the effect of dopamine in five infants in a low output state following cardiac operations.[1] The infants responded to dopamine, but the response was different from that observed in adults. Heart rate, systemic arterial pressure and cardiac index all increased. No significant changes were noted in right atrial pressure, left atrial pressure, pulmonary arterial pressure, systemic and pulmonary vascular resistances, and stroke volume. Despite the high dose of dopamine used in this study, no arrhythmia was observed.

Driscoll and colleagues studied the effect of dopamine in 24 older children in shock for various reasons.[2] The children ranged in age from 2 days to 18 years (mean: 39 months). The dose of dopamine was 0.3 to 25 µg/kg/min. A favorable response was determined as a 15% increase above control level in systolic arterial pressure and an increase in urine production. Thirteen of the patients responded favorably. The main problem in 4 of the 24 patients was infection; 2 of these 4 children survived. The other 20 children had congenital heart disease; 18 developed shock postoperatively. Seven of these 20 children survived. Dopamine increased systolic blood pressure from 69 ± 4 to 81 ± 4 mm Hg and increased the mean urinary output from 0.8 ± 0.2 to 2.7 ± 0.8 ml/kg/hour. None of the 4 children in whom dopamine was ineffective survived.[2]

Personal experience in pediatric intensive care units indicated that at least a transient response to dopamine was observed in more than 80% of 19 infants and children in shock.

Animal experiments revealed that dopamine may be ineffective in increasing cardiac output in the presence of pulmonary hypertension resulting from causes other than left ventricular dysfunction.[15] However, it was shown that dopamine may increase the pulmonary artery pressure.[16,17] These findings raised the question whether infants and children with congenital heart diseases, who have developed secondary pulmonary vascular disease, would benefit from dopamine. Some authorities even suggest that dopamine may be contraindicated in the presence of elevated pulmonary vascular resistance.

Use in Neonates

Relatively few data are available on the effect of dopamine in sick neonates.[13,18,19] The effect resembles in general those observed in older children and in adults. Driscoll, et al.,[18] reported that dopamine, isoprenaline, and dobutamine increased heart rate to the same extent in the newborn dog. Dopamine, however, increased cardiac output more effectively. Dopamine and dobutamine increased mean systemic arterial blood pressure whereas isoprenaline decreased it. Hoge et al.,[19] reported that low doses of dopamine in mature newborn lambs increased cardiac output and decreased systemic vascular resistance without altering heart rate. The decrease in systemic vascular resistance may be secondary to the increase in cardiac output.

Durmmond, et al.,[3] studied the effect of dopamine in neonatal lambs aged 12 to 24 hours. The drug increased pulmonary vascular resistance by about 50% and systemic vascular resistance by 99%. The pulmonary circulation was responsive only to higher doses of dopamine than those required for affecting the systemic circulation. Left atrial pressure increased sharply at doses of 50 μg/min or higher. Asymptomatic bradyarrhythmia occurred in 9 of 12 studies of neonates who received dopamine at doses of 50 to 200 μg/min and disappeared with higher doses. It was concluded that the effect of dopamine in neonates is complex and differs in various vascular beds.

Perinatal asphyxia can cause myocardial depression with hemodynamic deterioration. DiSessa and co-workers studied the cardiovascular effects of dopamine at an infusion rate of 2.5 μg/kg/min in 14 severely asphyxiated neonates.[5] The echocardiographically determined shortening fraction and the mean velocity of circumferential fiber shortening increased when compared to preinfusion values, whereas placebo-treated neonates showed no change. Systolic blood pressure rose during treatment with dopamine, and a smaller rise of diastolic pressure was also observed. Heart rate and echocardiographically measured systolic time intervals were not altered. Thus, low doses of dopamine increase cardiac performance and raise systolic blood pressure in severely asphyxiated neonates.[5] Dopamine may be important for cardiocirculatory support in such children.

Effect of Maturity on Drug Response

The stage of maturity affects the cardiovascular response to dopamine. Driscoll and associates reported that, in the neonatal canine ventricular myocardium, the dopamine-induced positive inotropic effect increased with increasing postnatal age.[20] The dose-response curve of the ventricular myocardium of a young puppy that had been given reserpine was similar to that of the ventricle of a rabbit that had received reserpine, whereas the dose-response curve of the ventricle of an older puppy that had been given reserpine was similar to that of the ventricle of a rabbit that had not received reserpine. These differences may have resulted from variations in the amount of norepinephrine available for release from nerve endings.[20]

Harris and Van Petten reported that the cardiovascular system of the unanesthesized fetal lamb responded to dopamine to a lesser extent than did that of the adult ewe.[21]

Lang and colleagues found that infants after corrective cardiac operations responded to dopamine, but this response was different from that observed in adults.[1] Because this series included only five infants, and because of the marked variability in the response to dopamine in adults, it is difficult to draw any conclusions from these findings.

The positive inotropic effect and other cardiovascular effects of dopamine are probably modified by maturity. Further studies are required before this modification is fully understood.

Combination with Other Drugs

Dobutamine

The combination of dopamine and dobutamine is discussed in Chapter 3.

Phenoxybenzamine

The rationale behind combining dopamine with phenoxybenzamine is to prevent the alpha-adrenergic action of dopamine by phenoxybenzamine and to encourage the beta-adrenergic and the specific ("dopaminergic") actions of dopamine. Kawamura and co-workers studied the effect of this combination in 27 infants and children, aged 8 months to 6 years, in whom withdrawal from cardiopulmonary bypass for low cardiac output was difficult.[22] Dopamine was given at 10 to 30 µg/

kg/min, after the additional administration of half of the initial dose of phenoxybenzamine, which was 0.5 to 1.0 mg/kg, given during the first half of cardiopulmonary bypass. With combined therapy, it was possible to withdraw the patient from cardiopulmonary bypass in a stable hemodynamic state and with an adequate urinary output.[22]

Digoxin

In children, digoxin and dopamine may be used together in conditions of cardiocirculatory collapse. No controlled studies have been performed.

Nitrates

I have observed significant hemodynamic improvement with the combined used of dopamine and intravenously administered nitroglycerin or isosorbide dinitrate. The rationale is to achieve the positive inotropic effect of dopamine and to abolish its peripheral vasoconstricting effect with the nitrates. The pediatric experience with intravenously administered nitrates is limited, but experience with nitroprusside is extensive. The combination of dopamine with nitroprusside may be beneficial in children with depressed myocardial contractility and peripheral vasoconstriction.

Clinical Pharmacology

Dopamine is effective by intravenous administration. When given orally, the drug is ineffective because it is metabolized by both monoamine oxidase and catechol-O-methyl transferase.

The effect of dopamine depends on the rate of infusion. In adults, at low infusion rates of 1.0 to 3.0 μg/kg/min, dopamine dilates the renal arterial bed and produces a slight positive inotropic effect. At rates of 5.0 to 10.0 μg/kg/min, the magnitude of the positive inotropic effect increases, a positive chronotropic effect is observed, and the peripheral vasoconstricting action becomes evident. At infusion rates higher than 10 μg/kg/min, the positive inotropic and peripheral vasoconstricting effects predominate. The renal vasodilatory effect is countered by the generalized vasoconstriction.

The maximal doses used in infants (30 to 40 μg/kg/min) are higher than those used in adults (up to 20 μg/kg/min). Therefore, it is possible that the ranges of doses at which the different effects are observed in infants are different from those in adults. Further studies in this field are required.

The onset of action of dopamine is rapid. It may be evident within minutes of initiation of infusion. Dopamine is rapidly metabolized, and its effect disappears within minutes of discontinuing the infusion.

Adverse Effects

Although the primary unfavorable side effects of dopamine are cardiovascular, the drug may also affect the central nervous system.

Cardiovascular Effects

The positive inotropic and chronotropic effects and the peripheral vasoconstricting effect of dopamine increase the myocardial oxygen consumption and may aggravate myocardial ischemia in patients with coronary artery disease. This effect is of little relevance in infants and children. Dopamine may also produce a hypertensive response. Like other sympathomimetic amines, dopamine has an arrhythmogenic potential. This potential is less than that of isoproterenol, but greater than that of amrinone and greater or equal to that of dobutamine. Dopamine-induced myocardial ischemia may enhance the arrhythmogenic effect produced by beta-adrenergic stimulation by dopamine and released endogenous catecholamines.

High infusion rates or extravasation of dopamine may cause ischemia and gangrene of extremities.[23-25] These adverse effects result from local vasoconstriction. They may be treated by local administration of alpha-adrenoreceptor blocking agents.

Other Effects

Dopamine may affect the central nervous system and may cause nausea and vomiting. It is not known how this effect is produced because dopamine does not cross the blood-brain barrier, and thus exogenously administered dopamine does not penetrate the brain.

Dosage and Administration

Dopamine is administered intravenously. The infusion rates used in adults are 2.5 to 20.0 µg/kg/min, and in infants and children, 1.0 to 30.0, or rarely even 40.0, µg/kg/min.

References

1. Lang, P., et al.: The hemodynamic effects of dopamine in infants after corrective surgery. J. Pediatr., *96*:630, 1980.
2. Driscoll, D.J., et al.: The use of dopamine in children. J. Pediatr., *92*:309, 1978.
3. Stephenson, L.W., et al.: Effects of nitroprusside and dopamine on pulmonary arterial vasculature in children after cardiac surgery. Circulation, *60 (Suppl. I)*: 104, 1979.
4. Fiddler, G.I., et al.: Dopamine infusion for the treatment of myocardial dysfunction associated with persistent transitional circulation. Arch. Dis. Child., *55*:194, 1980.
5. DiSessa, T.G., et al.: The cardiovascular effects of dopamine in the severely asphyxiated neonate. J. Pediatr., *99*:772, 1981.
6. McDonald, R.H., Jr., et al.: Augmentation of sodium excretion and blood flow by dopamine in man. Clin. Res., *11*:248, 1963.
7. McDonald, R.H., Jr., et al.: Effect of dopamine in man: glomerular filtration rate and renal plasma flow. J. Clin. Invest., *43*:1116, 1964.

8. Tsai, T.H., et al.: Effects of dopamine and methyldopamine on smooth muscle and on the cardiac pacemaker. J. Pharmacol. Exp. Ther., *156*:310, 1967.
9. Leier, C.V., et al.: Comparative systemic and regional haemodynamic effects of dopamine and dobutamine in patients with cardiomyopathic heart failure. Circulation, *58*:446, 1978.
10. Holzer, J., et al.: Effectiveness of dopamine in patients with cardiogenic shock. Am. J. Cardiol., *32*:79, 1973.
11. Rosenblum, R., et al.: Cardiac and renal haemodynamic effects of dopamine in man. Clin. Res., *18*:326, 1970.
12. Beregevich, J., et al.: Dose-related hemodynamic and renal effects of dopamine in congestive heart failure. Am. Heart J., *87*:550, 1974.
13. Durmmond, W.H., et al.: Cardiopulmonary dopamine dose response in chronically catheterized neonatal lambs, (Abstract.) Circulation, *62 (Suppl. III)*:25, 1980.
14. Maekawa, K., et al.: Comparison of dobutamine and dopamine in dogs with acute myocardial infarction. (Abstract.) Am. J. Cardiol., *49*:1037, 1982.
15. Marx, G.R., et al.: Response to dopamine in rats with acute and chronic pulmonary hypertension. (Abstract.) Am. J. Cardiol., *49*:939, 1982.
16. Harrison, D.C., et al.: The pulmonary and systemic circulatory response to dopamine infusion. Br. J. Pharmacol., *37*:618, 1969.
17. Holloway, E.L., et al.: Acute circulatory effects of dopamine in patients with pulmonary hypertension. Br. Heart J., *37*:482, 1975.
18. Driscoll, D.J., et al.: Comparative hemodynamic effects of isoproterenol, dopamine and dobutamine in the newborn dog. Pediatr. Res., *13*:1006, 1979.
19. Roge, C.L., et al.: Cardiovascular actions of isuprel, dopamine, and dobutamine in mature newborn lambs. (Abstract.) In World Congress of Pediatric Cardiology. London, June 2-6, 1980.
20. Driscoll, D.J., et al.: Inotropic response of the neonatal canine myocardium to dopamine. Pediatr. Res., *12*:42, 1978.
21. Harris, W.H., and Van Petten, G.R.: The effects of dopamine on blood pressure and heart rate of the unanesthetized fetal lamb. Am. J. Obstet. Gynecol., *130*:211, 1978.
22. Kawamura, M., et al.: Combined use of phenoxybenzamine and dopamine for low cardiac output syndrome in children at withdrawal from cardiopulmonary bypass. Br. Heart J., *43*:388, 1980.
23. Alexander, C.S., et al.: Pedal gangrene associated with the use of dopamine. N. Engl. J. Med., *293*:591, 1975.
24. Greene, S.I., and Smith, J.W.: Dopamine gangrene. N. Engl. J. Med., *294*:114, 1976.
25. Greenlaw, C.W., and Mull, L.W.: Dopamine induced ischemia. Lancet, *2*:555, 1977.

Chapter 3

Dobutamine

Dobutamine is a synthetic sympathomimetic amine with a potent positive inotropic effect. It was introduced over 10 years ago, and since then it has been investigated for treatment of congestive heart failure and shock. In adults, this agent is effective in the short-term management of patients with congestive heart failure and, to some extent, in long-term treatment as well, by repeat intravenous administration. It is also effective in treatment of cardiogenic shock in adults. In children, dobutamine is used mainly to treat cardiogenic and septic shock and has not been evaluated for treatment of chronic congestive heart failure. The beneficial effects of dobutamine in adults include an increase in cardiac output and arterial pressure and a decrease in pulmonary capillary wedge pressure without a significant change in heart rate. Unlike dopamine, dobutamine in low doses does not have a direct renal vasodilatory effect. In children, the hemodynamic profile of the drug may be different from that of adults, mainly in the effect on pulmonary capillary wedge pressure.

Structure

Dobutamine is 4-[2-(3-(p-hydroxy-phenyl-1-methylpropylamino) ethyl]-pyrocatechol hydrochloride. The molecule resembles that of dopamine.

Hemodynamic Effects

In adults, dobutamine has been studied primarily in patients with acute hemodynamic deterioration after myocardial infarction or chronic congestive heart failure. The hemodynamic changes produced by dobutamine are attributed mainly to its positive inotropic effect. They include increases in myocardial contractility, cardiac output, stroke volume, ejection fraction, and systemic arterial pressure and decreases in systemic and pulmonary capillary wedge pressure, with minimal to moderate acceleration of heart rate.[1-3] The hemodynamic improvement is evident both at rest and during exercise.[4]

The reduction in systemic vascular resistance during treatment with low to moderate doses of dobutamine probably results from a decrease in the enhanced sympathetic activity in patients with congestive heart failure. The decrease in sympathetic activity results from the overall hemodynamic improvement.[5]

Some investigations reported that the sudden hemodynamic improvement produced by dobutamine was sustained for several days of continuous treatment in about 67% of the patients with chronic congestive heart failure.[6,7] In 40% of these patients, sustained improvement was observed for 10 weeks. Some patients treated by repeat infusions of dobutamine for 5 hours each week during 24 weeks showed significant improvements in exercise performance and clinical condition, possibly because of a conditioning effect.[8] Continuous infusion for more than 3 days may result in the development of hemodynamic tolerance, however.[9] The tolerance may be attributed to down-regulation of beta-adrenoreceptors.

Dobutamine should be used with caution in mechanically ventilated patients because the reduction of systemic vascular resistance and pulmonary capillary wedge pressure may predispose these patients to systemic hypertension.[10]

Dobutamine has no direct effect on the coronary arteries. The increase in myocardial oxygen consumption resulting from the positive inotropic and chronotropic effects of dobutamine, however, may decrease the coronary vascular resistance and may increase coronary blood flow. The dobutamine-induced increase in myocardial oxygen consumption rarely causes overt myocardial ischemia, even in patients with coronary artery disease.[11]

The general hemodynamic improvement may also improve renal function, evident as increases in urinary flow and sodium concentration.[7] Unlike dopamine at low doses, dobutamine has no direct renal vasodilatory effect.

Young Age Groups

The hemodynamic effects of dobutamine in young age groups have been evaluated in a few animal and human studies. In general, the effects of the drug in young subjects are similar to those in adults. Therefore, dobutamine may play a role in the management of congestive heart failure and shock in infants and children. Although the drug has not been evaluated in the whole spectrum of hemodynamic disturbances, it increases cardiac output and, to some extent, systemic arterial pressure. The effect on pulmonary capillary wedge pressure is controversial and may differ from that observed in adults.

Driscoll and associates reported that, in anesthetized puppies with open chests, dobutamine increased cardiac output.[12] This phenomenon occurred at a much lower increase in heart rate than that produced by isoproterenol in achieving a similar increase in cardiac output. Systemic arterial blood pressure was increased, and renal blood flow was not altered. Dopamine raised arterial pressure to a greater extent than dobutamine.

In another study, Driscoll and colleagues evaluated the effect of dobutamine in 12 children with congenital heart disease during diagnostic cardiac catheterization.[13] Dobutamine was given at 2 infusion rates of 2 and 7.75 µg/kg/min, each for 10 min. At the higher infusion rate, the drug increased the cardiac index from 3.5 to 4.7 L/min/m^2, systemic arterial pressure from 109/61 to 151/74 mm Hg, mean arterial pressure from 80 to 104 mm Hg, and stroke index from 38 to 49 ml/beat/m^2. Pulmonary capillary mean blood pressure decreased from 8 to 6 mm Hg. All the changes were statistically significant. The lower dose of dobutamine produced similar, although less pronounced changes. Heart rate, pulmonary and right atrial mean blood pressure, and systemic and pulmonary vascular resistance were unchanged with either dose of dobutamine.[13]

As evident from the foregoing data, this agent is of special benefit in the treatment of patients in shock. Perkin and co-workers studied the hemodynamic effects of dobutamine in 33 infants and children in cardiogenic or septic shock.[14] The drug was administered at infusion rates of 2.5, 5.0, 7.5, and 10.0 µg/kg/min. It increased cardiac index, left ventricular stroke work index, and pulmonary capillary wedge pressure, and it decreased the systemic ateriolar resistance index. Heart rate, mean systemic arterial pressure, mean pulmonary arterial pressure, right atrial pressure, and pulmonary arteriolar resistance index were little changed. These data were further analyzed according to the cause of shock, the age of the patients, and hemodynamic parameters. It was concluded that dobutamine is a useful drug in the management of children in shock, especially in those older than 12 months in cardiac failure not complicated by severe hypotension.[14]

An important adverse hemodynamic effect of dobutamine in this series was the increase in pulmonary capillary wedge pressure, which led to pulmonary edema in at least one patient. It is difficult to understand the mechanism of this effect. Possible causes are pulmonary venoconstriction, which has been observed in animals given dobutamine, or diminished left ventricular compliance. This effect may limit the use of dobutamine in infants and children with pulmonary congestion or pulmonary hypertension.

The effects of dobutamine in infants and children with chronic congestive heart failure, caused either by endomyocardial diseases or by mechanical lesions, are yet to be studied. Dobutamine may not produce hemodyamic improvement in the presence of hypovolemia or in patients with severe, fixed, left ventricular outflow tract obstruction, such as valvar or subvalvar aortic stenosis.

Mechanism of Action

The most important effect of dobutamine is its positive inotropic effect, exerted by direct stimulation of beta-adrenoreceptors. At low doses, dobutamine has a peripheral vasoconstrictor effect because of stimulation of alpha-adrenoreceptors. At high doses, usually higher than the pediatric dose, dobutamine produces peripheral vasodilation.[15, 16] Dobutamine also increases the heart rate at these doses.

Comparison with Other Positive Inotropic Agents

The effects of dobutamine in adults are comparable to or are even superior to those of other positive inotropic agents. No comparative studies have been conducted in children, and data should be derived from studies in adults and young animals.

Dopamine

Dobutamine can increase cardiac output in a manner similar to that of dopamine. Dobutamine may be superior to dopamine in that it has a less arrhythmogenic effect and produces a smaller acceleration in heart rate and a greater decrease in pulmonary capillary wedge pressure[1-3] Dopamine may be better in patients with impaired renal function, however, because it has a direct vasodilatory effect on the renal vasculature. Dopamine may also be superior in mechanically ventilated patients in cardiogenic shock; dobutamine decreased systemic vascular resistance and pulmonary capillary wedge pressure to a greater extent than dopamine.[10] In mechanically ventilated patients, such effects may cause systemic hypotension. In my experience, some adults in cardiogenic shock, whether receiving mechanical ventilation or not, failed to respond to dopamine, but responded to dobutamine.

No comparative studies have been conducted in infants and children. Driscoll and associates compared the hemodynamic effects of dopamine and dobutamine in the newborn dog.[12] Both agents produced a significant increase in cardiac output and systemic arterial mean blood pressure and a moderate increase in heart rate. Dopamine increased renal arterial blood flow, whereas dobutamine did not alter this parameter.

From these data, it may be concluded that dobutamine is at least as effective as dopamine in increasing cardiac output. It may be tried in children in shock or congestive heart failure in whom dopamine has failed.

Isoproterenol

Isoproterenol is the inotropic agent used most commonly for treatment of cardiogenic shock in children. Isoproterenol is more effective, on a weight basis, than dobutamine in increasing cardiac output, but it has the disadvantage of accelerating heart rate to a much greater extent than dobutamine. Comparative studies of both agents in infants and children have not been reported. Driscoll and colleagues compared the hemodynamic effects of isoproterenol and dobutamine in the newborn dog.[12] They found that isoproterenol produced a much greater increase in heart rate than dobutamine, to achieve a similar elevation in cardiac output. Systemic arterial mean blood pressure was increased by dobutamine, but decreased by isoproterenol. Renal artery blood flow was not altered by dobutamine and was decreased by isoproterenol.

Prenalterol

No studies on the effect of this new beta-1-adrenoreceptor agonist in children have been reported. In adults, prenalterol may be more effective than dobutamine.[17]

Salbutamol

Dobutamine can produce a greater hemodynamic improvement than salbutamol in patients with elevated left ventricular filling pressure.[18] No comparative studies in children have been reported.

Combinations with Other Drugs

Dopamine

Combined treatment with dobutamine and dopamine may be superior to treatment with high doses of either agent alone. Dobutamine has the advantage of increasing cardiac output without elevating systemic vascular resistance, but it does not have a direct renal vasodilatory effect. At low doses, dopamine dilates the renal arteries, but at higher doses, it produces peripheral vasoconstriction. Therefore, it is reasonable to use low doses of dopamine together with low to high doses of dobutmine in patients with congestive heart failure or those in shock. This combination is preferred over a higher dose of dobutamine in mechanically ventilated patients, in whom excessive reduction of pulmonary capillary wedge pressure is undesirable. In my experience, in adults with congestive heart failure and hypotension, significant hemodynamic improvement is produced by the combination of low doses (up to 5 μg/kg/min) of dopamine and low to high doses of dobutamine (5 to 15 μg/kg/min), titrated according to the patient's response.

Nitroprusside

Nitroprusside is used in children to treat hypertensive emergencies, but not congestive heart failure. In adults with congestive heart failure, however, the combination of dobutamine and nitroprusside may produce a greater increase in cardiac output and a greater decrease in pulmonary capillary wedge pressure than either drug alone.

Nitrates

In my experience, the combination of dobutamine with intravenously administered nitrates, such as nitroglycerin and isosorbide dinitrate, may produce hemodynamic improvement in patients with congestive heart failure who are not responsive to either dobutamine or nitrates alone. The experience with nitrates in children is limited.

Clinical Pharmacology

Dobutamine is effective only by intravenous administration. Its effect, evident within minutes of the initiation of the infusion, disappears within several minutes of the termination of the infusion. A correlation between the rate of infusion and the drug's effect has been demonstrated in children.[13] In adults, infusion rates higher than 17 to 20 μg/kg/min produce no further hemodynamic improvement.

Dobutamine is metabolized and excreted in the urine as conjugates and other inactive metabolites. The elimination half-life is about 3 minutes.[19]

Side Effects

The side effects of dobutamine include adverse cardiovascular effects such as potentiation and provocation of arrhythmias, acceleration of heart rate, and rarely, in patients with coronary artery disease, myocardial ischemia. In children in shock, an increase in pulmonary capillary wedge pressure, leading in at least one case to the development of pulmonary edema, has been reported.[14] Other adverse effects, including headache, nausea, dyspnea, and palpitations, have occurred in up to 3% of the patients.

Dosage and Administration

Dobutamine is given only intravenously. In children, infusion rates range from 2 to 10 μg/kg/min. In adults, the usual infusion rate is 5 to 15 μg/kg/min.

References

1. Tuttle, P.R., and Mills, J.: Dobutamine, development of a new catecholamine to selectively increase cardiac contractility. Circ. Res., 36:185, 1975.

2. Loeb, H, Bredakis, J., and Gunnar, R.: Superiority of dobutamine over dopamine for augmentation of cardiac output in patients with chronic low output cardiac failure. Circulation, 55:375, 1977.
3. Leier, C.V., Webel, J., and Bush, C.A.: The cardiovascular effects of the continuous infusion of dobutamine in patients with severe cardiac failure. Circulation, 56:468, 1977.
4. Maskin, C.S. et al.: Failure of dobutamine to increase exercise capacity despite hemodynamic improvement in severe chronic heart failure. Am. J. Cardiol., 51:177, 1983.
5. Berkowitz, C., et al.: Comparative responses to dobutamine and nitroprusside in patients with chronic low output cardiac failure. Circulation, 56:918, 1977.
6. Unverferth, D.V., et al.: Long-term benefit of dobutamine in patients with congestive cardiomyopathy. Am. Heart J., 100:622, 1980.
7. Slutsky, R., Watkins, J., and Costello, D.: Radionuclide evaluation of the systolic blood pressure/end-systolic volume relationship: response to pharmacologic agents in patients with coronary artery disease. Am. Heart J., 105:53, 1983.
8. Leier, C.V., et al.: Drug-induced conditioning in congestive heart failure. Circulation, 65:7, 1982.
9. Unverferth, D.V., et al.: Tolerance to dobutamine after a 72 hour continuous infusion. Am. J. Med., 69:262, 1980.
10. Leier, C.V., et al.: Comparative systemic and regional hemodynamic effects of dopamine and dobutamine in patients with cardiomyopathic heart failure. Circulation, 58:466, 1978.
11. Warltier, D.C., et al.: Redistribution of myocardial blood flow distal to a dynamic coronary arterial stenosis by sympathomimetic amines. Am. J. Cardiol., 48:269, 1981.
12. Driscoll, D.J., et al.: Comparative hemodynamic effects of isoproterenol, dopamine, and dobutamine in the newborn dog. Pediatr. Res., 13:1006, 1979.
13. Driscoll, D.J., et al.: Hemodynamic effects of dobutamine in children. Am. J. Cardiol., 43: 581, 1979.
14. Perkin, R.M., et al.: Dobutamine: a hemodynamic evaluation in children with shock. J. Pediatr., 100:977, 1982.
15. Robie, N.W., et al.: In vivo analysis of adrenergic receptor activity of dobutamine. Circ. Res., 34.663, 1974.
16. Holloway, G.A., and Frederikson, E.L.: Dobutamine, a new beta agonist. Anesth. Analg., 53:616, 1974.
17. Richard, C, et al.: Combined hemodynamic effects of dopamine and dobutamine in cardiogenic shock. Circulation, 67:620, 1983.
18. Fowler, M.B., et al.: Comparison of haemodynamic responses to dobutamine and solbutamol in cardiogenic shock after acute myocardial infarction. Br. Med. J., 284:73, 1982.
19. Kates, S.E., and Leier, C.V.: Dobutamine pharmacokinetics in severe heart failure. Clin. Pharmacol. Ther., 24:537, 1978.

Chapter 4

Isoproterenol (Isoprenaline)

Isoproterenol is a potent beta-adrenoreceptor agonist. It was first synthesized in 1940,[1] and since then it has been used experimentally and clinically for cardiocirculatory support, predominantly in cases of severely symptomatic bradycardia. Until recently, the drug was the sympathomimetic amine of choice in infants and children.

Structure

Isoproterenol is DL-beta-[3,4,-dihydroxy-phenyl]-alpha-isopropyl-aminoethanol. The L-isomer is much more potent than the D-isomer.

Pharmacologic Properties

This drug is a potent beta-adrenoreceptor agonist without an effect on alpha-adrenoreceptors. This effect results in acceleration of heart rate and relaxation of vascular, bronchial, and gastrointestinal smooth muscles.

Hemodynamic Effects

Isoproterenol exerts positive chronotropic and inotropic and a peripheral vasodilatory effect. Cardiac output is increased because of increases in heart rate and contractility. Systolic pressure is unchanged or is elevated, and diastolic pressure is reduced. At high doses of the drug mean arterial pressure may fall.

The vasodilatory effect is partially selective. It increases renal blood flow in patients in shock, but reduces it in normotensive patients. Vasodilation occurs mainly in skeletal muscles, but also in mesenteric arteries. The isoproterenol-induced tachycardia results not only from beta-adrenoreceptor stimulation, but also from withdrawal of vagal tone due to the fall in mean arterial pressure.[2]

Until recently, isoproterenol was the sympathomimetic amine of choice in infants and children. In adults, it was replaced by dopamine and dobutamine, which produce a similar or greater positive inotropic effect with less acceleration of heart rate. In adults with coronary artery disease, it is especially important to avoid excessive acceleration of heart rate, and therefore, isoproterenol was replaced by more modern sympathomimetic amines. Because this problem is less significant in children, isoproterenol was used in pediatric practice until recently. The benefits of dopamine and dobutamine have been appreciated by pediatric cardiologists, and these agents have largely replaced isoproterenol in the treatment of severe circulatory decompensation. Isoproterenol is still the sympathomimetic amine of choice in cases of severe symptomatic bradycardia.

Effect on Pulmonary Function

Isoproterenol relaxes bronchial smooth muscle and relieves spontaneous or drug-induced bronchoconstriction. This effect cannot be used for long-term treatment of bronchial asthma because of rapid development of tolerance.

Effect on Primary Pulmonary Hypertension

Short-term administration of isoproterenol produces at least a transient decrease in pulmonary arterial pressure and pulmonary vascular resistance in patients with primary pulmonary hypertension.[3] A recent report has described a young patient with primary pulmonary hypertension who had noted relief of symptoms and improvement in exercise capacity and pulmonary hemodynamics during 6 years of therapy with sublingual isoproterenol.[4]

Hormonal and Metabolic Effects

By beta-adrenoreceptor stimulation, isoproterenol raises blood glucose levels. This increase and direct beta-adrenergic stimulation of pancreatic beta cells enhance insulin secretion. Like other beta-adrenoreceptor agonists, isoproterenol increases lipolysis and plasma levels of free fatty acids.

Clinical Pharmacology

Isoproterenol can be administered intravenously, by inhalation, sublingually, or orally. After oral administration, absorption is inconsistent, and the drug undergoes first-pass hepatic metabolism, which results in low and inconsistent systemic bioavailability.

The elimination half-life of the drug is short, and the effect is terminated within minutes of discontinuance of infusion. The drug is metabolized by catechol-O-methyl transferase and monoamine oxidase.

Side Effects

Such effects include tachycardia, cardiac arrhythmias, aggravation of ischemia, palpitations, headache, myocardial necrosis, and hypotension.

References

1. Konzett, H: Neue broncholytisch hochwirksame Körper der adrenalinreihe. Naunyn Schmiedebergs Arch. Exp. Pharmakol. Pathol., *197*:27, 1940.
2. Arnold, JMO and McDevitt, D.G.: Contribution of the vagus to the haemodynamic responses following intravenous boluses of isoprenaline. Br. J. Clin. Pharmacol., *15*:423, 1983.
3. Shettigar, U.R., et al.: Primary pulmonary hypertension: favorable effect of isoproterenol. N. Engl. J. Med., *295*:1414, 1976.
4. Pietro, D.A., et al.: Sustained improvement in primary pulmonary hypertension during six years of treatment with sublingual isoproterenol. N. Engl. J. Med., *310*:1032, 1984.

Chapter 5

Bipyridine Derivatives

Two bipyridine derivatives, amrinone and milrinone, have been clinically investigated for treatment of congestive heart failure. Both have positive inotropic and peripheral vasodilatory effects. Their mechanism of action differs from that of all other known positive inotropic agents. The use of bipyridine derivatives in newborns with congestive heart failure is controversial, but these drugs may play some role in the treament of newborns with pulmonary hypertension.

Amrinone is a bipyridine derivative with positive inotropic and peripheral vasodilatory properties in the presence or absence of congestive heart failure. In adults with congestive heart failure, amrinone produces hemodynamic and symptomatic improvement when given alone or in combination with other positive inotropic agents, diuretic agents, or vasodilators. It may be given to children in whom all other forms of treatment for congestive heart failure have failed. The drug is contraindicated, however, in neonates and in small infants because animal studies show that, at these early stages of life, amrinone may have a negative inotropic effect.

Studies of oral amrinone have been recently terminated because of poor results. Milrinone is now being evaluated for oral use.

Structure of Amrinone

Amrinone is 5-amino(3,4'-bipyridine)-6(1H)-one.

Hemodynamic Effects of Amrinone

The most important hemodynamic actions of amrinone are its positive inotropic effect and its peripheral vasodilatory effect. The positive inotropic effect has been demonstrated in isolated myocardial preparations of various animal species and in myocardium of human subjects obtained during cardiac surgical procedures. The human myocardium is more sensitive than the animal myocardium to the effect of amrinone.[1-4] Amrinone also has a direct peripheral vasodilatory effect. It does not depend on vascular innervation; this effect has also been demonstrated by direct injection of the drug to an isolated, denervated canine hindlimb. Amrinone dilates both systemic and pulmonary arteries.[3,5,6]

In patients with congestive heart failure, amrinone augments cardiac contractility. This effect is due to the direct positive inotropic effect of amrinone, as well as to sympathetic activation resulting from amrinone-induced peripheral vasodilation. In these patients, amrinone usually increases left ventricular dP/dt maximum, ejection fraction, and cardiac index and decreases peripheral vascular resistance, left ventricular end-diastolic pressure, and right atrial pressure. The heart rate is usually not altered, or it is slightly increased, and mean systemic arterial pressure is either unchanged or is slightly reduced.[7-9]

Hemodynamic improvement was also observed in patients already treated with digitalis and diuretics. This improvement was associated with relief of symptoms and an increase in exercise tolerance.

In patients with congestive heart failure, amrinone increased the renal plasma flow and the glomerular filtration rate.[10]

The beneficial effect of amrinone was sustained throughout long periods of treatment.

The mechanism of action of amrinone is unknown, but it does not operate by means of adrenergic receptors, like sympathomimetic amines, or by sodium-potassium-activated adenosine triphosphatase. Inhibition of phosphodiesterase or changes in calcium balance may play a role in the positive inotropic effect of amrinone. The positive inotropic effect of amrinone is additional to that produced by other positive inotropic agents.

Young Age Groups

Several preliminary animal studies showed that amrinone may not produce a positive inotropic effect in the fetus and newborn.[6,11] Binah and associates studied the effect of amrinone on systemic arterial pressure and dP/dt in newborn, young, and adult dogs.[12] These researchers found that the effect of amrinone on myocardial contractility changes with growth and development. Binah and co-workers also evaluated the effect of amrinone on the contractility and electrophysiologic features of isolated cardiac muscle of newborn to 96-day-old beagle dogs. The effect of amrinone on myocardial contractility was age related. A significant decrease of contractility of right ventricular trabecular and papillary muscles was observed in the 0-to-3-day-old puppies. In contrast, amrinone augmented contractility obtained from the 4-to-10-day-old puppies. The extent of the positive inotropic effect became greater through day 96 of life. That the negative inotropic effect of amrinone was not associated with changes in the action potential plateau suggests that the slow inward (calcium) current is not involved in the mechanism of this effect. Because of these findings, the drug is currently contraindicated in newborns with congestive heart failure.

Effect of Amrinone on Pulmonary Hypertension

Amrinone reduced pulmonary arterial resistance and pressure in one of seven adult patients with primary pulmonary hypertension.[13]

It was recently shown that bypiridine derivatives, particularly milrinone, but also amrinone, may be useful in managing neonatal hypoxic pulmonary vasoconstriction, especially in the presence of myocardial depression. Coe and colleagues studied the effect of amrinone on pulmonary arteriolar resistance in conscious newborn lambs.[14] After induction of hypoxic pulmonary vasocontriction and return to normoxia, bolus injections of amrinone, 100 to 1000 µg/kg (30 min apart), were given into the right pulmonary artery. Hypoxia increased pulmonary artery pressure by 45% and pulmonary arteriolar resistance by 52%. Amrinone reduced these levels by 17 and 24%, respectively. It also reduced systemic vascular resistance by 16% and increased cardiac output by 11%, heart rate by 11%, and left ventricular dP/dt by 40%.[14]

No studies of amrinone have been conducted in human newborns with pulmonary hypertension.

Electrophysiologic Effects of Amrinone

Amrinone slightly increases the maximum rate of phase 0 depolarization and slightly prolongs the duration of action potential.[15] It may prolong or shorten the P-R interval and may increase the spontaneous sinus rate.[16] Amrinone can be safely administered to patients with intraventricular conduction disturbances.[17]

Clinical Pharmacology of Amrinone

Amrinone is effective by both intravenous and oral administration. The effect of the drug becomes evident within several minutes from intravenous injection. After oral administration, the drug is absorbed rapidly from the gastrointestinal tract, with peak plasma levels and hemodynamic effects achieved within 0.5 to 3.0 hours.[10]

The volume of distribution is about 1.5 L/kg, and therapeutic plasma levels range between 0.5 and 4.0 µg/ml.[18, 19] Amrinone is eliminated by urinary excretion of the unchanged drug (up to 40%) and by hepatic metabolism.[19, 20]

Side Effects of Amrinone

Amrinone therapy is associated with a high incidence of side effects.

Cardiovascular Effects

Amrinone has a slight arrhythmogenic potential,[17, 21] even though it is not a sympathomimetic amine or a digitalis glycoside. High doses of amrinone may cause hypotension.[22] In patients with coronary artery disease, amrinone may aggravate ischemia by increasing the myocardial oxygen demand.

Other Effects

Gastrointestinal disturbances are the most common adverse effects of amrinone. Thrombocytopenia, a potentially deleterious complication, is common.[22,23] Disturbances of hepatic function, a viral-like illness, and reduction in tear secretion may occur.

Dosage and Administration of Amrinone

Intravenous Administration

Bolus injections of 100 to 1000 µg/kg were used in newborn lambs.

Oral Administration

Doses of 2 to 4 mg/kg, given 2 to 3 times daily, have been given.

References

1. Evans, D.B., et al.: In vitro and in vivo cardio-stimulant actions of amrinone and prenalterol. (Abstract.) Pharmacologist, 22:287, 1980.
2. Onuaguluchi, G., and Tanz, R.D.: Cardiac effects of amrinone on rabbit papillary muscle and guinea pig Langendorf heart preparations. J. Cardiovasc. Pharmacol., 3:1342, 1981.
3. Alousi, A.A., et al.: Cardiotonic activity of amrinone- Win 40680 (5-amino-3,4'-bipyridine-6(1H)-one). Circ. Res., 45:666, 1979.
4. Alousi, A., et al.: Comparative inotropic activity of amrinone in isolated human atria and cat atria and papillary muscle. (Abstract.) J. Mol. Cell. Cardiol., 11(Suppl. 1):2, 1979.
5. Millard, R.W., et al.: Direct vasodilator and positive inotropic actions of amrinone. J. Mol. Cell. Cardiol., 12:647, 1980.
6. Alousi, A., and Helstosky, A.: Amrinone: a positive inotropic agent with a direct vasodilatory activity in the canine isolated perfused hind-limb preparation. (Abstract.) Fed. Proc., 39:855, 1980.
7. Benotti, J.R., et al.: Haemodynamic assessment of amrinone: a new inotropic agent. N. Engl. J. Med., 299:1373, 1978.
8. LeJemtel, T.H., et al.: Amrinone: a new non-glycosidic, non-adrenergic cardiotonic agent effective in the treatment of intractable myocardial failure in man. Circulation, 59:1098, 1979.
9. Wilmshurst, P.T., et al.: Haemodynamic effects of intravenous amrinone in patients with impaired left ventricular function. Br. Heart J., 49:77, 1983.
10. LeJemtel, T.H., et al.: Sustained beneficial effects of oral amrinone on cardiac and renal function in patients with severe congestive heart failure. Am. J. Cardiol., 45:123, 1980.
11. Alousi, A.A., and Farah, A.E.: Reply to letter to the editor. Circ. Res., 46:888, 1980.
12. Binah, O., et al.: Developmental changes in the effects of amrinone on cardiac contraction. Am. J. Cardiol., 49:993, 1982.
13. Rich, S., et al.: Comparative actions of hydralazine, nifedipine and amrinone in primary pulmonary hypertension. Am. J. Cardiol., 52:1104, 1983.
14. Coe, J., et al.: Bypyridine products lower pulmonary arteriolar resistance (PAR) function in newborn lambs. AHA 1984.
15. Honerjager, P., et al.: Involvement of cyclic AMP in the direct inotropic action of amrinone. Naunyn Schmiedebergs Arch. Pharmac., 318:112, 1981.

16. Kodama, I., et al.: Effects of amrinone on the transmembrane action potential of rabbit sinus node pacemaker cells. Br. J. Pharmacol., *80*:511, 1983.
17. Naccarelli, G.V., et al.: Amrinone: electrophysiologic effects. AHA 1983.
18. Kullberg, M.P., et al.: Amrinone metabolism. Clin. Pharmacol. Ther., *29*:394, 1981.
19. Rocci, M.L., et al.: Amrinone pharmacokinetics after single and steady state doses in patients with chronic cardiac failure. Clin. Pharmacol. Ther., *33*:260, 1983.
20. Alousi, A.A., and Dobreck, H.P.: Amrinone. *In* New Drugs Annual: Cardiovascular Drugs. Edited by Alexander Scriabine. New York, Raven Press, 1983.
21. Leier, C.V., et al.: Amrinone therapy for congestive heart failure in outpatients with idiopathic dilated cardiomyopathy. Am. J. Cardiol. *52*:304, 1983.
22. Wilmshurst, P.T., and Webb-Peploe, M.M.: Side effects of amrinone therapy. Br. Heart J., *49*:447, 1983.
23. Wynne, J., et al.: Oral amrinone in refractory congestive heart failure. Am. J. Cardiol., *45*:1245, 1980.

Section II
CALCIUM ANTAGONISTS

The introduction of calcium antagonists to clinical practice is perhaps the most important advance in cardiovascular drug therapy since the introduction of beta-adrenoreceptor blocking agents. Calcium antagonists inhibit the slow inward calcium current and decrease the availability of intracellular calcium.

The intracellular calcium ion is an important mediator of contractility and is a link between electrical excitation and mechanical contraction. Calcium antagonists, also called calcium entry blockers, are, therefore, uncouplers of excitation and contraction because they depress muscular contractility without altering the amplitude and configuration of the action potential. The decreased contractility is evident in the myocardium as a negative inotropic effect and in the peripheral vasculature as a vasodilatory effect. The combination with a negative inotropic effect is especially suitable for treatment of hypertension and angina pectoris. Intracellular calcium also affects the generation and conduction of cardiac impulses. Therefore, certain calcium antagonists have also significant electrophysiologic and antiarrhythmic effects.

The introduction of calcium antagonists has changed cardiovascular drug therapy in adults. These agents are used to treat systemic hypertension, ischemic heart disease, cardiomyopathy, arrhythmias, pulmonary hypertension, and other diseases. Most of this progress has not reached pediatric cardiovascular therapy. The most important use of calcium antagonists in children is for termination of supraventricular arrhythmias. A few cases of systemic and pulmonary hypertension and cardiomyopathy treated by calcium antagonists have been studied. The three most important calcium antagonists clinically used today are verapamil, nifedipine, and diltiazem. Verapamil is the only calcium antagonist in common use in pediatric cardiovascular therapy.

Chapter 6

Verapamil

Verapamil is the first agent whose cardiovascular effects were recognized to result from its calcium-antagonist properties. When it was first studied over 30 years ago, verapamil was considered to be a beta-adrenoreceptor blocking agent,[1] a concept proved to be inaccurate.

In adults, verapamil has been used for treatment of angina pectoris, arrhythmias, especially supraventricular arrhythmias, hypertension, and hypertrophic cardiomyopathy. The drug is effective for these conditions and it is one of the three most widely used calcium antagonists; the others are nifedipine and diltiazem.

In children, the experience with verapamil is more limited. The drug has been used in many children with arrhythmias and hypertrophic cardiomyopathy and in a few young hypertensive patients, with good results. In reviewing the effects of verapamil in children, however, one must refer to some of the findings obtained from studies in adults.

Structure

Verapamil is a synthetic papaverine derivative.

Mechanism of Action

The therapeutic effects of verapamil are exerted mainly by its calcium-antagonist (slow-channel blocking) properties. Thus, verapamil inhibits calcium-dependent processes and thereby produces electrophysiologic changes and suppression of myocardial and smooth-muscle contractility.

Verapamil was originally considered to be a sympathetic inhibitor. Beta-adrenergic blockade probably plays little or no role in the effect of the drug; however, alpha-adrenergic blockade may be the mechanism of verapamil-induced inhibition of platelet activation produced by epinephrine.[1] The slowing of heart rate by verapamil may partially result from nonspecific inhibition of the sympathetic nervous system.[2,3]

Electrophysiologic Effects

Verapamil inhibits the electrophysiologic properties dependent on calcium current. Therefore, the drug mainly affects the slow-response action potential, in the sinoatrial and atrioventricular nodes. This effect is predominantly evident in the prolongation of conduction in the atrioventricular node, which is the most important mechanism of the antiarrhythmic properties of verapamil. The drug also affects those phases of the fast-response action potential that depend on calcium current, especially the plateau phase.

Sinoatrial Node

The effect of verapamil on the sinoatrial node is the net result of its direct depressant effect, of the sympathetic stimulation induced by the peripheral vasodilatory effect, and, perhaps, of sympathetic inhibition. In adults and children, these effects usually cause slight slowing of heart rate at rest or at any given level of submaximal exercise, but not at maximal exercise.[4-7] This effect is accentuated by concomitant administration of beta-blocking agents. Verapamil does not alter the sinoatrial nodal recovery time or sinoatrial conduction in patients with a normal sinoatrial node.

Atria

Verapamil usually has no effect on the electrophysiologic properties of the atria. High doses may affect intra-atrial conduction, as evident by prolongation of the duration of the P wave and by conversion of some cases of atrial flutter to atrial fibrillation.

Atrioventricular Node

The most important electrophysiologic effect of verapamil is prolongation of conduction time in the atrioventricular node. Animal experiments have shown that therapeutic concentrations of the drug prolong the A-H and P-R intervals by up to 25%. High concentrations of the drug prolonged these intervals up to appearance of high-degree atrioventricular block in 50% of the dogs studied; the H-V interval was not altered.[8]

Similar prolongation of the P-R and A-H intervals was also observed in healthy volunteers and in patients with heart diseases.[9-11] The extent of prolongation of the P-R interval was directly related to the pretreatment level of this interval.

In 1979, Shakibi and colleagues first performed invasive electrophysiologic studies in children treated with verapamil and found prolongation of atrioventricular nodal conduction. Electrocardiograms of several children with various arrhythmias showed prolongation of the P-R interval during sinus rhythm by intravenously or orally administered verapamil.[12]

The P-R interval was prolonged after administration of verapamil in all 9 children and adolescents with hypertrophic cardiomyopathy reported by Spicer and associates.[14] The mean P-R interval of 142 ± 12 msec before verapamil increased to 177 ± 24 msec after verapamil.

In 1 of 4 children with automatic atrial ectopic tachycardia, verapamil produced a second-degree atrioventricular block, and another patient had a junctional escape rhythm.[15]

In 2 of 16 infants with paroxysmal supraventricular tachycardia, verapamil produced long atrioventricular dissociation, and in another 2 patients, the drug caused cardiac arrest.[16]

Verapamil also delayed retrograde conduction in the atrioventricular node in most patients studied.

Accessory Atrioventricular Pathways

Verapamil does not usually affect retrograde ventriculoatrial conduction in accessory pathways. Its effect on antegrade conduction is variable. It may accelerate, inhibit, or not alter antegrade accessory pathway conduction.[17] In any case, the effect on the accessory pathway is much less than that on the atrioventricular node. In a recent study of 14 patients, several of them under the age of 18 years, verapamil prolonged the retrograde effective refractory period of the accessory pathway by about 30 to 70 msec.[18]

Ventricles

Verapamil does not usually affect the electrophysiologic properties of the ventricles. The H-V, QRS, and QTC intervals are not much altered in patients treated with verapamil. One report noted a 35% reduction in the amplitude of T waves at maximal concentration of verapamil.[10]

Effect on Arrhythmias

Verapamil has been used for termination and prevention of arrhythmias for more than 20 years. Because the main electrophysiologic effect of verapamil is on the atrioventricular node, it is especially effective in arrhythmias arising in that node or incorporating it into a re-entrant cycle. Therefore, the drug is especially useful in patients with supraventricular arrhythmias; rarely, it is also effective in those with ventricular arrhythmias.

Sinus Tachycardia

Verapamil effectively slows heart rate in patients with sinus tachycardia.[19]

Supraventricular Tachycardia

Verapamil terminates up to 90% of cases of re-entrant supraventricular tachycardia in adults and children.[20-24] Because most cases of supraventricular tachycardia involve a mechanism of re-entry, verapamil is usually effective in this arrhythmia in clinical practice.

In adults, four types of responses of supraventricular tachycardia to intravenous administration of verapamil have been observed: (1) abrupt termination of the tachycardia; (2) slowing of the rate of tachycardia, followed by termination; (3) various changes in the cycle length of the arrhythmia; and (4) appearance of a few premature ventricular beats prior to termination of the tachycardia.[25-27]

In several studies, the effect of verapamil on supraventricular tachycardia was specifically evaluated in infants and children. Porter and co-workers reported that intravenous verapamil terminated supraventricular tachycardia in all five patients with atrioventricular node re-entry and in two patients with atrioventricular node-Kent re-entry, but the drug was ineffective in all four patients with an atrial ectopic focus and in two patients with a junctional ectopic focus.[28] In both patients with juntional ectopic tachycardia, verapamil produced excessive peripheral vasodilation and hypotension, and resuscitation was required. These investigators recommended that until further data are available, patients with this arrhythmia should not receive verapamil.[28] In this study, oral verapamil prevented recurrences of the arrhythmia in three of four children with atrioventricular node re-entry and in one of two children with atrioventricular node-Kent re-entry and was ineffective in the one child with atrial ectopic focus.

Shahar and colleagues, of the Sheba Medical Center, summarized the treatment of paroxysmal supraventricular tachycardia in infants and children with verapamil.[29] These workers studied 14 infants and children, 9 of them under 2 years of age, with 53 episodes of paroxysmal supraventricular tachycardia. Stable sinus rhythm was obtained in 49 of 53 episodes (92.4%) immediately or within 60 sec of intravenous administration of verapamil. The drug was equally effective in infants and children. It terminated all 26 episodes in patients with structural anomalies and 17 of 18 episodes in patients with Wolff-Parkinson-White syndrome. Three of the four patients in whom verapamil failed to terminate the arrhythmia were under 6 weeks of age, and the fourth patient was 5 months of age. Two patients, treated with propranolol prior to administration of verapamil, had sinus bradycardia or atrioventricular block after receiving verapamil.[29]

The use of intravenous verapamil to terminate supraventricular tachycardia in early infancy is controversial. Several investigators have observed that, in some infants under 6 months of age, supraventricular tachycardia is especially resistant to conversion by verapamil, even at high doses.[28, 29] This resistance may result from incomplete development of the atrioventricular node in these young infants. Despite these findings, I recommend that verapamil may be tried even in young infants with this arrhythmia. This recommendation is based on my own experience, as well as on the favorable results obtained by Greco and associates in a large group of infants, many of them less than a month old.[16] Good results were also obtained by Soler-Soler and co-workers in 14 infants with a mean age of 4.4 months.[24] Moreover, a case of fetal supraventricular tachycardia successfully terminated by administration of digitalis and verapamil to the mother has been reported.[30]

Soler-Soler and colleagues studied the effect of verapamil, 1 to 2 mg intravenously over 30 sec, in 14 infants (mean age 4.4 months) with paroxysmal supraventricular tachycardia.[24] No infant had associated heart disease. Within a minute of injection of the drug, sinus rhythm was obtained in 28 of 29 episodes of the arrhythmia (96.5%). Bein and associates reported that intravenous administration of verapamil obtained sinus rhythm in all 70 attacks of supraventricular tachycardia in children aged 4 days to 14 years.[21] Greco and co-workers reported that 15 of 16 children up to 12 years of age who were admitted to a hospital for the first or second time in their life with supraventricular tachycardia responded to intravenous verapamil (93%).[16] In children with recurrent paroxysmal supraventricular tachycardia, 27 of 29 episodes of the arrhythmia responded to verapamil.

Verapamil can also be effective in cases of ectopic supraventricular tachycardia, as in two children reported by Sapire and colleagues.[13] These children received long-term oral therapy.

Several investigations have suggested that verapamil is the drug of choice for treatment of supraventricular tachycardia in infancy and childhood. This recommendation is based on: (1) high rate of success; (2) rapid onset of action; (3) relative safety; and (4) lack of serious arrhythmias if D.C. cardioversion is required following administration of the drug.

Electrophysiologic studies with short-term drug testing usually predict the response to verapamil. If it is not possible to perform such studies immediately, however, it is justifiable to administer the drug without prior electrophysiologic studies, to terminate supraventricular tachycardia.

Atrial Fibrillation and Flutter

Verapamil slows the ventricular response in patients with atrial fibrillation or flutter. This effect has been observed in adults as well as in children.[31] Less commonly, verapamil may convert these arrhythmias to sinus rhythm. In patients with atrial fibrillation and Wolff-Parkinson-White syndrome, verapamil may accelerate the ventricular rate.[32]

Sapire and associates reported that verapamil failed to terminate the arrhythmia in a child with atrial flutter.[13]

Ventricular Arrhythmias

Verapamil is rarely effective in adult patients with ventricular arrhythmias resistant to other antiarrhythmic agents. No studies on the use of this drug in ventricular arrhythmias in children have been reported.

Electrocardioversion after Verapamil Administration

An important advantage of verapamil is that electrocardioversion may be safely performed even several minutes after intravenous administration of the drug. Soler-Soler and co-workers evaluated the feasibility of electrocardioversion 5 to 7 minutes after intravenous administration of verapamil.[33] Forty-nine consecutive patients with atrial fibrillation or flutter were studied. Patients with congestive heart failure, acute myocardial infarction, sinus node dysfunction, or heart rates under 70 beats/min were excluded. In 6 patients, 8 complications occurred: 4 cases of hypotension, 2 of junction escape rhythm, and 2 of junctional tachycardia. The study suggested that electrocardioversion can be safely performed during the clinical action of verapamil.

Comparison with other Antiarrhythmic Drugs

Verapamil is considered to be the drug of choice for short-term control of supraventricular tachycardia in infants and children. Recently, however, it was suggested that adenosine or adenosine triphosphate may be preferable for pediatric patients with this arrhythmia.[16] Only a few comparative studies of the efficacy of these three agents were reported, and it is important to compare the properties of these drugs.

All three drugs depress the sinus and atrioventricular nodes. Verapamil acts by inhibition of the slow inward calcium current. The effects of adenosine and adenosine triphosphate are mediated by depression of the slow inward calcium current, by increase of potassium conductance, by some indirect antiadrenergic effects,[33a] and possibly also by a vagal effect. The efficacy of these three drugs in supraventricular tachycardia results from their effect on the atrioventricular node.

As described in the previous sections of this chapter, verapamil terminates at least two-thirds of paroxysms of supraventricular tachycardia in infants and children; the success rate of adenosine and adenosine triphosphate is higher in adults. Greco and colleagues compared the effects of adenosine triphosphate and verapamil in a group of 62 children with paroxysmal supraventricular tachycardia.[16] Both drugs similarly suppressed the arrhythmia in 90% of cases. Digitalis was effective in only 60 to 70%.[16]

Verapamil suppresses the arrhythmia within minutes of intravenous administration, but suppression by the other drugs may be even more rapid. Verapamil has the advantage of termination of the arrhythmia without producing marked sinus bradycardia, prevention of early recurrences, and low incidence of adverse effects, but it has the disadvantage of a negative inotropic effect, and it may cause hypotension and death, especially in patients with left ventricular dysfunction. Because most pediatric patients who are treated with verapamil have normal left ventricular function, this adverse effect is limited.

Adenosine and adenosine triphosphate have an elimination half-life of less than a minute. Therefore, even if they cause hemodynamic deterioration, it is of short duration. These drugs, however, have the disadvantage of not preventing recurrences and of a high incidence of cardiovascular side effects including sinus arrest, sinus bradycardia, and conduction disturbances. This subject is further discussed in Chapter 31.

Effect on Hypertrophic Cardiomyopathy

In the last decade, verapamil was successfully used for treatment of hypertrophic cardiomyopathy in adults and children. The use of verapamil for this condition was first described by Kaltenbach and associates in 1976.[34] Verapamil produced hemodynamic improvement and symptomatic relief, and it may also have had some antiarrhythmic effect.

Hemodynamic Effects

The hemodynamic improvement produced by verapamil in patients with hypertrophic obstructive cardiomyopathy includes decreases in left ventricular systolic outflow gradient and end-diastolic pressure and better diastolic filling of the heart. The abnormal relationships between the early and late filling phases in patients with hypertrophic cardiomyopathy are reverted toward normal with verapamil. Heart rate and cardiac index are only minimally altered.

In several series, verapamil altered both systolic and diastolic hemodynamic parameters, whereas in other studies, only diastolic or systolic parameters were altered. For example, Kaltenbach and co-workers reported that intravenous verapamil decreased left ventricular systolic pressure by 10% and end-diastolic pressure by 20%; the pressure gradient remained unchanged.[34] Rosing and associates reported that verapamil decreased the left ventricular outflow tract gradient at rest from 94 ± 14 to 49 ± 14 mm Hg and reduced the left ventricular filling pressure only in those patients with elevated pretreatment levels.[35] Bonow and colleagues reported that verapamil did not alter parameters of systolic function, but did improve diastolic function, as evident by an increase in left ventricular filling rate, in patients with hypertrophic cardiomyopathy.[36] These series included several patients under 18 years of age.

Spicer and co-workers studied the short-term hemodynamic effects of verapamil in 9 children and adolescents with hypertrophic cardiomyopathy.[14] The mean age of these patients was 10.3 years. Verapamil was given as a bolus injection of 0.1 mg/kg, followed by a 20-min continuous infusion of 0.007 mg/kg/min. Hemodynamic measurements were obtained at rest and at maximal supine bicycle exercise before and 15 minutes after verapamil administration.

At rest, verapamil increased the mean cardiac output from 3.3 ± 0.9 to 3.7 ± 0.9 L/min/m^2 and decreased left ventricular end-diastolic pressure from 19.3 ± 8.1 to 14.5 ± 6.9 mm Hg. In 6 patients with left ventricular outflow systolic pressure gradient, verapamil decreased the gradient from 17.5 ± 7.2 to 5.2 ± 4.5 mm Hg. At maximal exercise, cardiac output increased from 6.5 ± 1.3 to 7.8 ± 1.8 L/min/m^2, left ventricular end-diastolic pressure decreased from 29.1 ± 10.1 to 19.3 ± 10.4 mm Hg, and left ventricular systolic outflow tract gradient decreased from 31.2 ± 10.5 to 1.75 ± 1.7 mm Hg.[14]

Porter and associates studied the hemodynamic effects of verapamil in 2 children.[28] One was a 16-year-old boy with hypertrophic cardiomyopathy and bronchial asthma who suffered syncopal episodes despite treatment with a cardioselective beta-blocking agent. Verapamil, administered intravenously at a rate of 0.021 mg/kg/min, decreased the left ventricular outflow tract gradient from 160 to 45 mm Hg. The other patient, a 4-year-old boy, had a gradient of 60 mm Hg at rest despite a myectomy performed 9 months previously. Verapamil, 0.014 mg/kg/min, decreased the gradient to 10 mm Hg.

Relief of Symptoms

Verapamil also produces symptomatic relief and increases exercise tolerance. Spicer and colleagues reported that, in children and adolescents with hypertrophic cardiomyopathy, intravenous administration of verapamil increased the total work performed from 1743 ± 1284 to 3168 ± 1643 kg/m.[14] In a later study, Spicer and associates evaluated the effect of long-term verapamil therapy in pediatric and young adult patients with hypertrophic cardiomyopathy.[36a] The study group consisted of 13 patients, aged 7 months to 19 years (mean 12 years) with echocardiographic demonstration of a nondilated, hypertrophic left ventricle. Verapamil was administered orally, at a dose of 5.2 ± 1.1 mg/kg/day (range 2.8 to 7 mg/kg/day), divided into 3 to 4 doses. The period of treatment was 13 ± 6 months (range 2 to 20 months).

The patients had significant symptomatic improvement while receiving verapamil therapy. The patients, or their parents, reported an improved sense of well-being. Dyspnea was present in all 13 patients before therapy. During therapy, it disappeared in 7 patients and diminished in the remaining 6, who reported increased exercise tolerance and decrease in frequency and extent of dyspnea. Eight patients had had angina pectoris before treatment. During verapamil treatment, 5 patients, followed for a mean period of 17.7 months, did not have angina at rest or during regular activity. The remaining 3 patients noted a decrease in frequency and severity of the angina. The dizziness and lightheadedness that occurred in 8 patients before treatment disappeared in 7 during treatment. Syncope occurred in 2 of the patients before treatment and disappeared in 1 patient during treatment. To the best of my knowledge, these results show the most significant symptomatic improvement reported with any drug in pediatric patients with hypertrophic cardiomyopathy.

In 6 of these patients, the intensity of the systolic murmur heard over the left ventricular outflow tract diminished during treatment; this finding indicates a decrease in pressure gradient. The electrocardiogram showed a decrease in left ventricular electromotive forces in 4 patients, an increase in 5, and no change in 4. These data should be interpreted in view of the well-known progressive course of left ventricular hypertrophy in children with hypertrophic cardiomyopathy. Seven patients had exercise-induced ST segment depression before treatment; five patients noted an improvement during verapamil treatment. Three of four patients had complete or partial suppression of exercise-induced premature ventricular beats during treatment; duration of exercise increased by about 20%.

Echocardiographic interventricular septal thickness adjusted for body size and age decreased from 106 ± 70 to 45 ± 52% of predicted normal values, and left ventricular posterior wall thickness decreased from 40 ± 45 to 5 ± 26% of predicted normal values after verapamil treatment. Systolic anterior motion of the anterior mitral leaflet disappeared in 5 of 8 patients, and midsystolic closure of the aortic valve disappeared in 4 of 8 patients.[36a] Left ventricular end-diastolic dimension was increased. This change may have resulted in diminution of left ventricular end-diastolic pressure.

Rosing and co-workers reported that oral administration of verapamil improved exercise capacity by 53% after 5 days of treatment in a group of 78 patients aged 13 to 77 years.[37] In this study, 63% of the patients treated for long periods with oral verapamil reported symptomatic improvement.

Selection of Patients

Selection of patients for treatment with verapamil is important. Patients with obstructive hypertrophic cardiomyopathy and without signs of congestive heart failure are especially suitable for verapamil treatment. Epstein and Rosing emphasized verapamil's potential for causing serious complications, especially in dyspneic patients with high pulmonary capillary wedge pressure.[38] Such is usually not the case in pediatric patients. Even in patients with congestive heart failure, verapamil may be beneficial. This effect was demonstrated by Eldar and colleagues, who described a patient with hypertrophic cardiomyopathy, high pulmonary capillary wedge pressure, and significant left ventricular outflow obstruction on whom propranolol had had deleterious effects and in whom verapamil produced hemodynamic and symptomatic improvement.[39]

Mechanism of Action

Several mechanisms have been suggested to explain the beneficial effect of verapamil in hypertrophic cardiomyopathy: (1) direct suppression of myocardial contractility, resulting in a reduction in left ventricular outflow gradient; (2) arterial vasodilation, reducing left ventricular systolic pressure;[40] (3) preload reduction, reducing left ventricular end-diastolic pressure and relieving dyspnea; the reduction in wall stress by this mechanism may contribute to the relief of angina pectoris; (4) direct improvement of diastolic properties of the heart; in a study of 15 patients with hypertrophic obstructive cardiomyopathy, some under 18 years of age, treated with verapamil, symptomatic improvement was not usually related to changes in left ventricular outflow gradient or in systolic function of the left ventricle and may have been related to improved diastolic function;[40a] and (5) decrease in heart rate, improving diastolic filling.

It is still controversial whether verapamil suppresses the arrhythmias associated with hypertrophic cardiomyopathy. In a recent study, McKenna and associates showed that verapamil did not reduce the incidence of arrhythmias in 19 patients with hypertrophic cardiomyopathy.[41]

In summary, verapamil produces a marked hemodynamic and symptomatic improvement in pediatric patients with hypertrophic cardiomyopathy and alters the natural course of this disease. It is not known, however, whether verapamil prevents, delays, does not alter, or worsens the stage at which hypertrophic cardiomyopathy is converted into dilated cardiomyopathy with accelerated development of congestive heart failure. Careful follow-up of children with hypertrophic cardiomyopathy treated with verapamil is required to detect the possible development of this stage of the disease.

Hemodynamic Effects

Verapamil has complex hemodynamic effects, including negative chronotropic and inotropic effects, peripheral vasodilation, a direct effect on the diastolic properties of the heart, sympathetic activation by peripheral vasodilation, a nonspecific sympathetic inhibitory effect, and possibly also effects mediated by release of hormones. The negative chronotropic effect of verapamil has been discussed earlier in this chapter. The peripheral vasodilatory effect produces a 20 to 25% decrease in systemic vascular resistance. This decrease is completely expressed as a decrease in systemic arterial pressure because the negative chronotropic and inotropic effects of verapamil prevent a compensatory increase in cardiac output. Verapamil reduces the rate-pressure product at rest and at any given level of submaximal exercise, but not at maximal exercise.[42–44]

The direct negative inotropic effect of verapamil has been demonstrated by studies of isolated myocardial preparations and by direct injection of the drug into the coronary arteries.[45] Intravenous administration of high doses of verapamil may also exert a negative inotropic effect.[46–48] This effect may produce or may aggravate congestive heart failure in patients with impaired myocardial function. One may see this effect in adults with coronary artery disease and in children with endomyocardial diseases or rarely, with myocardial anomalies. In patients with normal or only slightly impaired myocardial function, the verapamil-induced sympathetic activation, resulting from peripheral vasodilation, is sufficient to counteract the direct negative inotropic effect.[6]

The improvement in diastolic function of the heart by verapamil is relevant mainly for patients with hypertrophic cardiomyopathy and is discussed under that heading.

Effects in Presence of Beta-Adrenergic Blockade

Most studies in adults indicate that intravenous administration of verapamil is contraindicated in patients receiving beta-adrenoreceptor blocking agents. Such agents, especially propranolol, are often given to children with recurrent supraventricular tachycardia. Therefore, intravenous verapamil cannot be used to convert episodes of acute supraventricular tachycardia to sinus rhythm in these patients.

Jackson and co-workers studied the hemodynamic effects of verapamil in the presence of beta-blockade in 12 puppies.[48a] At infusion rates of 125 μg/kg/min verapamil, a regimen of verapamil and propranolol decreased cardiac output, mean blood pressure, and heart rate and prolonged the PR interval to a greater extent than did the administration of verapamil alone. Left atrial pressure rose, whereas pulmonary arterial pressure and regional left ventricular shortening were little altered. Seven of the 12 puppies developed severe bradycardia associated with a marked decrease in cardiac output after receiving verapamil and propranolol combined. The bradycardia responded only to infusion of calcium gluconate. It was concluded that, in the presence of beta-adrenoreceptor blockade, verapamil has a marked cardiodepressant effect.[48a] Diltiazem, which has similar antiarrhythmic properties, produced less negative inotropic effect than verapamil in these puppies.

Effect on Systemic Hypertension

Verapamil was extensively studied for the treatment of systemic hypertension in adults. Several investigators reported a marked antihypertensive effect, associated with slowing of heart rate, particularly during the day.[49-52] The doses used in adults were 240 to 480 mg daily, in 3 to 4 divided doses. The mechanism of the antihypertensive effect of verapamil is, probably, peripheral vasodilation combined with negative inotropic and chronotropic effects. That heart rate is not increased by reflex sympathetic stimulation induced by peripheral vasodilation is an important advantage of verapamil over other vasodilators, including other calcium antagonists such as nifedipine.

When it is used as the only antihypertensive agent, verapamil does not produce fluid retention. Therefore, tolerance to the antihypertensive effect of verapamil does not develop during long-term therapy. Verapamil also improved the diastolic function of hypertrophied left ventricles in hypertensive patients in one report.[53]

No controlled studies of verapamil in hypertensive children have been reported. This agent should be kept in mind, however, as a possible alternative to conventional therapy.

Effect on Pulmonary Hypertension

Several calcium antagonists have been given to patients with pulmonary hypertension; results with some of these agents have been good. Therefore, it is important to emphasize a study suggesting a potentially deleterious effect of verapamil in this condition. Young and associates reported that, in experimental acute pulmonary vasoconstriction induced by prostaglandin $F_2 \alpha$, verapamil increased pulmonary vascular resistance from 7.3 ± 1.3 to 8.1 ± 1.4 mm Hg/L/min.[54] This increase is not significant, but in this model, nifedipine completely blocked pulmonary vasoconstriction. At present, I advise against administering verapamil to children with pulmonary hypertension.

Effect on Angina Pectoris

A most important indication for the oral administration of verapamil in adults is angina pectoris. Like other calcium antagonists, verapamil is effective in patients with stable angina pectoris, coronary spasm, and intermediate coronary syndromes when it is given alone or in combination with other antianginal drugs. In several double-bind, randomized, placebo-controlled cross-over studies, verapamil decreased the frequency of spontaneous anginal episodes, the severity of pain, the amplitude of ST segment deviations, and the need for nitroglycerin, and it increased exercise tolerance.[6, 55-58] The efficacy of the drug is sustained during long periods of treatment; no tachyphylaxis is reported.[59] There is marked interpatient variability in response.[60] The antianginal effect of verapamil is comparable to that of the beta-blocking agents. The combination of verapamil with beta-blockers may produce adverse effects. Verapamil, injected into the coronary arteries or given systemically, can relieve and may prevent spontaneous and induced coronary spasm.[61, 62]

Clinical Pharmacology

Verapamil is rapidly and almost completely absorbed from the gastrointestinal tract after oral administration. Maximal plasma concentration is achieved within 45 minutes of taking an oral dose.[63, 64] However, the systemic bioavailability of the drug is low, about 20 to 35%, because of extensive first-pass hepatic metabolism.[63-65] The liver is probably the only site of first-pass metabolism of the drug, as evident by 100% bioavailability in a patient with a mesocaval shunt bypassing the liver,[66] as well as by increased bioavailability to 50% in patients with hepatic cirrhosis.

The volume of distribution of verapamil is about 5 L/kg in adults.[11] In a group of children aged 7 to 18 years, the steady-state volume of distribution was 279 L/kg.[67]

In adults, the antianginal and electrophysiologic effects of verapamil correlated with the plasma concentration of the drug in many studies.[64, 68-70] Different concentrations are required to achieve specific effects, however. For example, in a study of patients with atrial fibrillation, higher plasma levels were needed for conversion to sinus rhythm than for control of ventricular rate.[71]

In a study of children with hypertrophic cardiomyopathy, neither electrophysiologic nor hemodynamic effects were related to plasma verapamil concentration.[14]

Verapamil is eliminated by hepatic metabolism. The most important metabolic pathways are N-dealkylation, O-demethylation, and conjugation. Only one of the metabolites, norverapamil, which is formed by N-demethylation of verapamil, has effects resembling those of the parent drug, although its potency is only 20% of that of the parent drug. The steady-state plasma concentration of norverapamil is about equal to that of the parent drug. More than 10 minor, pharmacologically inactive metabolites have been identified. The metabolites and 4% of the dose in the unchanged form are excreted in the urine.[68]

In adults, the elimination half-life of a single intravenous dose of verapamil is about 3 to 7 hours and that of a single oral dose is 3 to 5 hours. Repeated oral administration of verapamil causes saturation of the hepatic metabolic pathways responsible for the elimination of the drug. Therefore, the hepatic clearance of verapamil decreases with repeated doses, and the elimination half-life is prolonged to 5 to 12 hours. After 6 to 10 consecutive doses, a steady state is achieved, and the elimination half-life is not further increased.[10, 11, 63, 66, 72, 73] In patients with renal dysfunction, the duration of action of verapamil is prolonged, probably because of accumulation of the active metabolite norverapamil.

Hesslein and colleagues studied the effect of age on pharmacokinetic parameters of verapamil in pediatric patients.[73a] These investigators studied 7 children ranging in age from 2.8 to 15.3 years (median age 10.8 years). All had supraventricular tachycardia controlled by long-term oral verapamil therapy at doses of 0.4 to 2.9 mg/kg (mean dose 1.36 mg/kg). These doses achieved plasma verapamil concentrations of 248 ± 117 ng/ml and plasma norverapamil concentrations of 64 ± 38 ng/ml. Several age-dependent kinetic parameters were found. Younger children had faster drug uptake, lower relative bioavailability, smaller volume of distribution, and slower elimination half-life than older children. Younger children also had a diurnal variation in drug kinetics. No age-dependent difference in distribution, half-life, or elimination rate was found.

The net effect of these changes is that higher and, perhaps, more frequent doses than currently recommended in younger children may be necessary. It is possible that some of the discrepancy between the high efficacy of intravenously administered verapamil in termination of arrhythmias and the lower efficacy of orally administered verapamil in preventing these arrhythmias in young children may result from inadequate dosing.

Side Effects

Verapamil is safe, especially during oral therapy. Cases of adult patients treated with this drug for up to 10 years have been reported. The long-term safety of oral verapamil in children has not been accurately determined. Intravenous administration of verapamil is associated with a higher incidence of serious side effects than oral administration.

Encouraging findings were observed in a recent study of chronic oral administration of verapamil in 13 children with hypertrophic cardiomyopathy who received the drug for up to 20 months.[36a] No side effects were observed in this group.

Cardiovascular Effects

Cardiovascular side effects appear in about 10% of adult patients treated with verapamil. In children, the incidence of cardiovascular side effects is lower, probably because the coronary arteries and myocardial function are almost always normal in children treated with verapamil. Therefore, the incidence of hemodynamic deterioration is lower than in adults.

In adults, deterioration of congestive heart failure and even development of acute pulmonary edema may be produced by verapamil.[58] Pedal edema unrelated to congestive heart failure may also develop. Studies of immature animals showed severe hypotension and reduction in cardiac output after high doses of verapamil.[74] In adults, verapamil is an antihypertensive agent.[75] In adults and children with hypertrophic cardiomyopathy, verapamil may cause marked hemodynamic deterioration. For example, 10 of 120 patients of all ages with this disease developed pulmonary edema after initiation of treatment with verapamil.[38] In 9 children and adolescents with hypertrophic cardiomyopathy studied by Spicer and co-workers, the mean arterial blood pressure decreased after verapamil administration;[14] however, no patient became symptomatic or had the infusion stopped because of hypotension.

One infant with supraventricular tachycardia who inadvertently received a dose of verapamil 3 times greater than recommended developed severe hypotension with shock.[24] Two other children with junctional ectopic tachycardia became severely hypotensive after intravenous verapamil administration.[15] In adults, hypotension developed in about 1.5% of the patients with supraventricular tachycardia treated with intravenous verapamil.[76, 77]

Electrophysiologic disturbances may occur in children treated with verapamil. For example, 2 of 23 infants with paroxysmal supraventricular tachycardia reported by Greco and associates developed cardiac arrest, and 2 others developed long atrioventricular dissociation after administration of verapamil.[16] From studies in adults, it is evident that the combination of verapamil and beta-blocking agents produces an additive prolongation of atrioventricular nodal conduction. The risk is increased even further by intravenous administration of these agents.

Flushing

Flushing may result from the peripheral vasodilatory effect of verapamil. Greco and colleagues observed this side effect in 3 of 23 infants treated with verapamil.[16] This complication was not observed in several other series of infants and children treated with intravenous or oral verapamil.

Constipation

Constipation is the most common complication of treatment with verapamil. It occurs in up to 25% of the patients receiving the drug for a short period,[7,78] as well as in up to 50% of those receiving the drug for long periods.[60] This adverse effect is easily controlled by laxatives.

Verapamil Overdose

Adverse cardiovascular effects resulting from verapamil overdose may be treated symptomatically or specifically with calcium. In animal experiments, an increase of serum calcium concentration to an average of 6.5 mEq/L abolished the adverse hemodynamic effects of verapamil. Further elevation was required to suppress the prolongation of the PR interval. Several investigators reported that infusion of calcium solutions reversed the adverse cardiovascular effects of verapamil overdose in adults.[79-82] In my experience, severe verapamil-induced hypotension in infancy and childhood responds to intravenous infusion of calcium chloride. If acute hypotension develops after the intravenous administration of verapamil, calcium chloride should be infused as a solution of 10% at a dose of 10 mg/kg, together with sodium chloride, 0.9% solution, 10 ml/kg. The administration of sodium chloride is effective only if calcium is given concomitantly or if the patient is hypercalcemic.

Two of the effects of verapamil, suppression of sinus rate and peripheral vasodilation, are resistant to calcium administration. Sinus bradycardia can be treated with atropine. Excessive vasodilation may require vasopressor amines. Isoproterenol may effectively control bradycardia, but in children in whom verapamil was used to treat arrhythmias, the administration of isoproterenol may be deleterious. Ventricular pacing may be required in extreme cases.

A few cases of successful treatment of the adverse cardiovascular effects of oral ingestion of high doses of verapamil have been reported. A 2-year-old boy developed atrioventricular dissociation and junctional rhythm after inadvertent ingestion of an unknown quantity of verapamil.[83] Administration of metaproterenol, a beta-adrenergic stimulator, and atropine resulted in rapid restoration of sinus rhythm. An 18-year-old youth developed this complication after ingestion of 2.0 g verapamil in attempted suicide; he responded slightly to atropine.[80] A 14-year-old girl developed atrioventricular nodal conduction disturbances and hypotension following ingestion of 2.4 g verapamil in attempted suicide; she responded promptly to infusion of calcium gluconate, 10%.[84]

A case of a young child with combined poisoning with a barbiturate and verapamil was reported in the German literature.[83] It is difficult to analyze the patient's symptoms in this case. Passal and Grespin reported the case of an 11-month-old girl who accidentally ingested 400 mg verapamil.[85] She developed coma, seizures, respiratory depression, bradycardia, and hypotension. This patient was successfully resuscitated with intravenous administration of normal saline solution, calcium chloride, isoproterenol, and dopamine.

A patient with hypertrophic cardiomyopathy who died suddenly during continuous electrocardiographic monitoring after 4 days of treatment with verapamil has been reported.[86] Analysis of the electrocardiographic tape showed a third-degree atrioventricular block followed by complete asystole.

During treatment with verapamil, the effect of calcium on myocardial contractility persists for 45 minutes, whereas the positive inotropic effect of calcium in animals and persons not treated with verapamil lasts less than 15 minutes. These findings indicate that the mechanism of the beneficial effect of calcium in myocardial depression from verapamil overdose is a specific competitive inhibition of verapamil.

While one is using atropine to treat sinus bradycardia or atrioventricular block induced by verapamil in patients in whom verapamil has terminated supraventricular tachycardia, tachycardia may recur and may produce a faster ventricular rate due to 1:1 atrioventricular nodal conduction.

Dosage and Administration

Verapamil is given intravenously and orally. In certain investigational protocols, the drug has been injected directly into the coronary arteries of human patients.

An intravenous injection of 0.1 mg/kg, over 30 to 120 sec, may be given and may be repeated twice more at 15-minute intervals, up to a total dose of 0.3 mg/kg if no adverse reactions develop. Higher doses or more rapid injection may cause hypotension or conduction disturbances. This dosage regimen is used to terminate supraventricular tachycardia.[28] In children with hypertrophic cardiomyopathy, a dose of 0.1 mg/kg as a bolus injection, followed by a 20-min continuous infusion of 0.007 mg/kg/min has been used. It is possible that lower doses may be adequate because these doses are actually for adults. Adult oral doses rarely exceed 480 mg daily. In children, oral doses of 2.5 to 7.0 mg/kg/day, in 3 to 4 divided doses, have been used.

Determination of Plasma Levels

Determination of plasma levels of verapamil is of limited value in monitoring treatment in children.

Verapamil

1. Fisher, C.A., et al.: Verapamil and diltiazem as antiplatelet agents: spectrum and mechanisms of activity. AHA 1983.
2. Livesley, B., et al.: Double blind evaluation of verapamil, propranolol and isosorbide dinitrate against a placebo in the treatment of angina pectoris. Br. Med. J., 2:375, 1973.
3. Reichek, N.: Long-acting nitrates in the treatment of angina pectoris. JAMA, 236:1399, 1976.
4. Frishman, W.H., et al.: Comparative effects of abrupt withdrawal of propranolol and verapamil in angina pectoris. Am. J. Cardiol., 50:1191, 1982.
5. Weiner, D.A., and Klein, M.D.: Verapamil therapy for stable exertional angina pectoris. Am. J. Cardiol., 50:1153, 1982.
6. Tan, A.T.H., et al.: Verapamil in stable effort angina: effects on left ventricular function evaluated with exercise radionuclide ventriculography. Am. J. Cardiol., 49:425, 1982.
7. Subramanian, B., et al.: Long-term antianginal action of verapamil assessed with quantitated serial treadmill stress testing. Am. J. Cardiol., 48:529, 1981.
8. Mangiardi, L.M., et al.: Electrophysiologic and hemodynamic effects of verapamil: correlation with plasma drug concentrations. Circulation, 57:366, 1978.
9. Koike, Y., et al.: Pharmacokinetics of verapamil in man. Res. Commun. Chem. Pathol. Pharmacol., 24:37, 1979.
10. Dominic, J.A., et al.: The pharmacology of verapamil. III. Pharmacokinetics in normal subjects after intravenous drug administration. J. Cardiovasc. Pharmacol. 3:25, 1981.
11. McAllister, R.G., and Kirsten, E.B.: The pharmacology of verapamil. IV. Kinetic and dynamic effects after single intravenous and oral doses. Clin. Pharmacol. Ther., 31:418, 1982.
12. Shakibi, J.G., et al.: Electrophysiologic effects of verapamil in children. Jpn. Heart J., 20:709, 1979.
13. Sapire, D.W., O'Riordan, A., and Black, I.F.S.: Safety and efficacy of short- and long-term verapamil therapy in children with tachycardia. Am. J. Cardiol., 48:1091, 1981.
14. Spicer, R.L., et al.: Hemodynamic effects of verapamil in children and adolescents with hypertrophic cardiomyopathy. Circulation, 67:413, 1983.
15. Porter, C.J., et al.: Effects of verapamil on supraventricular tachycardia in children. Am. J. Cardiol., 48:487, 1981.
16. Greco, R., et al.: Treatment of paroxysmal supraventricular tachycardia in infancy with digitalis, adenosine-5'-triphosphate, and verapamil: a comparative study. Circulation, 66:504, 1982.
17. Harper, R.W., et al.: Effects of verapamil on the electrophysiologic properties of the accessory pathway in patients with the Wolff-Parkinson-White syndrome. Am. J. Cardiol., 103:459, 1982.
18. Wu, D., et al.: Effects of oral verapamil in patients with atrioventricular reentrant tachycardia incorporating an accessory pathway. Circulation, 67:426, 1983.

19. Schamroth, L.: Immediate effects of intravenous verapamil on atrial fibrillation. Cardiovasc. Res., 5:419, 1971.
20. Schamroth, L., Krikler, M.D., and Garrett, C.: Immediate effects of intravenous verapamil in cardiac arrhythmias. Br. Med. J., 1:660, 1972.
21. Bein, G., and Wolf, D.: The treatment of supraventricular paroxysmal tachycardia in infants and children with verapamil. Cardiol. Pneumol., 9:151, 1971.
22. Hills, E.: Improveratril and bronchial asthma. Br. J. Clin. Pharmacol., 24:116, 1970.
23. Musto, B., et al.: Trattamento acuto della tachicardia sopraventricolare e del flutter con verapamil, in eta pediatrica. G. Ital. Cardiol., 94:368, 1979.
24. Soler-Soler, J., et al.: Effect of verapamil in infants with paroxysmal supraventricular tachycardia. Circulation, 59:876, 1979.
25. Talano, J.V., and Tommaso, C.: Slow channel calcium antagonists in the treatment of supraventricular tachycardia. Prog. Cardiovasc. Dis., 25:141, 1982.
26. Vohra, J., et al.: Verapamil induced premature ventricular beats before reversion of supraventricular tachycardia. Br. Heart J., 36:1186, 1974.
27. Feigl, D., and Ravid, M.: Electrocárdiographic observations on the termination of supraventricular tachycardia by verapamil. Electrocardiography, 12:129, 1979.
28. Porter, C.-B.J., et al.: Verapamil: an effective calcium blocking agent for pediatric patients. Pediatrics, 71:748, 1983.
29. Shahar, E., et al.: Verapamil in the treatment of paroxysmal supraventricular tachycardia in infants and children. J. Pediatr., 98:323, 1981.
30. Wolf, F., et al.: Prenatal diagnosis and therapy of fetal heart anomalies: with a contribution on the placental transfer of verapamil. J. Perinat. Med., 8:203, 1980.
31. Waxman, H.L., et al.: Verapamil for control of ventricular rate in paroxysmal supraventricular tachycardia and atrial fibrillation or flutter: a double-blind randomized cross-over study. Ann. Intern. Med., 94:1, 1981.
32. Gulamhusein, S., et al.: Acceleration of the ventricular response during atrial fibrillation in the Wolff-Parkinson-White syndrome after verapamil. Circulation, 65:348, 1982.
33. Soler-Soler, J., et al.: Electroversion after verapamil administration. Chest, 2:225, 1983.
33a. Belardinell, L., et al.: Chronotropic and dromotropic effects of adenosine. In Regulatory Function of Adenosine. Edited by R.M. Berne, et al. Boston, Martinus Nijhoff, 1983, p. 377.
34. Kaltenbach, M., Hopf, R., and Keller, M.: Calciumantagonistische therapie bei hypertrophobstrukriver Kardiomyopathie. Dtsch. Med. Wochenschr., 101:1284, 1976.
35. Rosing, D.R., et al.: Verapamil therapy: a new approach to the pharmacologic treatment of hypertrophic cardiomyopathy. Circulation, 60:1201, 1979.
36. Bonow, R.O., et al.: Effects of verapamil on left ventricular systolic function and diastolic filling in patients with hypertrophic cardiomyopathy. Circulation, 64:787, 1981.
36a. Spicer, R.L., et al.: Chronic verapamil therapy in pediatric and young adult patients with hypertrophic cardiomyopathy. Am. J. Cardiol., 53:1614, 1984.
37. Rosing, D.R., et al.: Verapamil therapy: a new approach to the pharmacologic treatment of hypertrophic cardiomyopathy. III. Effects of long-term administration. Am. J. Cardiol., 48:545, 1981.
38. Epstein, S.E., and Rosing, D.R.: Verapamil: its potential for causing serious complications in patients with hypertrophic cardiomyopathy. Circulation, 64:437, 1981.
39. Eldar, M., et al.: Obstructive hypertrophic cardiomyopathy with left-sided cardiac failure: improvement after verapamil treatment. Am. J. Cardiol., 53:644, 1984.
40. Kaltenbach, M., et al.: Treatment of hypertrophic obstructive cardiomyopathy with verapamil. Br. Heart J., 42:35, 1979.
40a. Hanrath, P., et al.: Influence of verapamil therapy on left ventricular isovolume relaxation time and regional left ventricular filling in hypertrophic cardiomyopathy. Am. J. Cardiol., 45:1258, 1980.
41. McKenna, W.J., et al.: Arrhythmia in hypertrophic cardiomyopathy. II. Comparison of amiodarone and verapamil in treatment. Br. Heart J., 46:173, 1981.

42. Sadick, N.N., et al.: A double-blind randomized trial of propranolol and verapamil in the treatment of effort angina. Circulation, 66:574, 1982.
43. Johnson, S.M., et al.: Double-blind, randomized, placebo-controlled comparison of propranolol and verapamil in the treatment of patients with stable angina pectoris. Am. J. Med., 71:443, 1981.
44. Leon, M.B., et al.: Clinical efficacy of verapamil alone and combined with propranolol in treating patients with chronic stable angina pectoris. Am. J. Cardiol., 48:131, 1981.
45. Walsh, R.A., Badke, F.R., and O'Rourke, R.A.: Differential effects of systemic and intracoronary calcium channel blocking agents on global and regional left ventricular function in conscious dogs. Am. Heart J., 341, 1981.
46. Singh, B.N., and Roche, A.H.G.: Effects of intravenous verapamil on hemodynamics Am. Heart J., 593, 1977.
47. Smith, H.J., et al.: Regional contractibility: selective depression of ischemic myocardium by verapamil. Circulation, 56:629, 1976.
48. Ferlinz, J., Easthope, J.L., and Aronow, W.S.: Effects of verapamil on myocardial performance in coronary disease. Circulation, 59:313, 1979.
48a. Jackson, W.L., et al.: Comparative hemodynamic effects of verapamil and diltiazem in conscious puppies. AHA 1984.
49. Gould, B.A., et al.: The 24-hour ambulatory blood pressure profile with verapamil. Circulation, 65:22, 1982.
50. Lewis, G.R.J., Morley, K.D., and Lewis, B.M.: The treatment of hypertension with verapamil. N. Z. Med. J., 87:351, 1978.
51. Leonetti, G., et al.: Antihypertensive and renal effects of orally administered verapamil. Eur. J. Clin. Pharmacol., 18:375, 1980.
52. Leeuw, P.W., et al.: Effects of verapamil in hypertensive patients. Calcium antagonism in cardiovascular therapy. 1981, 233–237.
53. Hanrath, P., and Kremer, P.: Effect of verapamil on abnormal left ventricular diastolic performance in patients with secondary left ventricular hypertrophy due to systemic hypertension. Calcium antagonism in cardiovascular therapy: experience with verapamil. 1981, 222–230.
54. Young, T.E., et al.: Comparative effects of nifedipine, verapamil, and diltiazem on experimental pulmonary hypertension. Am. J. Cardiol., 51:195, 1983.
55. Haas, H., and Hartfelder, G.: α-isopropyl-α-(N-methyl-N-homoveratryl-aminopropyl)-3-4 dimethoxyphenylacetonitril), eine Aulstanz mit coronasgefassen Eigenschaften. Arzneimittelforsch., 12:549, 1962.
56. Neumann, M., and Luisada, A.A.: Double-blind evaluation of orally administered iproveratril in patients with angina pectoris. Am. J. Med. Sci., 251:552, 1966.
57. Brodsky, S.J., et al.: Treatment of stable angina of effort with verapamil: a double-blind, placebo-controlled randomized crossover study. Circulation, 66:569, 1982.
58. Pine, M.B., et al.: Verapamil versus placebo in relieving stable angina pectoris. Circulation, 65:17, 1982.
59. Weiner, D.A., et al.: Efficacy and safety of verapamil in patients with angina pectoris after 1 year of continuous, high-dose therapy. Am. J. Cardiol., 51:1251, 1983.
60. Scheidt, S., et al.: Long-term effectiveness of verapamil in stable and unstable angina pectoris. Am. J. Cardiol., 52:1185, 1982.
61. Solber, L.E., et al.: Prinzmetal's variant angina—response to verapamil. Mayo Clin. Proc., 53:256, 1978.
62. Winniford, M.D., et al.: Verapamil for Prinzmetal's variant angina: a long-term, double-blind, randomized trial. Circulation, 66(Suppl. 2):477, 1982.
63. Schomerus, M., et al.: Physiological disposition of verapamil in man. Cardiovasc. Res., 10:605, 1976.
64. McAllister, R.G., and Kirsten, E.B.: The pharmacology of verapamil. IV. Pharmacokinetic and drug effects after single intravenous and oral doses in normal subjects. Clin. Pharmacol. Ther., 31:418, 1981.
65. Eichelbaum, M., et al.: The metabolism of ^{14}C-verapamil in man. Drug Metab. Dispos., 7:145, 1979.

66. Woodcock, B.G., et al.: Direct determination of verapamil in cardiac patients. Clin. Pharmacol. Ther., *30*:52, 1981.
67. Wagner, J.G., et al.: Prediction of steady-state verapamil plasma concentrations in children and adults. Clin. Pharmacol. Ther., *32*:172, 1982.
68. Eichelbaum, M., et al.: Effects of verapamil on P-R intervals in relation to verapamil plasma levels following single IV and oral administration and during chronic treatment. Klin. Wochenschr., *58*:919, 1980.
69. McAllister, R.G., Bourne, D.W.A., and Dittert, L.W.: The pharmacology of verapamil. I. Elimination kinetics in dogs and correlation of plasma levels with effects on the electrocardiogram. J. Pharmacol. Exp. Ther., *202*:38, 1977.
70. Mangiardi, L.M., et al.: Hemodynamic and electrophysiologic effects of verapamil: correlations with drug plasma levels. Circulation, *57*:366, 1978.
71. Klein, H.O., and Kaplinsky, E.: Verapamil and digoxin: their respective effects on atrial fibrillation and their interaction. Am. J. Cardiol., *50*:894, 1982.
72. Kates, R.E., et al.: Pharmacokinetics of verapamil in patients with chronic atrial fibrillation. Circulation, *62(suppl. 3)*:183, 1980.
73. Kates, R.E., et al.: Verapamil disposition kinetics in chronic atrial fibrillation. Clin. Pharmacol. Ther., *30*:44, 1981.
73a. Hesslein, P., et al.: Age-dependent verapamil kinetics affect pediatric oral dose requirements: an Abstract. Submitted to the First International Symposium on Cardiovascular Pharmacology, Geneva 1985.
74. Gibson, R., et al.: The comparative electrophysiologic and hemodynamic effects of verapamil in puppies and adult dogs. Dev. Pharmacol. Ther., *2*:104, 1981.
75. Pedersen, O.L.: Does verapamil have a clinically significant antihypertensive effect? Eur. J. Clin. Pharmacol., *13*:21, 1978.
76. Sacks, H., and Kennelly, B.M.: Verapamil in cardiac arrhyhmias. Br. Med. J., *2*:716, 1972.
77. Witchitz, S., et al.: Accidents cardiovasculaires au cours des traitements par le verapamil: à propos de 6 observations. Nouv. Presse Med., *4*:337, 1975.
78. Andreasen, F., et al.: Assessment of verapamil in the treatment of angina pectoris. Eur. J. Cardiol., *2*:443, 1975.
79. Perkins, C.M.: Serious verapamil poisoning: treatment with intravenous calcium gluconate. Br. Med. J., *2*:6145, 1978.
80. Candell, J., et al.: Acute intoxication with verapamil. Chest, *75*:200, 1979.
81. Moroni, F., and Mannaioni, P.F.: Calcium gluconate and hypertonic sodium chloride in a case of massive verapamil poisoning. Clin. Toxicol., *17*:395, 1980.
82. Ahattori, V.T., Mandel, W.J., and Peter, T.: Calcium for myocardial depression from verapamil. N. Engl. J. Med., *305*:238, 1982.
83. Beitzke, A., and Grubbauer, H.M.: Vergiftung mit Isoptin (Verapamil). Padiatr. Padol., *11*:570, 1976.
84. Da Silva, O.A., et al.: Verapamil acute self-poisoning. Clin. Toxicol., *14*:361, 1979.
85. Passal, D.B., and Grespin, F.H., Jr.: Verapamil poisoning in an infant. Pediatrics, *73*:543, 1984.
86. Perrot, B., et al.: Verapamil: a cause of sudden death in a patient with hypertrophic cardiomyopathy. Br. Heart J., *51*:352, 1984.

Chapter 7

Nifedipine

Nifedipine is a 1,4-dihydropyridine with calcium antagonistic properties. It is the most widely used calcium antagonist in adults, for whom it is prescribed mainly for treatment of coronary arterial spasm, stable angina pectoris, and systemic and pulmonary hypertension. The drug has also been under investigation for secondary prevention of myocardial infarction, peripheral vascular diseases, and other conditions in adults. In children, nifedipine is useful in the treatment of pulmonary hypertension, and in the future, this agent may also play a role in the treatment of systemic hypertension and hypertropic cardiomyopathy. Because the experience with this drug in children is limited, the primary purpose of this chapter is to familiarize the pediatrician with its potential applications.

Structure

Nifedipine is 4-(2'-nitrophenyl)-2,6-dimethyl-3,5-dicarbomethoxy-1,4-dihydropyridine.

Hemodynamic Effects

The hemodynamic effects of nifedipine have been studied primarily in adult human subjects and in animals. The two main actions of this drug are a direct negative inotropic effect and a peripheral vasodilatory effect. By blocking the slow calcium current, nifedipine inhibits the calcium-dependent electromechanical coupling and thereby exerts a direct negative inotropic effect. This phenomenon has been directly demonstrated as a nifedipine-induced decrease in contractility of isolated papillary muscles,[1] as well as in isolated cardiac preparations.[2] In several studies, selective injection of nifedipine into the coronary arteries of human subjects produced a significant decrease in contractility, measured by radiographic evaluation of radiopaque markers inserted to the heart and a decrease in maximal left ventricular rate of development of pressure (dP/dt_{max}).[3-6] The direct depression of myocardial contractility was more prominent in ischemic than in nonischemic zones.[7,8] Systemic administration of nifedipine produces a potent systemic vasodilatory effect that stimulates the sympathetic nervous system. This activation more than compensates for the direct negative inotropic effect of the drug.

Inhibition of the calcium-dependent electromechanical coupling in vascular smooth muscle results in relaxation of vascular walls. Nifedipine thereby produces a potent vasodilatory effect, which is most prominent in the arterial vascular bed. Thus, nifedipine reduces systemic vascular resistance and cardiac afterload. This effect causes a compensatory increase in heart rate. In the intact heart, myocardial contractility is not changed or is even increased by systemic administration of nifedipine.[3, 9-11] In patients with coronary artery disease, nifedipine improves global and regional myocardial function.[12] The combination of peripheral vasodilation and direct negative intropic effect results in a fall in systemic arterial pressure. This fall is proportional to the pretreatment level of blood pressure. In normotensive patients, the reduction in arterial pressure is minimal.

In patients without congestive heart failure or coronary artery disease, nifedipine produces little change in left ventricular filling pressure. In patients with congestive heart failure, however, left ventricular filling pressure is reduced by nifedipine. Nifedipine prevents exercise-induced elevation in left ventricular filling pressure in patients with coronary artery disease. Nifedipine also improves the diastolic properties of the heart, mainly in patients with congestive heart failure.[14]

Effect on Coronary Arteries

The effect of nifedipine on the coronary arteries in adults is one of the most important therapeutic actions of this drug. Nifedipine dilates the large and small coronary arteries in animals, in healthy human subjects, and in patients with coronary artery disease. For example, Schultz and co-workers reported that the intravenous administration of 1 mg nifedipine increased the diameter of nonstenotic epicardial coronary arteries by 18.1%.[15] In another study, sublingual nifedipine dilated stenotic coronary segments by about 30% in almost half the cases.[16] Nifedipine is not a selective coronary vasodilator because the decrease in systemic resistance produced by the drug is almost equal to the decrease in coronary resistance. In coronary spasm, however, nifedipine has a selective effect. It was recently shown that nifedipine dilates fewer coronary segments and to a lesser extent than nitroglycerin.

Effects in Neonates

Coe and associates evaluated the effect of nifedipine in newborn lambs.[17] A bolus injection of nifedipine increased the pulmonary artery pressure by 16% and the pulmonary arteriolar resistance by 16%; this increase was greater than that produced by the vehicle alone. Nifedipine decreased cardiac output by 7%, systemic vascular resistance by 38%, and left ventricular dP/dt by 50%.

In this same study, hypoxic pulmonary vasoconstriction was not prevented by pretreatment with nifedipine. Hypoxia after pretreatment with nifedipine increased pulmonary arteriolar resistance by 45% and decreased systemic vascular resistance by 7%. It was concluded that nifedipine and its vehicle constrict the pulmonary arterioles of the newborn lamb and have a negative inotropic effect. The effects of nifedipine and vehicle were additive. Coe and associates recommended that nifedipine should not be used in the management of neonatal pulmonary hypertension, especially that due to hypoxia.[17]

Effect on Angina Pectoris

In adults, nifedipine was effective in treating all types of angina pectoris. In patients with stable angina pectoris due to coronary artery disease, nifedipine reduces the frequency and extent of spontaneous anginal episodes and the frequency and extent of ST-segment depression. It prolongs exercise tolerance and reduces the magnitude of ST-segment depression at any given work load.[18-21] In a multicenter, double-blind, placebo-controlled study conducted in the United States, nifedipine, 60 mg daily, decreased the required intake of nitroglycerin by about 50%, decreased the frequency of spontaneous anginal episodes by about 50 to 60%, and increased exercise tolerance, without a significant change in the rate-pressure product.

Nifedipine was also effective in the treatment and prevention of coronary artery spasm, as confirmed by direct demonstration during angiocardiographic and ergonovine testing, as well as by long-term clinical studies.[22,23] Stone and colleagues reported that the antianginal efficacy of nifedipine is greatest in patients with a component of coronary spasm.[24]

Several mechanisms have been suggested to account for the antianginal effect of nifedipine, but no single, predominant mechanism has been established. The drug is beneficial in patients with angina because it improves the oxygen supply-demand ratio. This effect is achieved by an increase in coronary arterial supply, by prevention of coronary spasm, dilation of normal and stenotic coronary arteries, and improvement of myocardial function. Myocardial oxygen demand is decreased by afterload reduction, by preload reduction, and possibly also by a direct myocardial "oxygen sparing" effect of the drug.

Effect on Pulmonary Hypertension

At present, the most important application of nifedipine in cardiovascular therapy in young age groups is in the treatment of pulmonary hypertension. Nifedipine has reduced elevated pulmonary pressure and vascular resistance in both primary and secondary pulmonary hypertension.[25-27] This effect has been clearly shown with short-term administration of the drug. For example, in 13 patients with secondary pulmonary hypertension, nifedipine, 20 mg sublingually, reduced pulmonary arterial pressure, whereas systemic vascular resistance, pulmonary wedge pressure, and arterial partial oxygen pressure remained unchanged. In another study, nifedipine, 20 mg sublingually, decreased pulmonary vascular resistance and increased cardiac output in all 8 patients with secondary pulmonary hypertension.[26] Two of these patients had Eisenmenger's syndrome.

Results at least comparably favorable have been obtained in patients with primary pulmonary hypertension. Olivari and co-workers reported marked improvement in 7 such patients within an hour of sublingual administration of 20 mg nifedipine.[28] Mean arterial pressure was reduced from 88.4 ± 9.7 to 72.6 ± 10.2 mm Hg, pulmonary arterial systolic pressure was reduced from 91.7 ± 13.9 to 76.8 ± 22.3 mm Hg, pulmonary arterial diastolic pressure fell from 41.3 ± 12.4 to 31.9 ± 12.3 mm Hg, mean pulmonary arterial pressure decreased from 58.1 ± 14.3 to 48.6 ± 16.3 mm Hg, pulmonary vascular resistance was reduced from 1070 ± 260 to 695 ± 266 dyne·sec·cm^{-5}, and systemic vascular resistance fell from 1505 ± 234 to 940 ± 172 dyne·sec·cm^{-5}. Cardiac index was increased from 2.6 ± 0.6 to 3.4 ± 0.8 L/min/m^2. In 2 of the patients in whom exercise testing was performed, exercise tolerance was increased by about 30%. Rubin and colleagues studied the hemodynamic effect of sublingual nifedipine, 10 to 20 mg, 15 to 30 min after administration.[29] The drug increased cardiac output from 3.6 ± 1.7 to 5.3 ± 2.8 L/min and decreased pulmonary vascular resistance from 1605 ± 787 to 1025 ± 540 dyne·sec·cm^{-5}, systemic vascular resistance from 2761 ± 1557 to 1591 ± 823 dyne·sec·cm^{-5}, and mean aortic pressure from 99 ± 19 to 85 ± 12 mm Hg. Right ventricular ejection fraction increased by 18%. One of the patients, however, developed a marked increase in pulmonary arterial pressure after a single dose of nifedipine.

Nifedipine was also effective in some of the patients treated for long periods. The largest series of long-term treatment of patients with primary pulmonary hypertension was reported by Rubin and associates.[29] Six patients were treated with nifedipine, 40 to 120 mg daily, for up to 14 months. The initial favorable hemodynamic response of an increase in cardiac output and a decrease in pulmonary vascular resistance was sustained in 5 of these 6 patients. Douglas reported that an initial favorable hemodynamic response in a woman with primary pulmonary hypertension was sustained for 6 months.[30] Other investigators reported cases of young patients with primary pulmonary hypertension in whom the initial beneficial effect of nifedipine was sustained for at least several months.[31-33]

Other investigators have reported less favorable results. For example, Klugmann and co-workers reported that long-term treatment with nifedipine had no beneficial effect in three patients with secondary pulmonary hypertension.[26] Another study suggested that the beneficial effect of nifedipine may not be generalized, but may rather be selective for patients with active pulmonary vasospastic disease. The occurrence of Raynaud's phenomenon may indicate the presence of such an active pulmonary vasospastic process.[34]

Rich and colleagues compared the effects of amrinone, hydralazine, and nifedipine in seven patients with primary pulmonary hypertension.[35] All these agents reduced pulmonary and systemic arterial pressures and increased cardiac output. In two of the patients, nifedipine reduced pulmonary resistance to a greater extent than systemic resistance. Amrinone and hydralazine primarily affected systemic resistance.

Fisher and co-workers reported that the effect of nifedipine in patients with secondary pulmonary hypertension was more potent than that of hydralazine.[34] The response to short-term administration of nifedipine predicted the patient's response to long-term therapy. Rozkovec and associates studied five patients with primary pulmonary hypertension.[36] Three of them, who had a favorable hemodynamic response to the short-term administration of nifedipine, 10 mg sublingually, had improved exercise tolerance after 3 months of treatment. The remaining patients, who did not improve after a single dose, did not show improvement with long-term treatment.

Three main problems are inherent in the use of nifedipine in patients with pulmonary hypertension. First is impairment of the ventilation-perfusion ratio. This effect was demonstrated in two patients treated with nifedipine,[37] but it is a well-known problem with conventional vasodilators as well. Second, in a considerable portion of the patients with pulmonary hypertension, nifedipine does not reduce the elevated pulmonary arterial pressure, despite a significant reduction in pulmonary vascular resistance. Finally, unlike the conventional vasodilators, nifedipine has a negative inotropic effect. This action may cause myocardial suppression and may limit the effect of the drug in patients with pulmonary hypertension. For example, Packer and colleagues reported that nifedipine and hydralazine similarly reduced systemic and pulmonary vascular resistance in patients with pulmonary hypertension.[38] Only nifedipine suppressed myocardial function, however, as evident from decreases in cardiac index and stroke volume. Suppression of right ventricular function by nifedipine was shown by an increase in right atrial pressure and a decrease in pulmonary arterial pressure.[38] Most of the patients with primary pulmonary hypertension in whom nifedipine was evaluated were young adults.

In summary, nifedipine may be tried in children and young adults with primary and secondary pulmonary hypertension. Hemodynamic evaluation is required at the initiation of treatment, to assess the results and to avoid continuing treatment in patients with an initially unfavorable response.

Effect on Hypertrophic Cardiomyopathy

Several findings suggest that nifedipine may be beneficial in hypertrophic cardiomyopathy. First, the negative inotropic effect of nifedipine may decrease myocardial contractility and left ventricular outflow pressure gradient. Second, nifedipine improves the myocardial oxygen supply-demand ratio and thereby eliminates the ischemic stimulus for hypertrophy. Third, calcium antagonists can affect cardiomyopathy in the hamster.

The experience with nifedipine in patients with hypertrophic cardiomyopathy is limited. Nifedipine, either alone or in combination with a beta-blocking agent, has decreased the resting left ventricular outflow gradient in some patients with hypertrophic obstructive cardiomyopathy.[39, 40]

The risk exists, however, that sympathetic activation due to peripheral vasodilation will augment myocardial contractility and will increase the pressure gradient. In one patient with hypertrophic cardiomyopathy and no pressure gradient at rest, administration of nifedipine produced a pressure gradient of 35 mm Hg.[40]

At present, I do not recommend the treatment of children with hypertrophic cardiomyopathy with nifedipine. Perhaps in the future nifedipine, possibly in combination with other drugs, will play some role in the treatment of these children.

Effect on Systemic Hypertension

In adults, nifedipine is effective in treatment of systemic hypertension. The mechanism of action is the selective dilating effect of the drug on resistance vessels. The acute hypertensive effect of nifedipine has been reported to correlate with the patient's pretreatment level of blood pressure and vascular resistance.[41, 42] This finding supports the suggested mechanism of a direct effect on the elevated peripheral vascular resistance. For example, Lund-Johansen and Omrik reported that, in hypertensive patients, nifedipine lowered arterial pressure at rest by approximately 17% and during exercise by approximately 15%.[43] This effect was due to a reduction of about 16% in peripheral vascular resistance. Moreover, the reduction of elevated arterial pressure by long-term treatment with nifedipine was shown to result from the same mechanism, as evident from repeated hemodynamic measurements at 3 weeks, 3 months, and 12 months of treatment.[41, 43]

Sublingual administration of nifedipine has lowered elevated blood pressure within 20 minutes. Long-term clinical studies have shown that nifedipine, administered orally in the form of capsules, 3 to 4 times daily, is effective in lowering both systolic and diastolic blood pressure, in the supine and standing positions, at rest and during exercise, alone or in combination with other antihypertensive drugs.[41, 44-46]

No attenuation of the effect of nifedipine has been observed with long-term treatment.[43] The drug has also been effective in the management of hypertensive crises. In my experience, nifedipine, given orally twice daily in the form of tablets, may be an effective antihypertensive agent in patients with resistant hypertension.

No formal studies of nifedipine administration in children with hypertension have been reported. By personal communication, however, I have collected data on isolated instances in which a favorable effect was achieved. At present, nifedipine should be tried with caution in children in whom other antihypertensive agents have failed.

Clinical Pharmacology

Nifedipine is currently available only for oral administration. More than 90% of the oral dose is absorbed from the gastrointestinal tract, at a rapid rate. The drug may be detected in the blood within about 2 min, and the maximal blood level is achieved within 30 min of sublingual administration. Nifedipine undergoes an extensive first-pass hepatic metabolism. Its metabolites are inactive. The effect of the drug correlates directly with its plasma level.

About 80% of the drug and its metabolites are excreted in the urine.

Side Effects

Acceleration of Heart Rate

Nifedipine increases heart rate, as a result of sympathetic activation by peripheral vasodilation. Rarely, the drug exacerbates angina pectoris in adults.

Congestive Heart Failure

The direct negative inotropic effect of nifedipine rarely causes congestive heart failure; at greater risk are patients concomitantly treated with beta-blocking agents.

Peripheral Edema

About 10% of patients treated with nifedipine develop peripheral edema, especially in the lower extremities. This edema is not related to congestive heart failure and probably results from dilation of renal arterioles and precapillary sphincters that increases renal filtration. This effect is uncommon in patients receiving less than 1 mg/kg.

Hypotension

Up to 5% of patients treated with nifedipine develop transient hypotension.

Gingival Hyperplasia

Gingival hyperplasia, resembling that seen in patients treated with phenytoin, may be caused by nifedipine. This effect has been observed in 4 of 2000 patients treated with nifedipine. The drug may also produce histologic changes in gums that appear to be clinically normal. Such changes include epithelial acanthosis, proliferation, reticulation and elongation of the rete pegs, and fibrosis of the lamina propria.

Flushing and Heat Sensation

These effects are encountered in up to 10% of patients treated with nifedipine and are probably related to vasodilation.

Other Effects

Palpitations, cholestasis, tremor, dizziness, and giddiness are uncommon side effects of this drug.

Dosage and Administration

In adults, daily oral doses of about 0.5 to 1.5 mg/kg in 3 to 4 divided doses are used. No guidelines exist for the use of nifedipine in children.

References

1. Bossert, F., and Vater, W.: Naturwissenschaften, 58:578, 1971.
2. Vater, W., et al.: Arzneimittelforsch., 22:1, 1972.
3. Fleckenstein, A., et al.: BAY a 1040: ein hochaktiver Ca-antagonistischer Inhibitor des elektromechanischen Koppelungsprocess in Warmbl Myokard. Arzneimittelforsch., 22:22, 1972.
4. Raff, K.H., Kosche, F., and Lochner, W.: Untersuchungen mit nifedipin, einer coronargefasse weiterenden Substanz mit schneller sublingualer Wirkung. Arzneimittelforsch., 22:33, 1972.
5. Serruys, P.W., et al.: Regional wall motion from radiopaque markers after intravenous and intracoronary injections of nifedipine. Circulation, 63:584, 1981.
6. Rousseau, M.F., et al.: Impaired early left ventricular relaxation in coronary artery disease: effects of intracoronary nifedipine. Circulation, 62:764, 1980.
7. Hugenholtz, P.G., et al.: Nifedipine in the treatment of unstable angina, coronary spasm and myocardial ischemia. Am. J. Cardiol., 47:163, 1981.

8. Abrahamsson, T., and Sjöquist, P.O.: Intracoronary nifedipine depresses left ventricular regional function more in ischemic than in non ischemic myocardium. AHA 1983.
9. Verdouw, P.D., Ten Cate, F.J., and Hugenholtz, P.G.: Effect of nifedipine on segmental myocardial function in the anesthetized pig. Eur. J. Pharmacol., 63:209, 1980.
10. Vater, W.: Myocardial oxygen consumption under the influence of nifedipine (Adalat) in the anaesthetized dog. In New Therapy of Ischemic Heart Disease. Edited by W. Lochner and G. Kronenberg. Berlin, Springer Verlag, 1975, p. 77.
11. Kissin, I., and Kilpatrick, J.V.: Effects of nifedipine on myocardial energy balance in experimental coronary vasoconstriction and occlusion. J. Cardiovasc. Pharmacol., 4:111, 1982.
12. Serruys, P.W., et al.: Influence of intracoronary nifedipine on left ventricular function, coronary vasomotility, and myocardial oxygen consumption. Br. Heart J., 49:427, 1983.
13. Zacca, N.M., et al.: Effect of nifedipine on exercise-induced left ventricular dysfunction and myocardial hypoperfusion in stable angina. Am. J. Cardiol., 50:689, 1982.
14. Lichtlen, P., et al.: Mechanism of various antianginal drugs: relationship between regional flow behaviour and contractility. In New Therapy of Ischaemic Heart Disease. Edited by A.D. Jatene and P.R. Lichtlen. Amsterdam, Excerpta Medica, 1976, p. 14.
15. Schultz, W., et al.: Active and passive changes in coronary artery diameters after vasodilatation: Fifth International Adalat Symposium. In New Therapy of Ischaemic Heart Disease and Hypertension. Edited by M. Kaltenbach and H.N. Neufeld. Amsterdam, Excerpta Medica, 1983, p. 309.
16. Rafflenbeul, W., and Lichtlen, P.R.: Release of residual vascular tone in coronary artery stenoses with nifedipine and glyceryl trinitrate: Fifth International Adalat Symposium. In New Therapy of Ischaemic Heart Disease and Hypertension. Edited by M. Kaltenbach and H.N. Neufeld. Amsterdam, Excerpta Medica, 1983, p. 300.
17. Coe, J.Y., et al.: Nifedipine elevates pulmonary arteriolar resistance (PAR) and depresses left ventricular (LV) function in unsedated newborn lambs. AHA 1984.
18. Ekelund, L.G., and Oro, L.: Antianginal efficiency of nifedipine with and without a beta-blocker, studied with exercise test: A double-blind randomized subacute study. Clin. Cardiol., 2:203, 1979.
19. Ekelund, L.G., Atterhog, J.H., and Melin, A.L.: Effect of nifedipine on exercise tolerance in patients with angina pectoris. In New Therapy of Ischemic Heart Disease: Proceedings of the First International Adalat Symposium. Edited by K. Hashimoto, E. Kinura, and T. Kobayarski. Tokyo, University of Tokyo Press, 1973, p. 144.
20. Moskowitz, R.M., et al.: Nifedipine therapy for stable angina pectoris: preliminary results of effects of angina frequency and treadmill exercise response. Am. J. Cardiol., 44:811, 1979.
21. Mueller, H.S., and Chahine, R.A.: Interim report of multicenter double-blind, placebo-controlled studies of nifedipine in chronic stable angina: symposium on nifedipine in angina pectoris. Am. J. Med., 71:645, 1981.
22. Bertrand, M.E., et al.: Treatment of spasm of the coronary artery with nifedipine. Eur. Heart J., 1(Suppl. B):65, 1980.
23. Tiefenbrunn, A.J., et al.: Nifedipine blockade of ergonovine-induced coronary arterial spasm: angiographic documentation. Am. J. Cardiol., 48:184, 1981.
24. Stone, P.H., et al.: Efficacy of nifedipine therapy in patients with refractory angina pectoris: significance of the presence of coronary vasospasm. Am. Heart J., 106:644, 1983.
25. Camerini, F., et al.: Primary pulmonary hypertensive effects of a calcium antagonist drug (nifedipine). Br. Heart J., 44:352, 1980.
26. Klugmann, S., Fioretti, P., and Camerini, F.: Acute hemodynamic effects of nifedipine in pulmonary hypertension. Circulation, 62(Suppl. III):503, 1980.
27. Simmonneau, G., et al.: Inhibition of hypoxic pulmonary vasoconstriction by nifedipine. N. Engl. J. Med., 304:1582, 1981.

28. Olivari, M.T., et al.: Beneficial hemodynamic and exercise response to nifedipine in primary pulmonary hypertension. ACC 1983.
29. Rubin, L.J., et al.: Treatment of primary pulmonary hypertension with nifedipine. Ann. Intern. Med., 99:433, 1983.
30. Douglas, J.S., Jr.: Hemodynamic effects of nifedipine in primary pulmonary hypertension. JACC, 2:174, 1983.
31. Saito, D., et al.: Primary pulmonary hypertension improved by long-term oral administration of nifedipine. Am. Heart J., 105:1041, 1983.
32. Wise, J.R., Jr.: Nifedipine in the treatment of primary pulmonary hypertension. Am. Heart J., 105:693, 1983.
33. De Feyter, P.J., Kerkkamp, J.J., and de Jong, J.P.: Sustained beneficial effect of nifedipine in primary pulmonary hypertension. Am. Heart J., 105:333, 1983.
34. Fisher, J., et al.: Nifedipine in pulmonary hypertension: importance of Raynaud's phenomenon. AHA 1983.
35. Rich, S., Ganz, R., and Levy, P.S.: Comparative actions of hydralazine, nifedipine and amrinone in primary pulmonary hypertension. Am. J. Cardiol., 52:1104, 1983.
36. Rozkovec, A., et al.: Value of acute vasodilator studies in management of primary pulmonary hypertension. AHA 1982.
37. Melot, C., et al.: Effects of nifedipine on ventilation/perfusion matching in primary pulmonary hypertension. Chest, 83:203, 1983.
38. Packer, M., et al.: Adverse hemodynamic and clinical effects of nifedipine in patients with primary pulmonary hypertension. ACC 1983.
39. Landmark, K., et al.: Haemodynamic effects of nifedipine and propranolol in patients with hypertrophic obstructive cardiomyopathy. Br. Heart J., 48:19, 1982.
40. Lorell, B.H., et al.: Modification of abnormal left ventricular diastolic properties by nifedipine in patients with hypertrophic cardiomyopathy. Circulation, 65:499, 1982.
41. Olivari, M.T., et al.: Treatment of hypertension with nifedipine, a calcium antagonistic agent. Circulation, 59:1056, 1979.
42. MacGregor, G.A., et al.: Circumstantial evidence that an abnormality of calcium transport may be important in essential hypertension. Clin. Sci., 60:6, 1981.
43. Lund-Johansen, P., and Omrik, P.: Haemodynamic effects of nifedipine in essential hypertension at rest and during exercise. J. Hypertension, 1:159, 1983.
44. MacGregor, G.A.: Discussion: Fifth International Adalat Symposium. In New Therapy of Ischaemic Heart Disease and Hypertension. Edited by M. Kaltenbach and H.N. Neufeld. Amsterdam, Excerpta Medica, 1983, p. 156.
45. Guazzi, M.D., et al.: Short- and long-term efficacy of a calcium-antagonistic agent (nifedipine) combined with methyldopa in the treatment of severe hypertension. Circulation, 61:913, 1980.
46. Thibonnier, M., Bonnet, F., and Corvol, P.: Antihypertensive effect of fractionated sublingual administration of nifedipine in moderate essential hypertension. Eur. J. Clin. Pharmacol., 17:161, 1980.

Chapter 8

Diltiazem

Diltiazem is a calcium antagonist recently developed in Japan and available in Europe and the United States. It has electrophysiologic properties resembling those of verapamil and hemodynamic properties resembling those of nifedipine. Diltiazem is now used for most of the conditions for which verapamil and nifedipine are prescribed. In adults, diltiazem has been effective in angina pectoris, especially variant angina resulting from coronary spasm, arrhythmias, hypertrophic cardiomyopathy, and systemic and pulmonary hypertension. The drug has also exerted a myocardial protective effect during ischemia.

The experience in children is limited, and no experience in infants has been reported. Diltiazem has been used in a few children and adolescents with supraventricular tachyarrhythmias, hypertrophic cardiomyopathy, and pulmonary hypertension. In the future, this agent may play some role in the treatment of systemic hypertension in young age groups.

Structure

Diltiazem is the d-*cis* isomer of 3 acetyloxy-2,3-dihydro-5-[2-(dimethylamino)-ethyl]-2-(P-methoxyphenyl)-1.5-benzothiazepine-4(SH)-one hydrochloride.

Mechanism of Action

Diltiazem, a calcium antagonist, acts by inhibiting the slow channels and the slow inward calcium current. Therefore, it affects processes that depend on calcium ions, such as myocardial and smooth cell contraction and slow-response action potential.

Electrophysiologic Effects

Diltiazem mainly affects electrophysiologic processes that depend on the inward calcium current, such as the slow-response action potential in the sinoatrial and atrioventricular nodes and the plateau phase of the fast-response action potential.

Microelectrode studies of His-Purkinje fibers and ventricular myocardium demonstrated that therapeutic concentrations of diltiazem decreased the amplitude of the plateau phase of the action potential. The drug also shortened the duration of this phase and thereby decreased the duration of the action potential.[1, 2] At high concentrations, diltiazem decreased the role of phase 0 action potential; this finding indicates some effect on the fast inward calcium current.[1]

As mentioned previously, diltiazem resembles verapamil in its electrophysiologic properties and nifedipine in its hemodynamic properties. The electrophysiologic effects of diltiazem occur at doses lower than those required to exert the hemodynamic effects of the drug.

Effect on the Sinoatrial Node

The effect of diltiazem on the sinoatrial node is the net result of the direct depressant effect and the sympathetic stimulation induced by peripheral vasodilation. Direct application of diltiazem to the sinoatrial node results in reduction of the spontaneous rate. In man, systemic administration of diltiazem usually causes a slight slowing, or no change, of heart rate. In animal experiments, the drug accelerated the spontaneous sinus rate by sympathetic stimulation and vagal withdrawal secondary to peripheral vasodilation.[3-7] In dogs with experimentally produced myocardial infarction, diltiazem prolonged the sinoatrial node recovery time.[8]

Effect on the Atria

Diltiazem does not usually have a significant effect on atrial conduction or effective refractory period.

Effect on the Atrioventricular Node

Diltiazem prolongs conduction in the atrioventricular node, as evident by prolongation of the AH and PR intervals. The drug also prolongs the effective and functional refractory periods of the atrioventricular node.[9, 10] For example, Jauernig and associates reported that diltiazem prolonged the AH interval by 67%.[11] The magnitude of the effect of diltiazem on the atrioventricular node is less than that of verapamil.

In patients with supraventricular tachycardia, diltiazem has slowed both anterograde and retrograde conduction in the atrioventricular node. Controversy exists over which of these effects predominates in termination of this arrhythmia by diltiazem.[11-14]

Effect on Accessory Atrioventricular Tracts

One report noted that diltiazem exerted a mild depressant effect on retrograde conduction in accessory atrioventricular tracts.[14] The drug had no effect on the refractoriness of these tracts.

Effect on the Ventricles

Diltiazem has no effect on intraventricular conduction and refractoriness, as evident by the lack of change in the duration of the HV and QRS intervals and the effective refractory periods of the His-Purkinje system and the ventricular myocardium.[8, 11, 15-17] Diltiazem has electrophysiologic effects on the ischemic myocardium, but this consideration is not usually applicable to children.

Effects on Arrhythmias

Like verapamil, diltiazem is especially effective in terminating and preventing supraventricular tachycardia and in controlling the ventricular rate in patients with atrial fibrillation or flutter.

Supraventricular Tachycardia

Diltiazem has terminated and prevented re-entrant supraventricular tachycardia by interfering in the tachycardia cycle at the atrioventricular node. Some series included older children and adolescents. For example, Yeh and co-workers studied 36 patients in a wide age range with supraventricular tachycardia.[14] In all of them, sustained supraventricular tachycardia could be induced; 24 of them had an accessory atrioventricular pathway, and the remaining 12 had intra-atrioventricular nodal re-entry. Diltiazem was given orally, 3 doses of 90 mg each, at 8-hour intervals. After the administration of diltiazem, 20 of 24 patients with accessory pathway lost the ability to induce or to sustain supraventricular tachycardia because of increased atrioventricular nodal refractoriness in 19 patients and because of increased retrograde accessory pathway refractoriness in 1 patient. Eight of the 12 patients with intranodal re-entrance lost the ability to induce or to sustain supraventricular tachycardia because of increased retrograde fast-pathway refractoriness in 6 patients and because of increased anterograde slow-pathway refractoriness in 2 patients.

On discharge from the hospital, 15 of the patients in the foregoing series were given prescriptions for oral diltiazem.[14] In 13 of these patients who had responded favorably to diltiazem during electrophysiologic studies, the drug prevented recurrences of the arrhythmia during a follow-up period of 5 ± 3 months. In 2 patients in whom diltiazem failed to prevent induction of supraventricular tachycardia, recurrences of the arrhythmia were observed during long-term treatment. Thus, electrophysiologic studies are effective in predicting the long-term clinical response to diltiazem.[14] The series reported by Yeh and colleagues did not include infants or small children, however.[14]

Several other investigators have reported excellent results with this drug in termination and prevention of supraventricular tachycardia in adults.[18, 19] Therefore, diltiazem appears to be a reasonable alternative to verapamil in children with supraventricular tachycardia unresponsive to verapamil and in children who are unable to tolerate verapamil.

Atrial Fibrillation and Flutter

In adults with atrial fibrillation and flutter, the effect of diltiazem appears to resemble that of verapamil. Diltiazem usually slows the ventricular response to the atrial arrhythmia and, uncommonly, may also convert the arrhythmia to sinus rhythm.[19, 20] No experience with diltiazem in children with atrial fibrillation or flutter has been reported, but it is reasonable to assume that this drug will resemble verapamil in the pediatric age group.

In summary, diltiazem is effective and safe in patients with a variety of supraventricular tachyarrhythmias. The clinically used intravenous doses required for termination or control of such arrhythmias usually have no adverse hemodynamic effects.

Hemodynamic Effects

The hemodynamic effects of diltiazem resemble those of nifedipine and verapamil and include a negative inotropic effect, a peripheral vasodilatory effect, and possibly also a direct effect on diastolic properties of the myocardium.

The negative inotropic effect of diltiazem has been demonstrated in isolated myocardial preparations. Intracoronary injection of diltiazem has also produced a transient attenuation of cardiac contractility.[21] Systemic administration to intact animals, to normal human subjects, and to patients with coronary artery disease but without marked impairment of pump function usually caused no myocardial depression; this effect resulted from sympathetic activation by peripheral vasodilation. By this mechanism, diltiazem occasionally even increased myocardial contractility, as evident by an increase in cardiac output and a decrease in pulmonary capillary pressure.[22-24] Diltiazem did not usually reduce blood pressure in normotensive subjects. In patients with congestive heart failure, diltiazem did not produce symptomatic deterioration,[25] and it even increased cardiac output and stroke work index by about 40%.[26] This agent should not be used for vasodilation in patients with congestive heart failure, however, because of its negative inotropic effect.

Effect on Hypertrophic Cardiomyopathy

Interest in the actions of diltiazem in patients with hypertrophic cardiomyopathy was raised by the finding that verapamil exerts beneficial hemodynamic and symptomatic effects in this condition, as well as by the recognition that impairment of diastolic properties of the heart plays an important role in the hemodynamic and clinical problems of patients with this disorder. Most investigators agree that diltiazem does not improve systolic function of the heart in patients with hypertrophic cardiomyopathy.[27-29] For verapamil, this question is still open. Diltiazem does improve the diastolic properties of the heart in these patients, however. For example, in a group of 11 patients with various types of hypertrophic cardiomyopathy, the intravenous administration of diltiazem shortened the abnormally prolonged isovolumic left ventricular relaxation time by about 30%.[27]

In another group of patients, the intravenous administration of diltiazem produced a sudden improvement in diastolic properties of the heart. This improvement was maintained during prolonged oral therapy.[28] In another group of 10 patients with hypertrophic cardiomyopathy, diltiazem inhibited the exercise-induced increase in left ventricular filling pressure.[29]

Most of the patients in these series were adults; infants and young children were not included in any of the series. It appears that diltiazem resembles verapamil in its beneficial effect in patients of all ages with hypertrophic cardiomyopathy.

Effects in the Presence of Beta-adrenergic Blockade in Young Ages

Most studies in adults indicate that the intravenous administration of verapamil is contraindicated in patients receiving beta-adrenoreceptor blocking agents. Propranolol is often given to pediatric patients with recurrent supraventricular tachycardia. Therefore, these patients cannot receive intravenous verapamil for conversion of acute episodes of the arrhythmia to normal sinus rhythm.

Because diltiazem has been suggested as an alternative to verapamil for management of supraventricular tachycardia in infants and children, one must determine whether the combination of diltiazem and beta-adrenoreceptor blocking agents will produce deleterious effects similar to those of verapamil combined with beta-adrenoreceptor blocking agents in young age groups.

Jackson and associates evaluated the effect of diltiazem given as a bolus injection after pretreatment with propranolol.[29a] Diltiazem alone produced no significant alterations in cardiac output, mean blood pressure, heart rate, and PR interval. Diltiazem given after propranolol caused a slight decrease in cardiac output and in mean blood pressure and a significant slowing of heart rate and prolongation of PR interval. Diltiazem had less of a negative inotropic effect than verapamil in these patients.[29a] These findings suggest that diltiazem may be superior to verapamil in pediatric patients receiving beta-adrenoreceptor blocking agents. This conclusion has to be confirmed, however, by studies of human patients.

Effects on Systemic Hypertension

Like other calcium antagonists, diltiazem is effective in treatment of systemic hypertension. It lowers systolic and diastolic blood pressure, both at rest and during exercise. This effect depends on the control level of blood pressure.[30, 31] One study found that the drug reduced elevated systolic blood pressure in up to 90% of patients with essential hypertension and reduced diastolic blood pressure in 66%.[32] In another study, the antihypertensive effect of diltiazem was sustained throughout prolonged treatment.[33] Diltiazem, administered intravenously, is also effective in hypertensive emergencies.[34] No experience has been reported in treatment of children with systemic hypertension with this drug, but in the future, the drug may play some role in the management of hypertension in pediatrics.

Effects on Pulmonary Hypertension

In patients with primary pulmonary hypertension, diltiazem may decrease pulmonary vascular resistance and pulmonary arterial pressure and may increase cardiac output.[35, 36] In one patient, these effects were sustained during a year of treatment. Diltiazem has an important advantage over other vasodilators in that it does not impair the ventilation-perfusion ratio or the pulmonary gas exchange.

Clinical Pharmacology

Diltiazem can be given intravenously or orally. It is rapidly absorbed from the gastrointestinal tract after oral administration. Diltiazem undergoes first-pass hepatic metabolism, which causes a marked intersubject variation in systemic bioavailability ranging between 13 and 74%.[37, 38] Peak plasma levels achieved with therapeutic doses range between 30 and 270 ng/ml. This peak level is reached within an hour from oral administration. In several patients, a second peak of plasma level has been observed.[10] With continued oral administration, the drug may accumulate (nonlinear kinetics).

Protein binding of diltiazem in the serum is about 80%. The elimination half-life of orally administered diltiazem is from 3 to 5 hours. The elimination of intravenously administered diltiazem is triexponential, and its terminal half-life is similar to that of oral diltiazem.[10] Diltiazem is eliminated by hepatic metabolism with urinary and biliary excretion of the metabolites.

Side Effects

The side effects of diltiazem are common, but usually mild. They include headache, pedal edema, sinus bradycardia, hypotension, and atrioventricular block.[39, 40]

Effects in Lactation

It is not clear whether diltiazem is excreted in human milk. At present, nursing mothers should avoid diltiazem.

Drug Interactions

Diltiazem has an additive depressant effect on the sinoatrial and atrioventricular nodes when given concomitantly with digoxin. Unlike verapamil, which has a similar effect but also elevates serum digoxin levels, diltiazem does not alter serum digoxin levels.[10] Therefore, diltiazem may be superior to verapamil in patients receiving digoxin.

Diltiazem and propranolol may have an additive depressant effect on heart rate and contractility.

Dosage and Administration

Oral Administration

In Japan, where the drug was developed, the usual adult dose is 30 mg 3 times daily. In the United States, doses of up to 120 mg 3 times daily are used. No recommendations on oral pediatric doses have been reported.

Intravenous Administration

A bolus injection of 0.25 mg/kg has been recommended. It may be followed by an infusion of 0.003 mg/kg/min.

References

1. Saikawa, T., Nagamoto, Y.Y., and Arita, M.: Electrophysiologic effect of diltiazem, a new slow channel inhibitor, on canine cardiac fibers. Jpn. Heart J., *18*:235, 1977.
2. Nakajima, H., et al.: Effect of diltiazem on electrical and mechanical activity of isolated cardiac ventricular muscle of guinea pig. Jpn. J. Pharmacol., *25*:383, 1975.
3. Subramanian, V.B., et al.: Comparison of the antianginal efficacy of four calcium ion antagonists with propranolol. Am. J. Cardiol., *49*:929, 1982.
4. Wagniart, P., et al.: Increased exercise tolerance and reduced electrocardiographic ischemia with diltiazem in patients with stable angina pectoris. Circulation, *66*:23, 1982.
5. Vouhe, P.R., et al.: Myocardial protection through cold cardioplegia with potassium or diltiazem. Circulation, *65*:6, 1982.
6. Millard, R.W., et al.: Differential cardiovascular effects of calcium channel blocking agents: potential mechanisms. Am. J. Cardiol., *49*:499, 1982.
7. Hossack, K.F., et al.: Divergent effects of diltiazem in patients with exertional angina. Am. J. Cardiol., *49*:538, 1982.
8. Naito, M., et al.: Electropharmacology of diltiazem in a chronic canine myocardial infarction, ventricular tachyarrhythmia model. ACC 1983.

9. Kawai, C., et al: Effect of nifedipine on atrioventricular conduction: clinical and experimental studies. In Adalat. New Experimental and Clinical Results. Edited by P. Puech and R. Krebs. Amsterdam, Excerpta Medica, 1979, p. 5.
10. Smith, M.S., et al.: Pharmacokinetic and pharmacodynamic effect of diltiazem. Am. J. Cardiol., 51:1369, 1983.
11. Jauernig, R., et al.: Suppressive effect of diltiazem in AV junctional reentrant tachycardia. ACC 1983.
12. Low, R.I., et al.: The effects of calcium channel blocking agents on cardiovascular function. Am. J. Cardiol., 49:547, 1982.
13. Taeymans, Y., et al.: A prospective randomized study of propranolol versus diltiazem in patients with unstable angina. AHA, 1982.
14. Yeh, S.J., et al.: Effects of oral diltiazem in paroxysmal supraventricular tachycardia. Am. J. Cardiol., 52:271, 1983.
15. Mitchell, L.B., et al.: Intracardiac electrophysiologic study of intravenous diltiazem and combined diltiazem-digoxin in patients. Am. Heart J., 103:57, 1982.
16. Oyama, Y., et al.: The effects of diltiazem hydrochloride on the cardiac conduction: a clinical study of His bundle electrogram. Jpn. Circ. J., 42:1257, 1978.
17. Kawai, C., et al.: Comparative effects of three calcium antagonists: diltiazem, verapamil and nifedipine on the sinoatrial node. AHA, 1982.
18. Rozanski, J.J., Zaman, L., and Castellanos, A.: Electrophysiologic effects of diltiazem hydrochloride on supraventricular tachycardia. Am. J. Cardiol., 49:621, 1982.
19. Betriu, A., et al.: Acute success of intravenous diltiazem in paroxysmal supraventricular tachyarrhythmias. ACC, 1982.
20. Betriu, A., et al.: Beneficial effect of intravenous diltiazem in the acute management of paroxysmal supraventricular tachyarrhythmias. Circulation, 67:88, 1983.
21. Kober, G., et al.: Linksventrikulare Funktion and Hamodynamik bei intrakoronarer und intravenoser Gabe von Diltiazem. In Calciumantagonisten zur Behandlung der Angina Pectoris, Hypertonie und Arrhythmie. Edited by F. Bender and K. Greef. Amsterdam, Excerpta Medica, 1982, p. 87.
22. Yasue, H., et al.: Pathogenesis and treatment of angina pectoris at rest as seen from its response to various drugs. Jpn. Circ. J., 42:1, 1978.
23. Low, R.I., et al.: Effects of diltiazem-induced calcium blockade upon exercise capacity in effort angina due to chronic coronary artery disease. Am. Heart J., 101:713, 1981.
24. Hossack, K.F., et al.: Divergent effects of diltiazem in patients with exertional angina. Am. J. Cardiol., 49:538, 1982.
25. Kinoshita, M., et al.: The effect of diltiazem hydrochloride upon sodium diuresis and renal function in chronic congestive heart failure. Arzneimittelforsch. 29:676, 1979.
26. Walsh, R.A., et al.: Salutary hemodynamic effects of intravenous and oral diltiazem in severe congestive heart failure. Circulation, 66 (Suppl. II):II-138, 1982.
27. Nagao, M., et al.: Effect of diltiazem on left ventricular isovolumic relaxation time in patients with hypertrophic cardiomyopathy. Jpn. Circ. J., 47:54, 1983.
28. Suwa, M., et al.: Effects of diltiazem, nifedipine and propranolol on systolic and diastolic function in hypertrophic cardiomyopathy. AHA 1983.
29. Nagao, T., et al.: Effects of diltiazem, a calcium antagonist, on regional myocardial function and mitochondria after brief coronary occlusion. J. Mol. Cell. Cardiol., 12:29, 1980.
29a. Jackson, W.L. et al.: Comparative hemodynamic effects of verapamil and diltiazem in conscious puppies. AHA 1984.
30. Lenz, K., and Magometschnigg, D.: Die hypotensive Wirkung von intravenos verabreichtem Diltiazem. In Calciumantagonisten zur Behandlung der Angina Pectoris, Hypertonie und Arrhythmie. Edited by F. Bender and K. Greef. Amsterdam, Excerpta Medica, 1981, p. 194.
31. Yamakado, T., et al.: Effects of diltiazem on cardiovascular responses during exercise in systemic hypertension and comparison with propranolol. Am. J. Cardiol., 52:1023, 1983.
32. Maeda, K., et al.: Clinical study on the hypotensive effect of diltiazem hydrochloride. Int. J. Clin. Pharmacol. Ther. Toxicol., 19:47, 1981.

33. Brandt, D., and Klein, W.:Dosiswirkungsbeziehung von Diltiazem bei Patienten mit essentieller Hypertonie. *In* Calciumantagonisten zur Behandlung der Angina Pectoris, Hypertonie und Arrhythmie. Edited by F. Bender and K. Greef. Amsterdam, Excerpta Medica, 1981, p. 202.
34. Rosenthal, J.: Die Behandlung der hypertensiven Krise mit Diltiazem. *In* Calciumantagonisten zur Behandlung der Angina Pectoris, Hypertonie und Arrhythmie. Edited by F. Bender and K. Greef. Amsterdam, Excerpta Medica, 1981, p. 227.
35. Kambara, H., et al.: Primary pulmonary hypertension: Beneficial therapy with diltiazem. Am. Heart J., *101*:230, 1981.
36. Crevey, B.J., et al.: Hemodynamic and gas exchange effects of intravenous diltiazem in patients with pulmonary hypertension. Am. J. Cardiol., *49*:578, 1982.
37. Piepho, R.W., et al.: Pharmakokinetik von Diltiazem. *In* Calciumantagonisten zur Behandlung der Angina Pectoris, Hypertonie and Arrhythmie. Edited by F. Bender and K. Greef. Amsterdam, Excerpta Medica, 1982, p. 59.
38. Bighley, L.D., Dimmitt, D.C., and McGraw, B.F.: Bioavailability of diltiazem hydrochloride formulation. (Abstract.) Clin. Res., *28*:587, 1980.
39. Strauss, W.E., et al.: Safety and efficacy of diltiazem hydrochloride for the treatment of stable angina pectoris: report of a cooperative clinical trail. Am. J. Cardiol., *49*:560, 1982.
40. Zelis, R.F., and Kinney, E.L.: The pharmacokinetics of diltiazem in healthy American men. Am. J. Cardiol., *49*:529, 1982.

Section III
VASODILATORS

Vasodilators are agents that dilate vascular segments, whether arterial or venous or both. They form the largest and perhaps most important group of drugs used for treatment of vascular diseases. Vasodilators are used for the following disorders: (1) systemic arterial hypertension, in which vasodilators act directly on the main hemodynamic abnormality in hypertension, the elevated systemic vascular resistance; (2) congestive heart failure, in which vasodilators reduce left ventricular afterload, by lowering systemic vascular resistance that is elevated by compensatory mechanisms in congestive heart failure; vasodilators thereby interfere with the cycle of congestive heart failure consisting of cardiac damage, leading to impairment of peripheral blood supply, leading to elevation of systemic vascular resistance in attempt to maintain perfusion pressure, leading to increased afterload and to additional impairment of cardiac performance; vasodilators also reduce preload by dilating the venous vascular bed; (3) ischemic heart disease and its manifestation such as angina pectoris, in which vasodilators improve the myocardial oxygen supply-demand ratio, by increasing coronary supply (by coronary vasodilation) and by decreasing coronary demand (by afterload and preload reduction); (4) left-to-right shunt, in which vasodilators reduce the resistance to left ventricular outflow and thereby reduce the magnitude of the shunt; (5) pulmonary hypertension, in which vasodilators produce hemodynamic improvement in pulmonary hypertension, probably by a direct decrease of the elevated pulmonary vascular resistance; and (6) peripheral vascular disease, in which vasodilators increase peripheral blood flow. In pediatric cardiovascular medicine, vasodilators are used for almost all these indications.

The vasodilators may be divided into several large groups, according to their mechanism of action: First are the direct-acting vasodilators. This group includes arterial dilators such as hydralazine, venodilators such as nitroglycerin and organic nitrates, and balanced vasodilators, which act similarly on arterial and venous vascular beds, such as nitroprusside. The next group comprises alpha-adrenoreceptor blocking agents. Systemic vasoconstriction is mediated by postsynaptic alpha-adrenoreceptors. Blockade of these receptors results in vasodilation.

The classic alpha-adrenoreceptor blocking agents such as phentolamine are of little use in modern cardiovascular therapy. The agents of this group in clinical use include prazosin, trimazosin, indoramin, and others. Most of these agents are balanced vasodilators. Another group comprises angiotensin-converting enzyme inhibitors. These agents block the vasoconstricting effect of the renin-angiotensin system by inhibiting conversion of angiotensin I to the potent vasoconstrictor angiotensin II. Captopril is the most widely used angiotensin-converting enzyme inhibitor. The remaining group consists of calcium antagonists, which inhibit the constriction of smooth muscle cells of vascular walls and myocardial cells by inhibiting the entry of calcium into the cells. Calcium is an important mediator of contractility, and reduction in the availability of intracellular calcium decreases the constriction of smooth cells of vascular walls and thereby results in vasodilation. The most important calcium antagonists are nifedipine, verapamil, and diltiazem. These agents are balanced vasodilators.

DIRECT-ACTING VASODILATORS

Chapter 9

Hydralazine

Hydralazine was the first arterial dilator to be used clinically. It is a direct-acting relaxant of vascular smooth muscle that affects the arterial vascular bed almost exclusively. It has been used for more than 30 years in the treatment of systemic arterial hypertension. Recently the drug was shown to be effective also in the treatment of chronic congestive heart failure, by the mechanism of afterload reduction. The use of hydralazine in such patients is still controversial because of the problems associated with this drug in coronary artery disease and because of the potential for drug tolerance.

The experience in children is limited. Several hypertensive children have been treated with hydralazine in combination with other antihypertensive agents. Hydralazine may also be effective in young patients with primary pulmonary hypertension, but in patients with pulmonary vascular obstructive disease secondary to congenital heart disease, hydralazine may be deleterious.

Perhaps the most important indication for hydralazine in children is the presence of a large ventricular septal defect with left-to-right shunt. It was recently shown that reduction of systemic vascular resistance by hydralazine decreases the magnitude of such a shunt. It is yet to be shown whether this effect, achieved by the short-term intravenous administration of hydralazine, can be sustained during long-term oral treatment.

In a few children with myocardial disease and congestive heart failure that is not adequately controlled by digoxin and diuretics, hydralazine, added to conventional treatment, produced hemodynamic and clinical improvement. In one child, this improvement was sustained throughout prolonged oral treatment. In children, hydralazine causes side effects common to all vasodilators, as well as some specific side effects such as systemic lupus erythematosus and neonatal thrombocytopenia.

Structure

Hydralazine is 1-hydrazinophthalazine.

Pharmacologic Properties

Hydralazine dilates the arterial vascular bed by direct relaxation of arteriolar smooth muscle. The drug has a minimal dilatory effect on the venous vascular bed. The arterial dilation is most pronounced in the coronary, splanchnic, and cerebral arteries. The mechanism of this direct vasodilation is unknown, but it may be related to chelation of trace metals important for cellular contraction. Results of animal and human studies suggest that hydralazine has also a positive inotropic effect.[1-3] This action could be a direct effect on the myocardium, or it may be a result of sympathetic activation by vasodilation. In at least one experimental study, hydralazine had no positive inotropic effect in an isolated myocardial preparation.[4]

Hemodynamic Effects

The most important hemodynamic effect of hydralazine is arterial dilation. This effect reduces peripheral vascular resistance and arterial pressure. Hydralazine also has some dilatory effect on the pulmonary arteries. The systemic vasodilation causes sympathetic activation, which results in acceleration of heart rate and enhancement of myocardial contractility. If hydralazine actually has a direct positive inotropic effect as well, as suggested by several investigators, it would further contribute to the increase in contractility.

The increases in heart rate and contractility and the decrease in systemic vascular resistance raise cardiac output. Occasionally, elevated left ventricular filling pressure is reduced.

The hemodynamic changes in patients with congestive heart failure, hypertension, and ventricular septal defect are described in detail in the following sections.

Effects on Congestive Heart Failure

Like other vasodilators, hydralazine is effective in patients with congestive heart failure. Its mechanism of action is peripheral vasodilation causing reduction of afterload. It is possible that the positive inotropic effects of hydralazine also contribute to the hemodynamic improvement. Most studies of hydralazine have been conducted in adults with chronic congestive heart failure. The typical hemodynamic response of these patients to intravenous administration of hydralazine is a decrease in systemic vascular resistance and, often, also of pulmonary artery pressure and increases in cardiac output and stroke work index by 10 to 50%. The most pronounced effects are the decrease in systemic resistance and the increase in cardiac output. Therefore, hydralazine is especially effective in patients with congestive heart failure who mainly have low cardiac output and is less effective in patients with dyspnea.[5-9] The reason is that hydralazine primarily dilates the arterial vasculature.

Hydralazine usually increases heart rate in patients with congestive heart failure. In patients with a rapid heart rate, however, the hemodynamic improvement may even decrease the heart rate. Because of this acceleration of heart rate, hydralazine is not recommended in patients with acute-onset congestive heart failure resulting from coronary artery disease.

The experience with hydralazine in infants and children with congestive heart failure that is not associated with ventricular septal defect is limited. Fried and co-workers reported a 12-year-old child who developed congestive heart failure due to adriamycin-induced myocardial damage.[10] The heart failure was initially controlled with digoxin and later with a combination of digoxin and diuretic agents. When this combination did not prevent further deterioration, hydralazine, 0.32 mg/kg, was injected intravenously over 2 minutes, and hemodynamic evaluation was performed. The pulmonary arterial oxygen saturation rose from 32 to 74%. Systemic arteriovenous oxygen difference was also improved. The cardiac index increased by 150%, from 1.13 to 2.87 L/min/m^2. Both systemic and pulmonary vascular resistances were reduced, but the reduction was greater in the systemic circulation. Because of this sudden improvement, the child was treated with hydralazine, given orally 3 times daily at doses of 20, 10, and 20 mg. Marked clinical and symptomatic improvement was observed and was sustained for the 4 months of follow-up.[10] Although the possibility of spontaneous regression of adriamycin-induced cardiomyopathy cannot be excluded, it is unlikely in this case because of the rapid improvement after initiation of treatment.

A less-favorable response was observed in a 4-year-old child with a dilated form of primary endocardial fibroelastosis. This patient had congestive heart failure that was slowly progressive despite treatment with digoxin and diuretics. He had low cardiac output and elevated systemic vascular resistance and pulmonary capillary wedge pressure. The administration of hydralazine caused a slight increase in cardiac output, but it produced marked hypotension, and treatment could not be continued. It is possible that, in this disease, the myocardium cannot adequately respond to the stimulus of peripheral vasodilation.

An important problem is the development of tolerance in some patients with congestive heart failure during long-term treatment with hydralazine. Several investigators reported that hemodynamic improvement produced by hydralazine was sustained throughout several months of treatment.[11, 12] Packer and colleagues reported, however, that tolerance to the hemodynamic effect of hydralazine developed in 11 patients with chronic congestive heart failure.[13] Hydralazine produced an initial hemodynamic and symptomatic improvement in these patients, but during continued treatment with the same doses, hemodynamic parameters and symptoms returned to pretreatment levels. Discontinuance of the drug did not produce deterioration of the patient's clinical status, and the initial response could not be restored, even by doses twice those used initially. The mechanism of this tolerance was not related to fluid retention, although such retention occurred in some patients. Because other vasodilators were effective in these patients, the tolerance appeared to be specific to hydralazine.[13] The mechanism of this tolerance is not known, but its site is most probably the receptor that interacts with hydralazine. The incidence of tolerance to hydralazine is yet to be confirmed.

Several attempts have been made to predict the long-term response to hydralazine by various parameters. Patients with severe hemodynamic impairment, and especially higher pulmonary capillary wedge pressure and right atrial pressure, are less likely to respond to the drug than those with mild or moderate impairment.[8,14] The pretreatment systemic vascular resistance is an important predictor of response; patients with higher systemic vascular resistance respond better to hydralazine.[15] This parameter is especially important in children with ventricular septal defect, large left-to-right shunt, and congestive heart failure, in whom the response to hydralazine closely correlates with the pretreatment levels of systemic vascular resistance.[16] Several other parameters, such as left ventricular dimensions, have been suggested. They are of little relevance in children, however. Only a limited correlation exists between the acute hemodynamic effect of hydralazine and the improvement in exercise tolerance.

Some investigators have suggested that only patients without progressive heart failure before initiation of treatment with hydralazine respond favorably to the drug.[14] Such was not the case, however, in the child reported by Fried and associates, who responded favorably despite progression of congestive heart failure before initiation of treatment.[10] Another problem is that not all patients with congestive heart failure respond to hydralazine. In several series, about one-third of the patients did not respond. This failure to respond is another reason that hemodynamic evaluation before treatment and short-term drug testing are required.

Whether prolonged treatment with hydralazine causes fluid and sodium retention is controversial, but several such cases have been reported.[12,13] Hydralazine increases renal blood flow and glomerular filtration rate in patients with congestive heart failure.[17,18] Excessive reduction of arterial pressure may impair renal function, however.

In summary, hydralazine produces hemodynamic and clinical improvement in many patients with congestive heart failure due to myocardial or coronary arterial disease. This improvement is usually sustained for long periods, but tolerance occasionally develops. Although the experience in children is limited, the drug appears to be promising, especially in patients with elevated systemic vascular resistance and symptoms of low cardiac output.

Hydralazine can be combined with other agents, such as digitalis and diuretics, to enhance their effect in congestive heart failure. The combination of hydralazine and nitrates produces a greater effect than either drug alone;[19] hydralazine dilates mainly the arterioles, whereas nitrates are potent venodilators. In patients with symptoms of low cardiac output, such as fatigue, and elevated left ventricular end-diastolic pressure, such as dyspnea, this combined therapy may be particularly effective.

Effects on Ventricular Septal Defect

Hydralazine was evaluated by several investigators in patients with ventricular septal defect. The rationale for this treatment is that reduction of systemic peripheral vascular resistance reduces left ventricular afterload, and if this effect occurs without a comparable reduction in pulmonary vascular resistance, the left-to-right shunt across the ventricular septal defect will decrease. Because hydralazine is a selective systemic arterial dilator, it may be superior to some other vasodilators in patients with this condition. This theory has been confirmed by animal studies showing that the magnitude of a left-to-right shunt across a ventricular septal defect is responsive to changes in systemic resistance.[20-22] Moreover, vasodilators that also produce venodilation and reduce preload may be deleterious in this condition. For example, Beekman and co-workers reported that the administration of nitroprusside, a balanced vasodilator, was associated with hemodynamic deterioration in infants with a large ventricular septal defect.[23] Therefore, hydralazine is a reasonable therapeutic choice in management of ventricular septal defect in patients with a large left-to-right shunt.

Despite the potential benefit, one of the first studies of hydralazine showed no improvement after administration of the drug to 5 children with large left-to-right shunts.[24] This group included children with shunts at various levels, however. In another study, hydralazine even increased the tendency to right-to-left shunting in patients with septal defects and pulmonary hypertension.[25] Better results were obtained in several more recent studies, which demonstrated acute hemodynamic improvement after intravenous administration of hydralazine. All these studies have been reported within the last 3 years.

In 1982, Beekman and colleagues reported a study of the effect of intravenous hydralazine, 0.2 mg/kg, in infants with a large ventricular septal defect.[26] The infants were 2.5 to 11 months old (mean 5.1 months). One of them had also a patent ductus arteriosus, and 5 had congestive heart failure. Hemodynamic measurements were made before and 5, 15, 25, and 35 min after hydralazine administration, and the hemodynamic changes were most pronounced at 35 min. Systemic blood flow increased from 4.5 ± 0.2 to 6.7 ± −0.5 L/min/m^2, whereas pulmonary blood flow was not altered. The pulmonary-to-systemic blood flow decreased by 32% from 3.4 ± 0.4 to 2.3 ± 0.2 L/min/m^2, and the absolute left-to-right shunt decreased by 24% from 10.8 ± 1.3 to 8.2 ± 1.2 L/min/m^2. Systemic vascular resistance decreased by about 25%, whereas pulmonary vascular resistance, aortic, pulmonary arterial and pulmonary capillary wedge pressures, heart rate, and oxygen consumption were not altered. Right atrial pressure decreased from 4.0 ± 0.6 to 2.4 ± 0.6 mm Hg. This finding was unexpected because hydralazine has a minimal venodilatory effect, if any. It may be secondary to afterload reduction. These authors concluded that, in infants with a large ventricular septal defect, hydralazine reduces the magnitude of the shunt, in relation to the decrease in systemic vascular resistance. This effect of short-term administration of hydralazine suggests that the drug may have also a long-term beneficial effect in infants and children with a large ventricular septal defect.

Nakazawa and associates studied the effect of hydralazine in 7 children[27] and, in a later study, in 17 infants and young children with a large ventricular septal defect.[16] Fourteen of the patients had isolated ventricular septal defect, 2 had also a patent ductus arteriosus, and 1 patient had a double-outlet right ventricle. These children ranged in age from 2 to 36 months, and 11 were less than a year old. The patients were divided into 2 groups. Group 1 comprised 14 patients with peak pulmonary arterial pressure greater than 75% of systemic pressure. This group was subdivided into group 1a, consisting of 6 patients with systemic vascular resistance of 20 u/m^2 or higher, and group 1b, which has 8 patients with a lower systemic vascular resistance. Group 2 comprised 3 patients with pulmonary arterial pressure lower than 75% of systemic pressure.

Intravenous administration of hydralazine, 0.3 mg/kg, reduced systemic vascular resistance in 15 of these 17 patients. The extent of reduction was related to the pretreatment level of systemic vascular resistance. The drug increased systemic blood flow from 3.7 ± 0.7 to 5.0 ± 0.8 L/min/m^2 and did not alter pulmonary blood flow. The ratio of pulmonary-to-systemic blood flow decreased from 3.6 ± 0.4 to 2.4 ± 0.2 L/min/m^2 in group 1a and increased from 2.6 ± 0.3 to 3.3 ± 0.5 L/min/m^2 in group 1b. The mean systemic arterial pressure for the 17 patients decreased from 69 ± 2 to 65 ± 2 mm Hg. The mean pulmonary arterial pressure decreased by 9 ± 4% in group 1 and by 17 ± 1% in group 2. The ratio between pulmonary and systemic blood flow after administration of hydralazine inversely correlated with pretreatment systemic vascular resistance in group 1 (r = −0.61, p = 0.2). Group 2 patients were excluded from this analysis.

Nakazawa and colleagues concluded that hydralazine can produce hemodynamic improvement evident by decrease in magnitude of shunting in some infants and young children with large ventricular septal defects.[16] The drug is especially beneficial in patients with high pretreatment systemic vascular resistance. This parameter may, therefore, be used to predict the response to hydralazine.

Thus, it appears that the ideal candidates for hydralazine are infants and children with a large ventricular septal defect, large left-to-right shunt, and high systemic vascular resistance. In patients with ventricular septal defect, pulmonary hypertension, elevated pulmonary vascular resistance, and normal or only slightly elevated systemic vascular resistance, hydralazine may reduce pulmonary vascular resistance more than systemic vascular resistance and may increase the left-to-right shunt, thereby causing hemodynamic deterioration.

In some patients, hydralazine does not reduce elevated pulmonary vascular resistance. For example, Fripp and co-workers reported that in two patients with pulmonary vascular obstructive disease secondary to congenital heart disease, hydralazine failed to lower the pulmonary vascular resistance.[28]

In summary, hydralazine can produce sudden hemodynamic improvement in patients with large ventricular septal defect, left-to-right shunt, and elevated systemic vascular resistance. The drug may be deleterious in patients with normal systemic resistance. Therefore, it is preferable to perform hemodynamic studies before initiation of treatment with hydralazine. It is unclear whether the beneficial effect is sustained during prolonged treatment.

Effects on Aortic Stenosis

Hydralazine may be effective in patients with valvar aortic stenosis, even though the site of maximal left ventricular afterload in these patients is the aortic valve and not peripheral arterioles. In a group of patients with mild aortic stenosis, hydralazine increased cardiac index by 50% and stroke volume index by 38%; it reduced systemic vascular resistance.[29] Hemodynamic improvement was also observed in several patients with moderate aortic stenosis and congestive heart failure.[30] Hydralazine should be avoided in patients with severe aortic stenosis.

Effects on Aortic Insufficiency

Afterload reduction can produce hemodynamic improvement in patients with aortic insufficiency. In a group of patients with severe aortic insufficiency and congestive heart failure, hydralazine, 0.3 mg/kg intravenously, reduced systemic vascular resistance by 44% and left ventricular end-diastolic pressure by 57% and it increased the forward cardiac index, stroke volume index, and ejection fraction.[31]

Effects on Mitral Insufficiency

Hydralazine produced sudden hemodynamic improvement in a group of patients with mitral insufficiency. This short-term effect was sustained for long periods in half the patients.[31, 32]

Effects on Pulmonary Vascular Diseases

Hydralazine dilates arterioles in the systemic and the pulmonary circulation. Several investigators have suggested that hydralazine effectively produces hemodynamic improvement, including reductions in pulmonary arterial resistance and pressure in adults with pulmonary hypertension and cor pulmonale of various causes. These findings in adults are controversial, however. In children, the limited experience indicates that hydralazine is of value only in increasing cardiac output; the drug does not reduce, and occasionally also increases, the pulmonary arterial pressure and resistance.

In 4 patients with primary pulmonary hypertension, hydralazine, 200 mg daily, reduced pulmonary vascular resistance from 17.5 to 7.7 U at rest and from 15.7 to 10.2 U during exercise. The drug did not alter pulmonary and systemic arterial pressures, and it increased cardiac output from 3.8 to 7.1 L/min/m^2 at rest and from 4.7 to 7.0 L/min/m^2 during exercise. This effect was observed after 2 days of treatment and was sustained for a follow-up period of up to 6 months.[33] In another 6 patients with primary pulmonary hypertension, hydralazine increased cardiac output and decreased the pulmonary and systemic vascular resistances.[34]

In contrast, McGoon and associates reported only an increase in cardiac output, without a decrease in pulmonary arterial pressure or resistance in patients with various pulmonary diseases and pulmonary hypertension (11 patients with primary pulmonary hypertension, 10 patients with parenchymal lung disease, and 6 patients with pulmonary emboli).[25]

In four children with intracardiac shunts, pulmonary hypertension, and elevated pulmonary vascular resistance, hydralazine did not alter cardiac output and pulmonary and systemic vascular resistance.[25] The decrease in systemic resistance was greater than that in pulmonary resistance, however, thereby promoting right-to-left shunting.[25]

Fripp and colleagues studied 2 children, a 3-year-old girl with D-transposition of the great arteries and patent ductus arteriosus, and a 6-year-old boy with patent ductus arteriosus.[28] The lesions were surgically corrected, and postoperative assessment revealed no residual shunting. The patients had pulmonary vascular obstructive disease secondary to the congenital cardiac anomaly. In both patients, the elevated pulmonary vascular resistance failed to decrease after administration of hydralazine; however, systemic vascular resistance decreased, cardiac output increased, and therefore the pulmonary arterial pressure was raised.

I recommend that hydralazine not be used at all, or only with great caution, in patients with pulmonary vascular disease secondary to congenital cardiac lesions. The drug is probably more effective and is safer in patients with primary pulmonary hypertension.

An important problem encountered with nitroprusside is vasodilation in areas of the lung that have poor ventilation. The ventilation-perfusion ratio and blood oxygenation are thereby impaired. With hydralazine, no change in arterial blood oxygenation has been observed in patients with pulmonary hypertension. Hemodynamic studies performed after the short-term administration of hydralazine in patients with pulmonary hypertension do not predict the long-term response to treatment.

Postoperative Use

Hydralazine is given intravenously to reduce elevated systemic vascular resistance early after cardiac operations.

Effects on Systemic Hypertension

Theoretically, hydralazine is an ideal antihypertensive agent because it lowers blood pressure by reducing elevated peripheral vascular resistance and thus acts directly on the major hemodynamic abnormality in hypertension. The effect of hydralazine when given alone, however, is limited by compensatory mechanisms such as sympathetic activation, acceleration of heart rate, enhancement of myocardial contractility, and fluid retention. Accumulation of fluid results from a direct renal effect or from activation of the renin-angiotensin system and can be controlled by the addition of a diuretic agent.

Hydralazine was introduced to the treatment of hypertension about 30 years ago. It is considered to be a third-line antihypertensive agent and is preferably used in combination with a diuretic agent and a beta-adrenoreceptor blocking drug. It can be used intravenously during hypertensive crises or orally for long-term therapy. Hydralazine may also be administered for diagnosis of renovascular hypertension because it increases the release of renin from the kidney with vascular disease more than from the contralateral kidney.

The experience with hydralazine in infants and children with hypertension is limited. It is effective mainly in older children. Plumer and colleagues studied the effects of various forms of treatment, including hydralazine, in 10 infants with systemic hypertension complicating umbilical arterial catheterization or renal artery stenosis.[35] The response to antihypertensive medication was generally poor. Five of the patients died. These investigators recommended prompt diagnostic evaluation and consideration of nephrectomy if the renal artery is occluded.

Comparison with Nitroprusside

Nitroprusside is the vasodilator most widely used in cardiovascular diseases in children. It differs from hydralazine in its balanced vasodilator effect (dilation of both arteries and veins); hydralazine is a selective arterial dilator. In addition to the hemodynamic effects resulting from this difference, hydralazine increases cardiac output to a greater extent than nitroprusside in patients with elevated pulmonary vascular resistance.[36]

Clinical Pharmacology

Hydralazine may be administered intravenously or orally. It is rapidly and almost completely absorbed from the gastrointestinal tract after oral administration. Maximal plasma levels may be reached within 1 to 3 hours of oral administration.[37, 38] These data are derived from studies in hypertensive patients. In patients with congestive heart failure, the magnitude and rate of absorption may be reduced. The systemic bioavailability of hydralazine is only 10 to 40% because the drug undergoes extensive first-pass hepatic metabolism. The systemic bioavailability is lower in fast acetylators, in whom the drug undergoes a more extensive metabolism, and is higher in slow acetylators.[38, 39] At high doses, the metabolic pathways are saturated, and bioavailability is higher. Bioavailability is also increased by concomitant administration of food.[37] Hydralazine is widely distributed in the body and concentrates mainly in arteries, kidneys, and liver. A difference in volume of distribution between younger and older hypertensive patients has been observed.[39–42] The plasma concentration of hydralazine correlates with its antihypertensive effect.

The onset of the antihypertensive effect of hydralazine is delayed by 15 min after intravenous administration. Hydralazine is bound by

85% to serum proteins. It is eliminated by hepatic metabolism and excretion in the urine of the metabolites, as well as a small amount of the unchanged drug. The elimination half-life is 3 to 4 hours.[39, 41]

Side Effects

Hydralazine produces side effects common to most vasodilators, as well as some specific side effects. In 20 to 30% of adults treated with hydralazine, the drug is discontinued because of adverse effects.

Cardiovascular Effects

Hydralazine usually accelerates heart rate, especially in patients with hypertension. This effect is mainly due to sympathetic activation by peripheral vasodilation. Marked tachycardia may require discontinuance of treatment or addition of a beta-adrenoreceptor blocking agent. Orthostatic hypertension may occur, particularly in patients with congestive heart failure. In infants and children with ventricular septal defect or congestive heart failure the heart rate is not much altered by intravenous hydralazine.[26]

Systemic Lupus Erythematosus

A hydralazine-induced syndrome resembling systemic lupus erythematosus develops in 3% of adult patients treated with 200 mg daily and in up to 20% of those receiving 400 mg or more daily.[43-46] Hydralazine is the second most common cause, after procainamide, of drug-induced systemic lupus erythematosus. Patients who do not develop symptoms and clinical signs may have serologic evidence of the disease, including antibodies to RNA, single-stranded DNA, and histones. These patients may develop severe anemia.[47] The symptoms and signs of systemic lupus erythematosus are reversed after discontinuance of the drug. This adverse reaction is more common in slow acetylators than in other patients.

Thrombocytopenia

Isolated thrombocytopenia associated with hydralazine treatment is a rare complication. Only a few cases have been reported in adults.[48, 49] A report of three cases of hydralazine-induced neonatal thrombocytopenia with an increased tendency for bleeding has been published by the Swedish Adverse Drug Reaction Committee.[50] The mothers of these patients had been treated with hydralazine for several months before delivery. The neonatal thrombocytopenia was transient, with complete recovery within a few weeks. No adverse reactions, including thrombocytopenia, were observed in the mothers.[50]

Agranulocytosis

Agranulocytosis is a serious, though rare, side effect of hydralazine.

Headache, Flushing, and Palpitations

These side effects occur frequently, especially during initiation of treatment. They result from the vasodilatory effect of hydralazine.

Other Effects

Peripheral neuropathy, drug fever, obstructive jaundice and hepatitis are rare complications of hydralazine therapy. Mild gastrointestinal disturbances are common. Anxiety, conjunctivitis, lacrimation, and nasal congestion may occur. Changes in arterial walls have been noted in animal studies. This effect is probably responsible for the increased mortality rate from aortic rupture in turkeys treated with hydralazine.[51]

Effects During Pregnancy and Lactation

Hydralazine crosses the placenta and is excreted in breast milk.[52] It may cause side effects in the neonate even in the absence of such effects in the mother.[50]

Interaction with Propranolol

Hydralazine has been used together with propranolol in several hypertensive children. In normal volunteers, hydralazine has doubled peak plasma concentration of propranolol, probably because of reduction of hepatic blood flow and hepatic clearance of propranolol.[53]

Dosage and Administration

Intravenous Administration

Doses of 0.2 to 0.3 mg/kg, injected over about a minute, have been used for short-term drug testing in infants and children.

Oral Administration

No recommended dosage regimen for oral administration of hydralazine in infants and children has been established. Adults should receive 100 to 400 mg daily, in 3 to 4 divided doses. Doses prescribed for patients with congestive heart failure are higher than for patients with hypertension. I suggest that for older children, doses of 50 to 75 mg daily be used. In smaller children and in infants, doses should be smaller and proportional to age.

References

1. Khatri, I., et al.: Direct and reflex cardiostimulatory effects of hydralazine. Am. J. Cardiol., *40*:38, 1977.

2. Leier, C.V. et al.: Positive inotropic effects of hydralazine in human subjects: comparison with prazosin in the setting of congestive heart failure. Am. J. Cardiol., 46:1039, 1980.
3. Rabinowitz, B., et al.: Effects of hydralazine on the adenylcyclase system of canine ventricular myocardium: evidence of an adrenergic mechanism. ACC 1982.
4. Chatterjee, K., and Rouleau, J.K.: Hemodynamic and metabolic effects of vasodilators, nitrates, hydralazine, prazosin and captopril in chronic ischemic heart failure. Acta Med. Scand., 210 (Suppl. 651):295, 1981.
5. Franciosa, J.A., Pierpont, G., and Cohn, J.N.: Hemodynamic improvement after oral hydralazine in left ventricular failure. Ann. Intern. Med., 86:388, 1977.
6. Stunkard, A., Wertheimer, L., and Redisch, W.: Studies on hydralazine: evidence for a peripheral site of action. J. Clin. Invest., 33:1047, 1954.
7. Rowe, G.G., et al.: Hemodynamic effects of 1-hydrazinophthalazine in patients with arterial hypertension. J. Clin. Invest., 34:115, 1955.
8. Walsh, W.F., and Greenberg, B.H.: Results of long-term vasodilator therapy in patients with refractory congestive heart failure. Circulation, 64:3, 1981.
9. Ablad, B.: A study of the mechanism of the hemodynamic effects of hydralazine in man. Acta Pharmacol. Toxicol., 20(Suppl. 1):53, 1963.
10. Fried, R., et al.: Use of hydralazine for intractable cardiac failure. J. Pediatr. 97:1009, 1980.
11. Unverferth, D.V., et al.: Regression of myocardial cellular hypertrophy with vasodilator therapy in chronic congestive heart failure associated with idiopathic dilated cardiomyopathy. Am. J. Cardiol., 51:1392, 1983.
12. Massie, B.M., Kramer, B., and Haughom, F.: Acute and long-term effects of vasodilator therapy on resting and exercise hemodynamics and exercise tolerance. Circulation, 64:6, 1981.
13. Packer, M., et al.: Hemodynamic characterization of tolerance to long-term hydralazine therapy in severe chronic heart failure. N. Engl. J. Med., 306:2, 1982.
14. Massie, B., et al.: Long-term vasodilator therapy for heart failure: clinical response and its relationship to hemodynamic measurements. Circulation, 63:2, 1981.
15. Wilson, J.R., et al.: Determinants of circulatory response to intravenous hydralazine in congestive heart failure. Am. J. Cardiol. 52:299, 1983.
16. Nakazawa, M., et al.: Significance of systemic vascular resistance in determining the hemodynamic effects of hydralazine on large ventricular septal defects. Circulation, 68:420, 1983.
17. LeJemtel, T., et al.: Hemodynamic and renal response to oral hydralazine therapy in severe heart failure. (Abstract.) Circulation, 45 (Suppl. III): III-9, 1979.
18. Cogan, J.J., et al.: Renal effects of nitroprusside and hydralazine in patients with congestive heart failure. Circulation, 61:316, 1980.
19. Massie, B., et al.: Hemodynamic advantage of combined administration of hydralazine orally and nitrates nonparenterally in the vasodilator therapy of chronic heart failure. Am. J. Cardiol., 40:794, 1979.
20. Synhorst, D.P., et al.: Hemodynamic effects of vasodilator agents in dogs with experimental VSD. Circulation, 54:472, 1976.
21. Tanenbaum, H., and Pfaff, W.: Effect of pressor amines on experimental intracardiac shunts and valvular regurgitation. Dis. Chest, 44:485, 1963.
22. Boucek, M.M., et al.: Effects of pranzosin and hydralazine on the hemodynamics of chronically instrumented lambs with ventricular septal defect (Abstract). Circulation, 62(Suppl III): III-115, 1980.
23. Beekman, R.H., et al.: Hemodynamic effects of nitroprusside in infants with a large ventricular septal defect. Circulation, 64:553, 1981.
24. Linday, L.A., et al.: Effect of vasodilators on left-to-right shunts in infants and children. Pediatr. Res., 14:447, 1980.
25. McGoon, M.D., et al.: Hemodynamic response to intravenous hydralazine in pulmonary hypertension patients. AHA 1982.
26. Beekman, R.H., et al.: Hemodynamic effects of hydralazine in infants with a large ventricular septal defect. Circulation, 65(3):523, 1982.

27. Nakazawa, M., et al.: Afterload reduction treatment for large ventricular septal defects. Dependence of haemodynamic effects of hydralazine on pretreatment systemic blood flow. Br. Heart J., 49:461, 1983.
28. Fripp, R.R., et al.: Oral hydralazine in patients with pulmonary vascular disease secondary to congenital heart disease. Am. J. Cardiol., 48:380, 1981.
29. Greenberg, B.H., and Massie, B.M.: Beneficial effects of afterload. Reduction therapy in patients with congestive heart failure and moderate aortic stenosis. Circulation, 61:6, 1980.
30. Massie, B., et al.: Hemodynamic and clinical responses to combined captopril-hydralazine therapy (Abstract). Circulation, 66(Suppl. II):210, 1982.
31. Greenberg, B.H., et al.: Beneficial effects of hydralazine on rest and exercise hemodynamics in patients with chronic severe aortic insufficiency. Circulation, 62:1,1980.
32. Greenberg, B.H., et al.: Arterial dilators in mitral regurgitation: effects on rest and exercise hemodynamics and long-term clinical follow-up. Circulation, 65:1, 1982.
33. Rubin, L.J., and Peter, R.H.: Oral hydralazine therapy for primary pulmonary hypertension. N. Engl. J. Med., 302:69, 1980.
34. Lupi-Herrera, E., et al.: The role of hydralazine therapy for pulmonary arterial hypertension of unknown cause. Circulation, 65:4, 1982.
35. Plumer, L.B., et al.: Hypertension in infants—a complication of umbilical arterial catheterization. J. Pediatr. 89:802, 1976.
36. Lee, K.Y., et al.: Effects of hydralazine and nitroprusside on cardiopulmonary function when a decrease in cardiac output complicates a short-term increase in pulmonary vascular resistance. Circulation, 68:299, 1983.
37. Melander, A., et al.: Enhancement of hydralazine bioavailability by food. Clin. Pharmacol., Ther., 22:104, 1977.
38. Shepherd, A.M.M., et al.: Hydralazine kinetics after single and repeated oral doses. Clin. Pharmacol. Ther., 28:804, 1980.
39. Reece, P.A. Gozamanis, I., and Zacest R.: Kinetics of hydralazine and its main metabolites in slow and fast acetylators. Clin. Pharmacol. Ther., 28:769, 1980.
40. Talseth, T.: Studies on hydralazine. III. Bioavailability of hydralazine in man. Eur. J. Clin. Pharmacol., 10:395, 1976.
41. Ludden, T.M., et al.: Hydralazine kinetics in hypertensive patients after intravenous administration. Clin. Pharmacol. Ther. 28:737, 1980.
42. Shen, D.D., et al.: Pharmacokinetics of hydralazine and its acid labile hydrazone metabolites in relation to acetylator phenotype. J. Pharmacokinet. Biopharm., 8:53, 1980.
43. Lunde, P.K.M., Frislid, K., and Hansteen, V.: Disease and acetylation polymorphism. Clin. Pharmacokinet., 2:182, 1977.
44. Perry, H.M., Jr., Sakamoto, A. and Tan, E.M.: Relationship of acetylating enzyme to hydralazine toxicity. J. Lab. Clin. Med., 70:1020, 1967.
45. Bing, R.F., et al.: Hydralazine in hypertension: is there a safe dose? Br. Med. J., 3:353, 1980.
46. Dustan, H.P., et al.: Rheumatic and febrile syndrome during prolonged hydralazine therapy. JAMA, 154:23, 1954.
47. Macleod, W.N.: Hydralazine. Scott. Med. J., 28:121, 1983.
48. Swedish Adverse Drug Reaction Committee: Notice No. 32, August 1980.
49. Böttiger, L.E.: Thrombocytopenia. II. Drug-induced thrombocytopenia. Acta Med. Scand., 191:541, 1972.
50. Widerlöv, E., et al.: Hydralazine-induced neonatal thrombocytopenia. N. Engl. J. Med.,303:1235, 1980.
51. Simpson, C.F., and Taylor, W.J.: Effect of hydralazine on aortic rupture induced by β-Aminopropionitrile in turkeys. Circulation, 65:4, 1982.
52. Liedholm, H., et al.: Transplacental passage and breast milk concentrations of hydralazine. Eur. J. Clin. Pharmacol., 21:417, 1982.
53. McLean, A.J., et al.: Interaction between oral propranolol and hydralazine. Clin. Pharmacol. Ther., 27:726, 1980.

Chapter 10

Nitroprusside

Nitroprusside, available as sodium nitroprusside, is a potent direct-acting vasodilator. It is a balanced vasodilator that affects the arterial and venous vascular beds similarly. In adults, the drug is used for treatment of congestive heart failure and hypertensive emergencies and in attempts to limit infarct size. The main indication for nitroprusside in pediatric cardiovascular therapy is in severe hypertension and hypertensive emergencies. This drug has the advantage of quick action, beginning several minutes from the initiation of the intravenous infusion. It is used also for short-term treatment of severe congestive heart failure.

Three factors limit the use of nitroprusside. First, the drug is not effective orally. Second, it has a potent hypotensive effect and consequently requires careful monitoring. Third, prolonged infusion may result in thiocyanate toxicity. This pharmacologic profile has determined the clinical use of nitroprusside. It is a drug of first choice for treatment of acute episodes of severe hypertension or peripheral vasoconstriction in children, but the duration of treatment should be as short as possible. At present, I do not think that nitroprusside should be given to children with ventricular septal defect.

Pharmacologic Properties

Nitroprusside is a direct-acting relaxant of smooth muscle, with high selectivity for vascular walls. Its mechanism of action at the cellular level is unknown. Nitroprusside also inhibits platelet aggregation,[1,2] an effect that may contribute to the therapeutic benefit of the drug.

Hemodynamic Effects

Nitroprusside is one of the most extensively studied vasodilators. Studies of this drug have played a major role in our understanding of the hemodynamic effects of vasodilators in normal subjects and in patients with hypertension or congestive heart failure. Although most of these studies were either animal experiments or hemodynamic studies in adults, they should be mentioned here to characterize the hemodynamic profile of the drug.

Effects in Patients without Congestive Heart Failure

In the absence of congestive heart failure, nitroprusside reduced peripheral vascular resistance to a similar extent in the arterial and venous beds, both in animal experiments and in studies of human patients. The vasodilation in the arterial bed reduces peripheral vascular resistance. Venodilation and dilation of the pulmonary vasculature reduce the left ventricular filling pressure. The reduction of this parameter is smaller than that observed in patients with congestive heart failure, who have an elevated left ventricular filling pressure.[3-9] Despite the arterial vasodilation, cardiac output is not increased or is even slightly decreased by peripheral venodilation, which limits heart rate by a reflex mechanism activated by peripheral vasodilation and mediated by the sympathetic nervous system. It lowers systemic arterial pressure in normotensive and hypertensive patients because of the reduction in peripheral resistance not associated with an increase in cardiac output.

Nitroprusside has no effect on myocardial contractility.[4] In this aspect, it is superior to several modern vasodilators, such as calcium antagonists, which have a negative inotropic effect.

Effects in Patients with Congestive Heart Failure

The hemodynamic effects of nitroprusside in patients with congestive heart failure result from the peripheral, balanced, vasodilatory action of this drug. These effects resemble those seen in patients without congestive heart failure; systemic vascular resistance is reduced by up to 50%, left ventricular filling pressure is reduced by up to 40%, and heart rate is not much altered, or it may be either slightly increased by reflex sympathetic activation or slightly reduced by general hemodynamic improvement. Unlike in patients without congestive heart failure, however, nitroprusside increases cardiac output by up to 60% in patients with congestive heart failure, largely because of an increase in stroke volume.[3, 10-12]

The favorable response is not uniform. About one-third of adult patients fail to show even a transient improvement. Obviously, patients with high peripheral vascular resistance and pulmonary capillary wedge pressure benefit maximally from nitroprusside.[10, 13]

The experience with nitroprusside is also extensive in pediatric patients with congestive heart failure. For example, Dillon and associates reported that nitroprusside produced marked improvement in 6 patients, aged 6 months to 28 years, with severe congestive heart failure.[14]

Because nitroprusside is a balanced vasodilator, its venodilatory effect can limit the benefit of the arteriolodilatory effect and may even cause hemodynamic deterioration. This phenomenon is especially evident in patients with low cardiac output who do not have a significant elevation of left ventricular filling pressure. Excessive reduction of this pressure by the drug may reduce cardiac output and may cause hemodynamic deterioration.

Pediatric Effects. The hemodynamic improvement induced by nitroprusside in adults with congestive heart failure has also been observed in children. For example, Beekman and co-workers evaluated the effect of a continuous infusion of nitroprusside, 2.0 µg/kg/min, in 7 children, aged 0.2 to 14.5 years, with severe left ventricular dysfunction or mitral regurgitation.[15] The drug increased cardiac index by an average of 33% and increased stroke index by 29%; pulmonary arterial wedge pressure decreased by 28%. A significant decrease of systemic vascular resistance was also observed. This early improvement was evident as symptomatic improvement in congestive heart failure when nitroprusside was replaced by oral vasodilators.[15] These findings confirm the results of studies in adults; nitroprusside, by its balanced peripheral vasodilatory effect, produces a hemodynamic improvement, including enhancement of cardiac function.

Lukes and colleagues studied a 16-year-old boy with congestive heart failure. His mean arterial pressure was 95 mm Hg, and nitroprusside reduced it to 70 mm Hg.[10] Left ventricular filling pressure was reduced from 35 to 23 mm Hg; cardiac output increased from 2.1 to 3.5 L/min. Systemic vascular resistance was reduced by about 50%. Stroke work index was increased to a significant degree.

Thus, it appears that nitroprusside may produce at least a transient hemodynamic improvement in children with congestive heart failure. This treatment has not become popular, however, because it is not commonly used in infants and children with this disorder.

Regional Effects

The effect of nitroprusside is not uniform for all vascular beds in the body. Nitroprusside dilates normal and stenotic coronary arteries.[16, 17] This effect is especially prominent in small coronary arteries, although the drug may also dilate large coronary arteries.[18] Nitroprusside, administered systemically, however, has reduced coronary blood flow despite its direct coronary dilatory effect.[19-21] Because this reduction was associated with generalized preload and afterload reduction, it was attributable to a reduction in myocardial oxygen consumption.

Controversial findings were obtained from studies evaluating the effect of nitroprusside on renal hemodynamics. Cogan and associates reported that nitroprusside increased renal blood flow by 33% and did not alter the glomerular filtration rate in patients with congestive heart failure.[22] In contrast, Leier and co-workers, studying another group of patients with congestive heart failure, reported that nitroprusside did not alter renal blood flow despite a decrease in renal vascular resistance because of decreases in systemic arterial pressure and in renal perfusion pressure.[23] These investigators also reported that nitroprusside produced vasodilation in the limb and increased limb blood flow in patients with congestive heart failure.[23]

Effects in Arterial Hypertension in Children

In the past 15 years, intravenous administration of nitroprusside has become conventional therapy for immediate control of severe hypertension and hypertensive emergencies in infants and children. The first report of the efficacy of this drug in hypertension in children and adolescents was published in 1969.[24] Six years later, a large-scale study of the efficacy of nitroprusside in 20 children with hypertensive crises of renal origin was published.[25] The patients were 7 to 17 years of age; 13 of them were boys. All had diastolic blood pressures above 110 mm Hg. Nitroprusside was infused at a rate of 14 μg/kg/min. Control of blood pressure was achieved in all patients within 1 to 20 minutes from initiation of treatment. All patients showed rapid improvement of signs of heart failure. Neurologic signs of distress disappeared in 16 of the 20 children within 24 to 48 hours of treatment. In the majority of these patients, the intravenous treatment was discontinued and was replaced by oral therapy. One patient showed no improvement and died of cerebral hemorrhage. With this short-term therapy, no undesirable effects were observed.[25]

Since these reports were published, many centers, including my own, have gained experience in the use of nitroprusside for control of severe hypertension in children. Most of this experience is unpublished because the number of cases in each center is small; a multicenter study has not been performed. Nonetheless, the drug is accepted as conventional therapy for this indication.

One of the most important limitations of nitroprusside is that it cannot be given orally. In most chapters on orally active vasodilators in this book, the effect of these agents has been compared to that of intravenous nitroprusside. The recommendations of the task force on blood pressure control in children state that "despite aggressive pharmacotherapy it is occasionally impossible to lower a preadolescent's blood pressure to acceptable levels on an outpatient basis. In these situations hospitalization is mandatory." One of the first drugs of choice in such cases is nitroprusside.

Patients who do not respond initially to oral therapy or even to some forms of intravenous therapy may be treated for a short period by nitroprusside; they may then respond better to oral therapy. For example, Adelman reported an infant with severe hypertension who failed to respond to furosemide, hydralazine, methyldopa, and diazoxide and who responded only to nitroprusside.[26] The patient's blood pressure was subsequently controlled by furosemide, hydralazine, and methyldopa.

Adelman and Russo studied a 12-year-old girl with malignant hypertension and severe renal failure who recovered significant renal function after aggressive control of blood pressure and the use of hemodialysis.[27] Nitroprusside was the cornerstone of antihypertensive treatment in this patient. The patient had a 6-week history of headaches, abdominal pain, fatigue, nausea, and vomiting. One week prior to hospital admission, passage of dark urine was observed. The patient's blood pressure was 260/180 mm Hg, and the serum creatinine level was 5.1 mg/dl. An intravenous pyelogram and a renal arteriogram revealed a stenotic right renal artery and a small right kidney.

The patient's elevated blood pressure was treated with hydralazine, methyldopa, hydrochlorothiazide, diazoxide, propranolol, and prazosin. It was controlled only after addition of nitroprusside to the combined therapeutic regimen, however. The blood pressure could not be maintained at an acceptable level when the dose of nitroprusside was tapered. A right nephrectomy was performed, and the patient was treated with hemodialysis. Her renal function improved, and hemodialysis was discontinued.

An important indication for nitroprusside is the need for rapid reduction of arterial blood pressure in patients with aortic dissection. In the pediatric age group, this event may complicate Marfan's syndrome.

Effects in Patients with Ventricular Septal Defect

Infants and children with a large left-to-right shunt may develop congestive heart failure. To evaluate the effect of short-term vasodilator therapy in such cases, Beekman and colleagues administered nitroprusside intravenously, at an initial infusion rate of 0.5 $\mu g/kg/min$ and at increments of 0.5 $\mu g/kg/min$, to 5 children with ventricular septal defect.[28] The mean age of the patients was 2.8 months. All had congestive heart failure, and the study was performed during cardiac catheterization. The drug increased the pulmonary-to-systemic flow ratio from 2.2 ± 0.2 to 3.4 ± 0.2, as a consequence of a marked decrease in systemic blood flow from 5.3 ± 0.7 to 3.6 ± 0.5 $L/min/m^2$. Pulmonary flow did not change much. Right atrial pressure decreased from 6.0 ± 1.4 to 2.8 ± 1.1 mm Hg. Mean pulmonary capillary wedge pressure decreased by 53%, from 10.2 ± 1.4 to 4.8 ± 1.4 mm Hg. Mean aortic pressure decreased from 63.6 ± 3.0 to 54.6 ± 2.1 mm Hg, and mean pulmonary arterial pressure decreased from 41.4 ± 6.2 to 32.0 ± 6.7

mm Hg. Systemic vascular resistance was paradoxically increased from 11.7 ± 1.6 to 15.4 ± 2.4 U.

These data indicate that, in infants with a large ventricular septal defect, nitroprusside increases the left-to-right shunt and decreases the systemic blood flow. These investigators suggested that maintenance of ventricular preload by administration of fluids may improve the response of these infants to nitroprusside.[28] It is difficult to make general conclusions from the study of Beekman and co-workers because ventricular function, cardiac output, and systemic vascular resistance were normal in the infants studied.[28] Until further studies have been conducted, however, I do not recommend the use of nitroprusside in infants with large ventricular septal defect and congestive heart failure.

Nitroprusside has caused hemodynamic improvement in patients with acute rupture of the intraventricular septum due to myocardial infarction.

Effects after Cardiac Surgical Procedures

After cardiac surgical procedures, severe peripheral vasoconstriction often prevents hemodynamic recovery and produces acute hypertensive episodes. Nitroprusside, by its vasodilatory effect, may produce an improvement in these conditions. The peripheral vasodilation also improves cardiac function and enhances cardiac recovery.[29] This improvement has also been seen in children operated on for correction of congenital and acquired heart diseases.

Benzing and colleagues studied the effect of nitroprusside in 11 children immediately after open heart procedures for congenital heart disease.[30] Only patients whose cardiac index was less than 2.0 L/min/m^2 and whose systemic vascular resistance exceeded 30 U were included in the study. The patients ranged in age from 1 to 12 years and were operated for ventricular septal defect, with or without pulmonic stenosis, atrial septal defect with pulmonic stenosis, anomalous pulmonary venous return, atrial septal defect, tetralogy of Fallot, and infundibular and valvar pulmonic stenosis. The investigators primarily wanted to evaluate the effect of afterload, and therefore they eliminated the effect of preload reduction by keeping the mean left atrial pressure at a constant level by blood transfusion. During infusion of nitroprusside, at a rate of 1.6 to 6.8 µg/kg/min, mean arterial pressure decreased by 18.6%, systemic vascular resistance decreased by 53.7%, and cardiac index increased by 76.9% None of the children died.

These authors suggested, and my colleagues and I have confirmed it in several cases, that nitroprusside may produce hemodynamic improvement in children after cardiac operations, with or without hypothermic cardioplegia, who have peripheral vasoconstriction, depressed myocardial contractility, and low cardiac output. These patients are especially suitable for treatment with nitroprusside because they usually require only short-term treatment. Patients who have both elevated systemic vascular resistance and high left ventricular filling pressure benefit most from nitroprusside.

Appelbaum and co-workers studied 16 infants under 18 months old within 3 hours of undergoing intracardiac surgical procedures.[31] The infants ranged in age from 2 weeks to 17 months. Four had tetralogy of Fallot, 4 had pulmonic stenosis, 3 had single ventricular septal defect, 2 had multiple ventricular septal defects, 1 had an infradiaphragmatic type of total anomalous pulmonary venous connection, and 1 had complete transposition of the great arteries. Initial mean arterial pressure and systemic vascular resistance were higher than normal in each infant (99 ± 17.2 mm Hg and 48 ± 18.1 U/m^2, respectively). Cardiac index was low, at 1.9 ± 0.48 L/min/m^2. Mean left atrial pressure was 11.4 ± 2.4 mm Hg, and right atrial pressure was 12.5 ± 3.1 mm Hg. Pulmonary vascular resistance was 8.6 U/m^2. Infusion of nitroprusside, at a rate that normalized mean arterial pressure, increased cardiac index by 17% and decreased left atrial pressure by 25% and right atrial pressure by 22%. Mean pulmonary arterial pressure decreased by 31%. When atrial pressures returned to initial levels after infusion of blood, nitroprusside increased cardiac index by another 24%. When infusion of nitroprusside was discontinued, cardiac index decreased to 116% of the initial value. Thus, nitroprusside has a favorable effect on cardiac output in infants with elevated arterial pressure early after intracardiac operations.

Adverse effects on blood gases may limit the use of nitroprusside in children after cardiac surgical procedures. This subject is further discussed in the section on adverse effects of nitroprusside.

Effects in Acute Myocardial Infarction

Although these studies are not relevant to the pediatric age group, nitroprusside has been evaluated in the last 15 years for treatment of acute myocardial infarction and its complications. The afterload and preload reduction by nitroprusside have been considered beneficial for limiting the infarct size and for treatment of hemodynamic complications such as congestive heart failure, rupture of the intraventricular septum, and mitral regurgitation. A recent review suggested that nitroprusside should not be used in the first 12 hours after acute myocardial infarction. If a patient's hemodynamic condition undergoes significant deterioration during this early phase and if nitroprusside is required, coronary arterial perfusion pressure should be maintained by an intraaortic balloon. In the later phases of necrosis and healing, nitroprusside may, by afterload or preload reduction, reduce the stress on the necrotic area and may improve the overall cardiac performance. Nitroprusside has not been generally accepted as conventional treatment of acute myocardial infarction.

Clinical Pharmacology

Nitroprusside is administered intravenously, and the onset of its action is within 1 to 20 minutes from the initiation of infusion. During administration, the infusion system should be protected from light because the drug is photosensitive.

The half-life of nitroprusside is short. Because it does not accumulate in vessel walls, its effect disappears within several minutes of termination of the infusion.

Nitroprusside is eliminated by metabolism in various tissues, and finally in the liver, to thiocyanate. This compound is excreted by the kidneys and may accumulate in patients with renal failure. This subject is further discussed in the next section of this chapter.

Adverse Effects

Treatment with nitroprusside is associated with some serious adverse effects that limit its use.

Toxicity

Prolonged infusion of high doses of nitroprusside may cause toxicity because of the accumulation of thiocyanate and cyanide.[32-36] The principal manifestations of this toxicity are dyspnea, convulsions, muscle spasms, rigidity, nausea, vomiting, disorientation, psychotic behavior, and bone marrow depression.

The biochemical pathway leading to this toxicity is formation of cyanide by interaction of nitroprusside with sulfhydryl groups. Cyanide is then rapidly metabolized in the liver by the enzyme rhodanase, and thiocyanate is liberated to the plasma. Thiocyanate is excreted almost exclusively by the kidney, with an elimination half-life of about a week in patients with normal renal function. Symptoms of thiocyanate toxicity begin to appear at plasma levels of 5 to 10 mg/dl. Plasma levels of thiocyanate should be monitored in patients treated with a continuous infusion of nitroprusside. If these levels exceed 12 mg/dl, treatment should be discontinued.[37]

Thiocyanate can be removed from the plasma by peritoneal dialysis. This technique may be used in severe cases of toxicity.

Impairment of Oxygenation

Some investigators have suggested that nitroprusside, and possibly other vasodilators as well, may reduce arterial blood oxygen tension and saturation.[23, 38, 39] This phenomenon has occasionally been noted with vasodilators other than nitroprusside; therefore, it has been attributed to the vasodilating effect and not to any specific effect of nitroprusside. Because the drug produces generalized vasodilation, it dilates pulmonary arterioles in areas of the lung that are not adequately ventilated and thus changes the ventilation-perfusion ratio and impairs arterial blood oxygenation. This problem may be significant in children recovering from cardiac operations, although the general hemodynamic improvement produced by the drug compensates for this impairment in the ventilation-perfusion ratio.

Because nitroprusside is usually given to critically ill patients, it is preferable to give a vasodilator that does not have such an effect on arterial oxygenation. The reader is referred to the other chapters in Section III of this book for comparative data.

Other Side Effects

Nitroprusside may provoke myocardial ischemia by reducing the coronary perfusion pressure. This effect is usually not relevant in children, but it may be important in adults with coronary artery disease. Like other vasodilators, nitroprusside may produce flushing and headache. It may also produce skin rashes. A single case of hypothyroidism in a patient treated with nitroprusside has been reported.[40]

Dosage and Administration

Nitroprusside is given only intravenously. The infusion rate in children is 0.25 to 6.5 µg/kg/min. Treatment should be initiated with low doses and increased by increments of about 0.5 µg/kg/min. If prolonged treatment is planned, monitoring of thiocyanate plasma levels should be performed. This dose should be titrated according to the hemodynamic response.

References

1. Saxson, A., and Kattlove, H.E.: Platelet inhibition by sodium nitroprusside, a smooth muscle inhibitor. Blood, 47:957, 1976.
2. Mehta, J., and Mehta, P.: Platelet function studies in heart disease. VI. Enhanced platelet aggregation formation activity in congestive heart failure: inhibition by sodium nitroprusside. Circulation, 60:497, 1979.
3. Pouleur, H., et al.: Effects of nitroprusside on venous return and central blood volume in the absence and presence of acute heart failure. Circulation, 61:2, 1980.
4. Chatterjee, K., et al.: Hemodynamic and metabolic responses to vasodilator therapy in acute myocardial infarction. Circulation, 48:1183, 1973.
5. da Luz, P.L., et al.: Hemodynamic and metabolic effects of sodium nitroprusside on the performance and metabolism of regional ischemic myocardium. Circulation, 52:400, 1975.
6. Merillon, I.P., et al.: Study of left ventricular pressure-volume relations during nitroprusside infusion in human subjects without coronary artery disease. Br. Heart J., 41:325, 1979.

7. Packer, M., et al.: Rebound hemodynamic events after the abrupt withdrawal of nitroprusside in patients with severe chronic heart failure. N. Engl. J. Med., *301*:1193, 1979.
8. Schlant, R.C., et al.: Studies on the acute cardiovascular effects of intravenous sodium nitroprusside. Am. J. Cardiol., *9*:51, 1962.
9. Cohn, J.N., et al.: Contrasting effects of vasodilators on heart rate and plasma catecholamines in patients with hypertension and heart failure. Clin. Res., *26*:547a, 1978.
10. Lukes, S.A., et al.: Haemodynamic effects of sodium nitroprusside in 21 subjects with congestive heart failure. Br. Heart J., *41*:187, 1979.
11. Thompson, D.S., et al.: Effects of sodium nitroprusside upon cardiac work, efficiency and substrate extraction in severe left ventricular failure. Br. Heart J., *46*:394, 1981.
12. Levin, R.I., et al.: The interaction of sodium nitroprusside with human endothelial cells and platelets: nitroprusside and prostacyclin synergistically inhibit platelet function. Circulation, *66*:1299, 1982.
13. Brownlee, K.A.: Statistical Theory and Methodology in Science and Engineering. New York, John Wiley, 1960.
14. Dillion, T.R. et al.: Vasodilator therapy for congestive heart failure. J. Pediatr., *96*:623, 1980.
15. Beekman, R.H., et al.: Vasodilator therapy in children: acute and chronic effects in children with left ventricular dysfunction or mitral regurgitation. Pediatrics, *73*:43, 1984.
16. Yeh, B.K., et al.: Sodium nitroprusside as a coronary vasodilator in man. Am. Heart J., *93*:610, 1977.
17. Patrick, T.A. et al.: Telemetry of left ventricular diameter and pressure measurements from un-restrained animals. J. Appl. Physiol., 37:276, 1974.
18. Macho, P., et al.: Effects of nitroglycerin and nitroprusside on large and small coronary vessels in conscious dogs. Circulation, *64*:1101, 1981.
19. Rowe, G.G., and Henderson, R.H.: Systemic and coronary hemodynamic effects of sodium nitroprusside. Am. Heart J., *87*:83, 1974.
20. Mann, T., et al.: Effect of nitroprusside on regional myocardial blood flow in coronary artery disease. Circulation, *57*:732, 1978.
21. Pagani, M., et al.: Hemodynamic effects of intravenous sodium nitroprusside in the conscious dog. Circulation, *57*:144, 1978.
22. Cogan, J.J., et al.: Renal effects of nitroprusside and hydralazine in patients with congestive heart failure. Circulation, *61*:316, 1980.
23. Leier, C.V., et al.: Central and regional hemodynamic effects of intravenous isosorbide dinitrate, nitroglycerin and nitroprusside in patients with congestive heart failure. Am. J. Cardiol. *48*:1115, 1978.
24. Loggie, J.M.H.: Hypertension in children and adolescents. II. Drug therapy. J. Pediatr., *74*:640, 1969.
25. Cordillo-Paniagua, G., et al.: Sodium nitroprusside treatment of severe arterial hypertension in children. J. Pediatr., *87*:799, 1975.
26. Adelman, R.D.: Neonatal hypertension. *In* Symposium on hypertension in children and adolescence. Pediatr. Clin. North Am., *25*:99. 1978.
27. Adelman, R.D., and Russo, J.: Malignant hypertension: recovery of renal function after treatment with antihypertensive medications and hemodialysis. J. Pediatr., *98*:766, 1981.
28. Beekman, R.H. et al.: Hemodynamic effects of hydralazine in infants with a large ventricular septal defect. Circulation, *65*:523, 1982.
29. Goodman, D.J., et al.: Effect of nitroprusside on left ventricular dynamics in mitral regurgitation. Circulation, *50*:1025, 1978.
30. Benzing, G., III, et al.: Nitroprusside after open-heart surgery. Circulation, *54*:467, 1976.
31. Appelbaum, A., et al.: Afterload reduction and cardiac output in infants early after intracardiac surgery. Am. J. Cardiol., *39*:445, 1977.
32. Fonzes-Diacon, H., and Carguet, J.: Sur la toxicité du nitroprussiate de soude. Bull. Soc. Chim., *29*:638, 1903.

33. Palmer, R.F., and Lasseter, K.: Sodium nitroprusside. N. Engl. J. Med., *292*:294, 1975.
34. Koch-Weser, J.: Hypertensive emergencies. N. Engl. J. Med., *290*:211, 1974.
35. Page, J.H., et al.: Cardiovascular actions of sodium nitroprusside in animals and hypertensive patients. Circulation, *11*:188, 1955.
36. Moraca, P.P., et al.: Clinical evaluation of sodium nitroprusside as a hypertensive agent. Anesthesiology, *23*:193, 1962.
37. Ahearn, D.J., and Crim, C.E.: Treatment of malignant hypertension with sodium nitroprusside. Arch. Intern. Med., *133*:187, 1974.
38. Pierpont, G., et al.: Effects of vasodilators on pulmonary hemodynamics and gas exchange in left ventricular failure. Am. Heart J., *99*:208, 1980.
39. Mookherjee, S., et al.: Hemodynamics, ventilatory and blood gas changes during infusion of sodium nitroferricyanide (nitroprusside). Chest, *72*:273, 1977.
40. Nourok, D.S., et al.: Hypothyroidism following prolonged sodium nitroprusside therapy. Am. J. Med. Sci., *248*:129, 1964.

Chapter 11

Nitroglycerin

Nitroglycerin, the most widely used nitrate, has been used for over 100 years for the treatment of angina pectoris in adults. The drug acts by direct peripheral and coronary vasodilation. Recently, it was found to be effective in the short-term treatment of congestive heart failure and hemodynamic disturbances complicating acute myocardial infarction.

Intravenously administered nitroglycerin has recently been suggested as the vasodilator of choice in the postoperative management of pediatric cardiac patients with pulmonary hypertension.

Pharmacologic Properties

Nitroglycerin is a direct-acting vasodilator. Its mechanism of action is not known. Nitroglycerin may act by release of the vasodilator prostacyclin, but this concept is controversial.

Hemodynamic Effects

Nitroglycerin dilates systemic veins and, to a lesser extent, arteries. It also has some vasodilatory effect on the pulmonary circulation. These effects decrease systemic arterial pressure and cardiac volumes. Nitroglycerin may increase ejection fraction in patients with a normal heart or with coronary artery disease but without congestive heart failure,[1] or it may not produce a change.[2] Nitroglycerin accelerates heart rate, secondary to sympathetic activation by peripheral vasodilation. In patients with congestive heart failure, the drug reduces the elevated left ventricular filling pressure and systemic vascular resistance and may increase cardiac output.[3,4]

The hemodynamic effects of nitroglycerin in patients with coronary artery disease are discussed in the following section of this chapter.

In patients with congestive heart failure, nitroglycerin produces hemodynamic and symptomatic improvement. The hemodynamic effects are more favorable in patients with higher pretreatment left ventricular filling pressure and lower cardiac output.[5-7] The drug is effective mainly for short-term treatment. Most patients with congestive heart failure treated with nitroglycerin for long periods probably develop hemodynamic tolerance.

Nitroglycerin exerts a dilatory effect on the pulmonary vasculature, primarily the veins. This phenomenon may partially account for the beneficial effect of the drug in pulmonary edema.

Ilbawi and co-workers studied 20 infants and children, aged 4 months to 6 years, who received intravenous nitroglycerin following intracardiac repair of congenital heart diseases.[8] Six of these patients had atrial septal defect, 11 had ventricular septal defect, and 3 had atrioventricular canal. All patients had a ratio of pulmonary-to-systemic flow greater than 2.5:1. In 14 patients, the preoperative pulmonary artery pressure was equal to the aortic pressure, and in 5 patients, the pulmonary vascular resistance was higher than 6 U. In the 6 patients with normal preoperative pulmonary artery pressure, intravenous nitroglycerin increased the cardiac index from 3.97 ± 0.61 to 4.30 ± 0.77 L/min/m^2 and reduced systemic vascular resistance from 1602 ± 359 to 1137 ± 305 dynes · sec · cm^{-5} and pulmonary vascular resistance from 175 ± 27 to 148 ± 28 dynes · sec · cm^{-5}. In the 14 patients with elevated preoperative pulmonary artery pressure, intravenous nitroglycerin increased the cardiac index from 3.06 ± 0.48 to 3.74 ± 0.45 L/min/m^2 and reduced systemic vascular resistance from 1635 ± 217 to 1294 ± 249 dynes · sec · cm^{-5} and pulmonary vascular resistance from 305 ± 78 to 214 ± 76 dynes · sec · cm^{-5}. The changes were most significant in the patients with elevated preoperative pulmonary artery pressure. Ilbawi and associates concluded that intravenous nitroglycerin is the vasodilator of choice in the postoperative management of the pediatric cardiac patient with pulmonary hypertension.[8]

Effects in Ischemic Heart Disease

Nitroglycerin is the cornerstone of treatment of angina pectoris. Sublingual administration of nitroglycerin is the most rapid therapeutic intervention for relief of anginal pain in patients with chronic stable angina pectoris, as well as in patients with some other forms of angina pectoris. Nitroglycerin also increases exercise capacity and decreases electrocardiographic ST-segment depression. The mechanism of action of nitroglycerin in angina pectoris may involve a peripheral vascular effect or a direct coronary effect. Direct dilation of large coronary arteries and collateral vessels improves the myocardial blood supply. Unlike other potent coronary dilators, nitroglycerin does not dilate coronary arterioles and therefore does not cause coronary steal from ischemic zones. Nitroglycerin can also abolish coronary spasm. Because this drug dilates peripheral arteries and veins, it thereby decreases peripheral vascular resistance and left ventricular filling pressure, two important determinants of myocardial oxygen demand. The decrease in left ventricular filling pressure improves perfusion of the subendocardial myocardium.

Recently, intravenously administered nitroglycerin was shown to reduce infarct size in patients with acute myocardial infarction. This phenomenon resulted from an improved myocardial oxygen supply-to-demand ratio, by mechanisms similar to those seen with nitroglycerin in angina pectoris.

Clinical Pharmacology

In patients with coronary artery disease, nitroglycerin is usually given sublingually or transcutaneously. For treatment of congestive heart failure, nitroglycerin is given intravenously; such is the case in infants and children with pulmonary hypertension following cardiac surgical procedures. Transcutaneous administration of nitroglycerin may play a role in treatment of congestive heart failure or pulmonary hypertension in infants and children.

Peak plasma levels of nitroglycerin are achieved within a few minutes of sublingual administration. These levels are usually 2 to 3 ng/ml.[9] The intravenous administration of therapeutic doses of nitroglycerin results in plasma levels of 1 to 65 ng/ml.[10] Nitroglycerin is not effective orally because of the drug's extensive first-pass hepatic metabolism.

The drug is eliminated by hepatic, and probably also by extrahepatic, metabolism. The metabolites, dinitrates and mononitrates, are excreted by the kidneys or are further metabolized to glycerol.[11] Nitroglycerin is eliminated from the plasma within 15 to 20 minutes of discontinuance of the infusion.

Side Effects

Nitroglycerin may cause hypotension, postural symptoms, and tachycardia. Headache, caused by cerebral vasodilation, is the most common side effect of nitroglycerin in adults.

Dosage and Administration

In infants and children, nitroglycerin is given intravenously at a dose of 5 µg/kg/min.

References

1. Ritchie, J.L., et al.: Radionuclide angiography: noninvasive assessment of hemodynamic changes after administration of nitroglycerin. Am. J. Cardiol., *43*:278, 1979.
2. Slutsky, R., et al.: Effect of nitrates on left ventricular size and function during exercise: comparison of sublingual nitroglycerin and nitroglycerin paste. Am. J. Cardiol., *45*:831, 1980.

3. Williams, D.O., et al.: Hemodynamic effects of nitroglycerin in acute myocardial infarction: decrease in ventricular preload at the expense of cardiac output. Circulation, 51:421, 1975.
4. Darby, T.D., et al.: Evaluation of sympathetic reflex effects on the inotropic action of nitroglycerin, quinidine, papaverin, aminophylline and isoproterenol. J. Pharmacol. Exp. Ther., 122:386, 1958.
5. Gold, H.K., et al.: Sublingual nitroglycerin in congestive failure following acute myocardial infarction. Circulation, 46:839, 1972.
6. Magrini, F., and Niarchos, A.P.: Ineffectiveness of sublingual nitroglycerin in acute left ventricular failure in the presence of massive peripheral edema. Am. J. Cardiol., 45:841, 1980.
7. Franciosa, J.A., et al.: Nitrate effects on cardiac output and left ventricular outflow resistance in chronic congestive heart failure. Am. J. Med., 64:207, 1978.
8. Ilbawi, M.N., et al.: Hemodynamic effects of intravenous nitroglycerin in postoperative pediatric cardiac patients. AHA 1984.
9. Armstrong, P.W., et al.: Blood levels after sublingual nitroglycerin. Circulation, 59:585, 1979.
10. Curfman, G.D., et al.: Intravenous nitroglycerin in the treatment of spontaneous angina pectoris: a prospective, randomized trial. Circulation, 67:276, 1983.
11. McNiff, E.F., et al.: Nitroglycerin. In Analytical Profiles of Drug Substances. Vol 9. Edited by K. Florey. New York, Academic Press, 1980.

Chapter 12

Minoxidil

Minoxidil, a direct-acting potent vasodilator, has been used successfully for the treatment of hypertension and congestive heart failure. Because the prolonged use of this drug is associated with unique cardiac and epicardial side effects, however, minoxidil administration is limited to emergency use in patients with severe hypertension refractory to other drugs or in patients who cannot tolerate other drugs. It is also used in patients with severe refractory congestive heart failure. Minoxidil is the first vasodilator introduced to clinical use after hydralazine, and minoxidil's long duration of action, 8 to 24 hours, provides an important clinical benefit.

Structure

The chemical structure of minoxidil is unique among cardiovascular drugs. It is 2,4-diamino-6-piperdinylpyrimidine-3-oxide.

Pharmacologic Properties

Minoxidil is a direct-acting vasodilator, with an effect predominantly on the arterial vasculature.[1]

Effects in Hypertension

Because of its direct vasodilatory activity, minoxidil lowers elevated peripheral resistance and controls hypertension. The antihypertensive effect was first shown by animal experiments,[2] and it was later confirmed by several clinical studies.[3-5] In combination with beta-blocking agents and diuretics, minoxidil controls hypertension refractory to other drugs.[3,6,7] Beta-blocking agents are required during the initiation of minoxidil therapy, to ovecome a compensatory mechanism; the need for beta-blocking agents diminishes during long-term minoxidil treatment.[8]

Minoxidil controls all degrees of hypertension, including severe hypertension. It is effective in children as well as in adults.[9-12] This drug is also useful in patients with severe childhood hypertension refractory to other antihypertensive agents.[9,10]

Discontinuance in Hypertensive Patients

Rebound hypertension may occur when minoxidil is abruptly discontinued. In 3 children treated with minoxidil, 40 to 50 mg daily for 1 to 3 years, sudden discontinuance of the drug caused rebound hypertension with hypertensive encephalopathy. The rebound hypertension correlated with the weekly dose and the rate of withdrawal, but not with the duration of treatment.[12] If discontinuance of minoxidil is indicated in hypertensive patients, the process should be gradual.

Comparison with Prazosin

The antihypertensive effect of prazosin was compared to that of minoxidil when added to atenolol, 100 mg daily, and chlorthalidone, 25 mg daily, in 12 patients whose blood pressure was not adequately controlled by this combination of beta-blocking and diuretic agents. Diastolic blood pressure was reduced to 95 mm Hg or less in 8 of 12 patients during treatment with minoxidil, 7.5 mg daily, and in 4 of the 12 patients during treatment with prazosin, 3 mg daily. Therefore, minoxidil was more effective than prazosin.

Effects in Congestive Heart Failure

Several short-term studies have shown that minoxidil exerts a beneficial effect in patients at rest who have chronic congestive heart failure, although the use of this drug is associated with fluid retention.[13-16] The improvement noted in these studies was mainly attributed to afterload reduction by arteriolar vasodilation and was manifested by increased cardiac output, decreased systemic resistance, and an absent or minimal effect on pulmonary pressure. For example, McKay and colleagues reported that, in 11 patients with severe chronic congestive heart failure, a single oral dose of minoxidil increased cardiac index by 63% and stroke volume index by 52% and decreased systemic vascular resistance by 38%.[16] Pulmonary capillary wedge pressure was reduced from 24 ± 8 to 21 ± 7 mm Hg. The average mean arterial pressure was not altered, but 1 patient developed significant hypotension. Eight patients received prolonged oral treatment and showed fluid retention; 4 of these patients noted an improvement with higher doses of diuretics.[16]

Minoxidil produced hemodynamic improvement both at rest and during exercise in 10 patients with severe chronic heart failure refractory to digitalis and diuretics.[17] Cardiac index at rest increased from 1.99 ± 0.38 to 2.64 ± 0.33 L/min/m^2 after short-term minoxidil administration. Cardiac index during symptom-limited maximal exercise increased from $2.88 \pm$ to 0.79 to 3.55 ± 0.84 L/min/m^2 after minoxidil administration. This increase was due to a rise in stroke volume because the change in heart rate was not significant. Systemic vascular resistance was decreased by minoxidil from 2050 ± 722 to 1325 ± 374 dynes · sec · cm^{-5} during maximal exercise. Left ventricular filling pressure, right atrial pressure, and pulmonary arterial pressure were little changed, but pulmonary vascular resistance decreased both at rest and during exercise. Maximal exercise oxygen consumption increased by about 10%. Exercise performance increased in terms of load and duration. Five of the patients continued follow-up treatment for 6 weeks, and all showed symptomatic improvement. These 5 patients all developed increased edema and required higher doses of diuretics, however. In 2 of the 10 patients studied, symptoms of ischemic heart disease worsened during treatment.[17]

Franciosa and Cohn reported that, in 18 patients with chronic left ventricular failure caused by ischemic heart disease or by primary cardiomyopathy, oral minoxidil produced marked hemodynamic improvement seen by an increase in cardiac index from 2.34 ± 0.14 to 2.95 ± 0.29 L/min/m^2 and a decrease in systemic vascular resistance from 19.6 ± 1.5 to 15.0 ± 1.3 U.[18] Heart rate rose slightly, and mean arterial pressure fell slightly. Right atrial, pulmonary arterial, and pulmonary capillary wedge pressures were not altered.

Packer and associates reported that 5 serial right-heart catheterizations in a 78-year-old man with severe congestive heart failure due to idiopathic cardiomyopathy showed the development of hemodynamic and clinical tolerance to hydralazine and captopril after favorable initial responses to both agents.[19] Minoxidil, 20 mg orally twice daily, had a sustained effect after 4 and 9 weeks of continued treatment, however. This finding suggests that tolerance is drug-specific, and minoxidil may be used in patients who develop tolerance to other vasodilators.[19] This particular patient also had a sustained response to nitroprusside.

Leddy and co-workers showed that minoxidil-induced improvements in hemodynamics and in left ventricular function persisted throughout a treatment period of 3 months.[20] No clinical efficacy was observed, however, possibly because of the induction of tachycardia.

The dose of minoxidil should be carefully titrated in patients with congestive heart failure, and patients should be examined twice weekly for the first 3 weeks, to prevent fluid retention.[17] Serial echocardiograms should be performed to detect pericardial effusion. The hemodynamic and clinical effects of minoxidil can be sustained throughout prolonged treatment.

The mechanism of fluid retention, which is a more serious problem with minoxidil than with other vasodilators, is not known. Perhaps the drug alters the intrarenal distribution of blood.

Comparison with Hydralazine

Both minoxidil and hydralazine are direct-acting arterial dilators.

Stein and colleagues compared the hemodynamic and clinical effects of minoxidil and hydralazine in 18 patients with severe chronic congestive heart failure.[21] Both agents increased cardiac index and lowered systemic vascular resistance. Fluid retention was greater with minoxidil than with hydralazine, but it was controlled by increasing the doses of diuretics. The long-term survivors showed symptomatic improvement with both agents.

Markham and associates reported that, in patients with congestive heart failure, the hemodynamic effects of minoxidil and hydralazine are similar.[22] Both drugs similarly increased cardiac index (minoxidil, from 1.65 ± 0.29 to 2.26 ± 0.40 L/min/m^2, and hydralazine, from 1.88 ± 0.61 to 2.34 ± 0.90 L/min/m^2), decreased systemic vascular resistance, increased heart rate, and did not alter pulmonary arterial, pulmonary capillary wedge, or right atrial pressures. These findings indicate that minoxidil is an arterial dilator. Fluid retention was greater with minoxidil than with hydralazine, despite similar effects on renal function, the renin-angiotensin system, or the sympathetic nervous system.

Comparison with Nitroprusside

Minoxidil is an arterial dilator, and nitroprusside is a balanced vasodilator. In patients with congestive heart failure, both agents increase cardiac index and decrease systemic vascular resistance. Minoxidil increases heart rate, however, whereas nitroprusside does not alter it. Pulmonary arterial and right atrial pressures are decreased by nitroprusside, but not by minoxidil. Nitroprusside decreases relative hepatomesenteric flow, when compared with minoxidil and hydralazine which increase it.

In one report, nitroprusside decreased plasma norepinephrine levels by 21%, whereas minoxidil increased these levels. Nitroprusside did not alter plasma renin activity; minoxidil increased it.[22]

Renal Effects

In studies of hypertensive patients, minoxidil did not alter renal blood flow or glomerular filtration rate, but it decreased urinary sodium excretion.[6,23] In patients with congestive heart failure, minoxidil increased renal blood flow by 8% and did not produce any other significant or consistent change in renal function.[22]

Neurohumoral Effect

By means of vasodilation, minoxidil activates both the sympathetic and the renin-angiotensin systems.[22] In some hypertensive patients, an apparent dissociation of aldosterone from plasma renin activity has been observed.[24] This effect has been attributed to changes in hepatic metabolism of aldosterone.

Clinical Pharmacology

In humans, over 95% of orally administered minoxidil is absorbed from the gastrointestinal tract. Absorption is rapid. The drug appears in the plasma within 30 minutes of oral administration, and its concentration reaches a peak within an hour. It does not bind to plasma proteins. About 90% of the absorbed drug is metabolized, mainly by conjugation with glucuronic acid. Its elimination half-life is about 4 hours, and almost all the absorbed amount is excreted in the urine, as conjugates, within 12 hours.[25]

Despite the short elimination half-life of minoxidil, its hypotensive effect may persist for up to 24 hours.[1,25] This phenomenon may result from persistence of the drug at receptor sites in vessel walls. In patients with congestive heart failure, the peak hemodynamic effect has been observed 5 hours after oral administration.

Adverse Effects

Minoxidil has adverse effects of two types: (1) nonspecific effects resulting from vasodilation; and (2) effects specific for minoxidil. The specific effects limit the use of this drug.

Pericardial Damage

Minoxidil can produce pericarditis or pericardial effusion. Several cases of pericardial involvement have been reported in patients treated with minoxidil.[5,26-30] In 1977, a report noted that hypertensive patients treated with minoxidil may have a high incidence of pericardial effusion.[31] In a prospective study, 2 of 22 patients treated with minoxidil had echocardiographically demonstrated pericardial effusion. In a retrospective review of 15 patients in whom minoxidil was discontinued, 7 patients with pericardial effusion and 1 patient with pericarditis were identified.[32] In 5 of these patients, the effusion disappeared when the drug was discontinued. Rechallenge with minoxidil produced recurrent pericardial effusion in 1 patient. Among 1869 patients who were included in experimental protocols, 91 cases of pericardial damage were found (4.8%).[33] In 21 of these patients, this disorder was manifested by pericardial tamponade, and 8 of them died. It was not possible to predict which patients would develop pericardial involvement. The reaction was not dose-dependent.[32,33] This adverse effect is considered to be an idiosyncratic reaction.

This complication may require limitation of the use of minoxidil. This adverse effect has been hypothetically related to impairment of renal function, but this theory is probably not correct.

Right Atrial Damage

In dogs treated with minoxidil, 1 mg/kg or more for a month, a species-specific lesion of the right atrium of the heart was observed.[34] The lesion was adjacent to the second atrial branch of the right coronary artery. Microscopically, extravasation of erythrocytes, atrophy of myocardial cells, accumulation of mast cells and macrophages with hemosiderin pigmentation, and proliferation of angioblasts and connective tissue were observed. This lesion was not found in humans. The vascular lesions were related to uremia. Nonspecific, papillary-muscle, myocardial lesions were found during animal experiments and autopsies of human patients.[34]

Electrocardiographic Changes

Nonspecific T-wave changes, such as flattening or inversion, have been reported in up to 60% of patients treated for long periods with minoxidil.[17] These manifestations may result from changes in left ventricular volume.

Hypertrichosis

Hypertrichosis occurs commonly in patients taking high doses of minoxidil.[35] It was observed in about 80% of a group of patients taking the drug for 1 year and is thought to result from an increase in blood flow to the skin.[36] This side effect usually appears during the 3 to 4 weeks of therapy and disappears within 2 to 3 months of discontinuance of the drug.

Effects Resulting from Vasodilation

Hypotension, tachycardia, sympathetic hyperactivity, and fluid and sodium retention result from the vasodilatory effect of minoxidil.[6, 37] These side effects are not serious enough to require discontinuance of the drug. Some of these effects may be controlled by concomitant administration of beta-blocking and diuretic agents.

If minoxidil is used alone, the fluid retention may not only compromise the antihypertensive effect of the drug, but may also precipitate left heart failure, especially in patients with impaired renal function.

Dosage and Administration

Congestive Heart Failure

Oral doses of 10 to 20 mg twice daily are used.

Hypertension

Oral doses of 2.5 to 20 mg twice daily are given. Certain patients require 50 mg daily or administration of the daily dose in 3 divided doses.

References

1. Pluss, R.G., et al.: Tissue distribution and hypotensive effects of minoxidil in normotensive rats. J. Lab. Clin. Med., 79:639, 1972.
2. Pettinger, W.A., and Mitchell, H.C.: Minoxidil—an alternative to nephrectomy for refractory hypertension. N. Engl. J. Med., 289:167, 1973.
3. Dargie, H.J., et al.: Minoxidil in resistant hypertension. Lancet, 2:515, 1977.
4. O'Malley, K., and McNay, J.: A method for achieving blood pressure control expeditiously with oral minoxidil. Clin. Pharmacol. Ther., 18:39, 1975.
5. Mehta, P., et al.: Severe hypertensives: treatment with minoxidil. JAMA, 233:249, 1975.
6. Gilmore, E., et al.: Treatment of essential hypertension with a new vasodilator in combination with beta-adrenergic blockage. N. Engl. J. Med., 282:521, 1970.
7. Dormois, J.C., et al.: Minoxidil in severe hypertension: value when conventional drugs have failed. Am. Heart J., 90:360, 1975.
8. Brunner, L.R., et al.: Need for beta-blockade in hypertension reduced with long-term minoxidil. Br. Med. J., 2:385, 1978.
9. Sinaiko, A.R., and Mirkin, B.L.: Management of severe childhood hypertension with minoxidil: a controlled study. J. Pediatr., 91:138, 1977.
10. Pennisi, A.F., et al.: Minoxidil therapy in children with severe hypertension. J. Pediatr., 90:813, 1977.
11. Makker, S.P.: Minoxidil in refractory hypertension. J. Pediatr., 86:621, 1975.
12. Makker, S.P., and Moorthy, B.: Rebound hypertension following minoxidil withdrawal. J. Pediatr., 96:762, 1980.
13. Chatterjee, K., et al · Combination vasodilator therapy for severe chronic congestive heart failure. Ann. Intern. Med., 85:467, 1976.
14. McKay, C., et al.: Improved cardiac performance by minoxidil in severe chronic congestive heart failure. (Abstract.) Circulation, 62:232, 1980.
15. Franciosa, J.A., and Cohn, J.N.: Hemodynamic effects of minoxidil in patients with left ventricular failure. Circulation, 60:231, 1979.
16. McKay, C.R., et al.: Minoxidil therapy in chronic congestive heart failure: acute plus long-term hemodynamic and clinical study. Am. Heart J., 104:575, 1982.
17. Nathan, M., et al.: Effects of acute and chronic minoxidil administration on rest and exercise hemodynamics and clinical status in patients with severe, chronic heart failure. Am. J. Cardiol., 50:960, 1982.
18. Franciosa, J.A., and Cohn, J.N.: Effects of minoxidil on hemodynamics in patients with congestive heart failure. Circulation, 63:652, 1981.
19. Packer, M., et al.: Sustained effectiveness of minoxidil in heart failure after development of tolerance to other vasodilator drugs. Am. J. Cardiol., 48:375, 1981.
20. Leddy, C.L., et al.: Sustained hemodynamic efficacy of minoxidil during long-term administration in chronic heart failure. ACC 1983.
21. Stein, L.: Randomized comparison of minoxidil and hydralazine in severe chronic congestive heart failure. ACC 1983.
22. Markham, R.V., Jr., et al.: Central and regional hemodynamic effects and neurohumoral consequences of minoxidil in severe congestive heart failure and comparison to hydralazine and nitroprusside. Am. J. Cardiol., 52:774, 1983.
23. Zins, G.R.: Alterations in renal function during vasodilator therapy. In Recent Advances in Renal Physiology and Pharmacology. Edited by L. G. Wesson and G. M. Fanelli. Baltimore, University Park Press, 1974, p. 165.

24. Gottlieb, T.B., et al.: Combined therapy with vasodilator drugs and beta-adrenergic blockade in hypertension: a comparative study of minoxidil and hydralazine. Circulation, 45:571, 1972.
25. Gottlieb, T.B., et al.: Pharmacokinetic studies of minoxidil. Clin. Pharmacol. Ther., 13:436, 1972.
26. Bennett, W.M.: Pericardial effusions associated with minoxidil. Lancet, 2:1356, 1977.
27. Connor, G., et al.: Double-blind comparison of minoxidil and hydralazine in severe hypertension. Clin. Sci. Mol. Med., 51(Suppl. 3):593, 1976.
28. Schacht, R.A., et al.: Severe hypertension in chronic renal failure treated successfully with minoxidil. Proc. Eur. Dial. Transplant. Assoc., 11:229, 1975.
29. Svahn, D.S.: Minoxidil and cardiac enlargement. JAMA, 240:1713, 1978.
30. Zacest, R., et al.: Clinical and haemodynamic effects of minoxidil in refractory hypertension. Drugs, 11(Suppl.):177, 1976.
31. Marques-Julio, A., et al.: Minoxidil in refractory hypertension: benefits, risks. Proc. Eur. Dial. Transplant. Assoc., 14:501, 1977.
32. Reichgott, M.: Minoxidil and pericardial effusion: an idiosyncratic reaction. Clin. Pharmacol. Ther., 30:64, 1981.
33. Martin, W.B., et al.: Pericardial disorders occurring during open label study of 1,869 severely hypertensive patients treated with minoxidil. J. Cardiovasc. Pharmacol., 2(Suppl. 2):S217, 1980.
34. Sobota, J.T., et al.: Minoxidil: right atrial cardiac pathology in animals and in man. Circulation, 62:376, 1980.
35. Eahart, R.N., et al.: Minoxidil induced hypertrichosis: treatment with calcium thioglycollate depilatory. South. Med. J., 70:442, 1977.
36. Campese, V.M., et al.: Treatment of severe hypertension with minoxidil: advantages and limitations. J. Clin. Pharmacol., 19:231, 1979.
37. Wilburn, R.L., et al.: Long term treatment of severe hypertension with minoxidil, propranolol and furosemide. Circulation, 52:706, 1975.

Chapter 13

Diazoxide

Diazoxide is a potent vasodilator used in the treatment of systemic and pulmonary hypertension. It is thought to act directly on vascular smooth muscle to decrease peripheral vascular resistance. The drug has no diuretic effect. It is used mainly intravenously, to treat patients with severe hypertension or hypertensive emergencies requiring rapid lowering of blood pressure. The most important use of diazoxide is in the rapid elimination of severe hypertension in hypertensive crisis. The drug has also been evaluated for use in congestive heart failure. Diazoxide has the dual advantages of a rapid onset and a long duration of action. Its use is limited by serious side effects, however, including hyperglycemia.

Structure

Diazoxide is a benzothiadiazine derivative. It is 7-chloro-1,2,4-benzothiadiazine-3-methyl-1,1-dioxide.

Pharmacologic Properties

Diazoxide is a potent direct vasodilator. Its effect is considered by most investigators to be independent of the autonomic nervous system.[1] Diazoxide is primarily a direct-acting vasodilator, but alpha-adrenergic blockade or beta-adrenergic stimulation may play a role in this effect.[2,3] Diazoxide may also inhibit the calcium current.

Hemodynamic Effects

Effects on Systemic Hypertension

Diazoxide is a potent antihypertensive agent, administered primarily by the intravenous route, for treatment of hypertensive emergencies. In several studies in adults, a dose of 300 mg or 5 mg/kg rapidly reduced severe hypertension.[4-6] This effect has also been confirmed in studies of severe essential and renal hypertension in children.[5,7] The reduction of blood pressure persists for up to 4 hours. The reductions in blood pressure produced by diazoxide are usually marked. For example, in the first clinical study of diazoxide, the drug, 2 mg/kg, reduced mean arterial pressure by 19 mm Hg.[8] In another study, diazoxide, 150 mg, lowered diastolic blood pressure of hypertensive patients by an average of greater than 30 mm Hg.[9]

Boerth and Long reported that, in 16 children aged 10 months to 13 years, diazoxide, 3 mg/kg, lowered diastolic blood pressure by an average of 30 mm Hg.[10] Diazoxide was effective, in combination with other antihypertensive agents, in a case of neonatal hypertension complicating umbilical artery catheterization.[11]

Tachycardia secondary to diazoxide-induced vasodilation is an important complication of this drug. Beta-blockade before administration of diazoxide effectively prevents the increase in heart rate, however.[12]

Diazoxide lowers arterial pressure by reducing peripheral vascular resistance. Cardiac output and stroke volume are usually increased. The coronary renal and splanchnic blood flow is increased.[13] Myocardial contractility, measured by left ventricular dP/dt, and right atrial pressure are usually increased by diazoxide.

Despite its structural relation to chlorothiazide, diazoxide has no diuretic effect. On the contrary, prolonged treatment with diazoxide may be associated with salt and water retention. This effect may result from compensatory mechanisms common to most vasodilators, including stimulation of renin secretion, which results in elevation of plasma renin activity.[14]

Effects on Primary Pulmonary Hypertension

Primary pulmonary hypertension is a disease of unknown cause, predominantly occurring in young women. No specific agent has been found to be effective in the long-term treatment of this condition. Klinke and Gilbert reported the case of a 19-year-old woman with primary pulmonary hypertension in whom injection of diazoxide into the pulmonary artery at the time of cardiac catheterization decreased pulmonary artery pressure and resistance and increased cardiac output; the patient subsequently received oral diazoxide and was followed for 6 months, with complete resolution of her symptoms (fatigue and dyspnea on effort).[15]

Diazoxide appears to act in primary pulmonary hypertension by direct pulmonary vasodilation, causing a secondary increase in cardiac output. That diazoxide increased the left ventricular stroke work index in the case reported by Klinke and Gilbert suggests a possible positive inotropic effect of this drug.[15]

Effects on Congestive Heart Failure

Like other vasodilators, diazoxide may be of value in the treatment of congestive heart failure. Massie and co-workers evaluated the effect of diazoxide in 9 patients with congestive heart failure refractory to conventional treatment and to other vasodilators.[16] At intravenous doses of 450 to 900 mg, diazoxide reduced systemic vascular resistance by up to 44%. Arterial pressure was not much altered, but the cardiac index rose by 64%, and the stroke volume index rose by 49%. These effects occurred rapidly. Pulmonary capillary wedge pressure declined more gradually, by a mean of 8 mm Hg. The hemodynamic improvement was sustained for about 10 hours. These findings indicate that intravenous diazoxide may be useful in the treatment of acute heart failure. To the best of my knowledge, no study of the use of oral diazoxide in congestive heart failure has been published.

Clinical Pharmacology

Diazoxide may be administered either intravenously or orally. The intravenous dose is given as a rapid injection because about 90% of the drug is bound to plasma proteins and the effect must be achieved before this binding occurs.[17, 18] Two studies showed, however, that administration of the drug over 10 or 30 minutes yielded results similar to those seen with administration of the drug over 10 and 30 seconds, respectively.[19, 20] The antihypertensive effect of diazoxide becomes evident soon after intravenous administration. Following oral administration, several days may pass before the maximal effect becomes evident. The reduction in blood pressure is dose-related.[10] The response to diazoxide varies from patient to patient.[21, 22]

Side Effects

Like other potent direct-acting vasodilators, diazoxide may cause tachycardia, palpitations, hypertension, and aggravation of myocardial ischemia. An important adverse effect of diazoxide is hyperglycemia. This effect, which limits the use of diazoxide to short-term treatment, may be prevented by propranolol administration.[23]

Dosage and Administration

Intravenous Administration

Currently, it is recommended to give diazoxide as a rapid intravenous injection of 5 mg/kg.[24, 25] This dosage is used in adults as well as in children.[5, 7] Lower doses may be effective, however, and it has been suggested that the dose be titrated in the range of 2 to 7.5 mg/kg. In children, the dose may be given in several repeated injections.[10] Slower infusions are also effective in adults and are probably safer than a rapid injection.[26]

Oral Administration

Doses of 5 mg/kg daily are given.

References

1. Rubin, A.A., et al.: Pharmacology of diazoxide, an antihypertensive, nondiuretic benzothiadiazine. J. Pharmacol. Exp. Ther., 136:344, 1962.
2. Dhazmana, K.M., et al: Peripheral cardiovascular effects, in the pithed rat, of compounds used in the treatment of hypertension. Br. J. Pharmacol., 46:508, 1972.
3. Taylor, J., and Green, R.D.: Evidence of an antagonistic action of diazoxide at alpha-adrenergic receptors in rabbit aorta. Eur. J. Pharmacol., 12:385, 1970.
4. Finnerty, F.A., Jr., et al.: Hypertensive vascular disease: the long-term effect of rapid repeated reductions of arterial pressure with diazoxide. Am. J. Cardiol., 29:377, 1967.
5. McLaine, P.N., and Drummond, K.N.: Intravenous diazoxide for severe hypertension in childhood. J. Pediatr., 79:829, 1971.
6. Mroczek, W.J., et al.: The importance of the rapid administration of diazoxide in accelerated hypertension. N. Engl. J. Med., 285:603, 1971.
7. Kohaut, E.C., et al.: Intravenous diazoxide in acute post-streptococcal glomerulonephritis. J. Pediatr., 87:795, 1975.
8. Kakaviatos, N., and Finnerty, F.A., Jr.: Preliminary observations on the value of diazoxide administered intravenously in man. Angiology, 13:541, 1962.
9. Miller, W.E., et al.: Management of severe hypertension with intravenous injections of diazoxide. Am. J. Cardiol., 24:870, 1969.
10. Boerth, R.C., and Long, W.R.: Dose-response relation of diazoxide in children with hypertension. Circulation, 56:1066, 1977.
11. Bauer, S.B., et al.: Neonatal hypertension: a complication of umbilical-artery catheterization. N. Engl. J. Med., 292:1032, 1975.
12. Huysmans, F.T.M., et al.: Combined intravenous administration of diazoxide and beta-blocking agent in acute treatment of severe hypertension or hypertensive crisis. Am. Heart J., 103:395, 1982.
13. Nayler, W.G., et al.: Some effects of the hypotensive drug, diazoxide, on the cardiovascular system. Am. Heart J., 75:223, 1968.
14. Vandongen, R., and Greenwood, D.M.: The stimulation of renin secretion by diazoxide in the isolated rat kidney. Eur. J. Pharmacol., 33:197, 1975.
15. Klinke, W.P., and Gilbert, M.B.: Diazoxide in primary pulmonary hypertension. N. Engl. J. Med., 302:91, 1980.
16. Massie, B.M., et al.: Beneficial hemodynamic effects of intravenous diazoxide in refractory congestive heart failure. Am. Heart J., 104:581, 1982.
17. Sellers, E.M., and Koch-Wesser, J.: Protein binding and vascular activity of diazoxide. N. Engl. J. Med., 281:1141, 1969.
18. Sellers, E.M., and Koch-Weser, J.: Influence of intravenous injection rate on protein binding and vascular activity of diazoxide. Ann. N.Y. Acad. Sci., 226:319, 1973.
19. Johnson, B.F., and Kapur, M.: The influences of rate of injection upon the effects of diazoxide. Am. J. Med. Sci., 263:481, 1972.
20. Crout, J.R., et al: Intravenous diazoxide in hypertension. (Abstract.) Clin. Res., 18:337, 1970.
21. Lockwood, C.H., et al.: Diazoxide therapy in hypertension. Am. J. Med. Sci., 246:312, 1963.
22. Johnson, B.F.: Diazoxide and renal function in man. Clin. Pharmacol. Ther., 12:815, 1971.
23. Sponer, G., et al.: Effect of beta-adrenoceptor blockade on the cardiovascular and hyperglycemic actions of diazoxide. Naunyn Schmiedebergs Arch. Pharmacol., 303:15, 1978.
24. Koch-Weser, J.: Diazoxide. N. Engl. J. Med., 294:1271, 1976.
25. Drug Commentary, Department of Drugs: Evaluation of diazoxide (Hyperstat I.V.). JAMA, 224:1422, 1973.
26. Garrett, B.N., and Kaplan, N.M.: Efficacy of slow infusion of diazoxide in the treatment of severe hypertension without organ hypoperfusion. Am. Heart J., 103:390, 1982.

ALPHA-ADRENORECEPTOR BLOCKING AGENTS

Chapter 14

Prazosin

Prazosin is a peripheral alpha-adrenoreceptor blocker, affecting mainly postsynaptic alpha-1-adrenoreceptors in the walls of blood vessels. The drug is a balanced vasodilator; it affects the arterial and venous vascular beds to the same extent. As with other modern alpha-adrenoreceptor blockers, prolonged treatment with prazosin is associated with no or minimal changes in heart rate, plasma catecholamine levels, and plasma renin activity. In adults, prazosin has been used primarily to treat systemic hypertension.

The experience with prazosin in children is limited. The cases of a few children with congestive heart failure who were successfully treated with prazosin have been reported. My colleagues and I have limited experience with prazosin in hypertension in adolescents and young adults. Prazosin has an important advantage in children because orally administered prazosin has a hemodynamic profile similar to intravenously administered nitroprusside, one of the few vasodilators widely used in infants and children.

Structure

Prazosin is a quinazoline derivative.[1]

Pharmacologic Properties

The most important effect of prazosin is competitive inhibition of postsynaptic alpha-1-adrenoreceptors. The drug has a high affinity for these receptors, but because its selectivity is relative, it may also inhibit alpha-2-adrenoreceptors, presynaptic as well as postsynaptic.[2] Alpha-1-adrenoreceptor blockade in vascular walls is the most important mechanism of prazosin-induced peripheral vasodilation. Prazosin is also a phosphodiesterase inhibitor.[3]

Hemodynamic Effects

Effects on Normal Circulation

In animal experiments, prazosin produced a peripheral and coronary vasodilatory effect and decreased arterial pressure, peripheral resistance, and left ventricular dimensions. In limited studies performed in healthy human subjects, prazosin dilated capacitance vessels and relaxed sympathetically mediated, peripheral venoconstriction.[4]

Effects on Congestive Heart Failure

Almost all studies of the effect of prazosin in congestive heart failure have been performed in adults. In patients with congestive heart failure, prazosin decreased peripheral vascular resistance by up to 50%. Smaller decreases were observed in mean systemic arterial pressure, right atrial pressure, left ventricular filling pressure, and pulmonary vascular resistance. Heart rate was not altered, was slightly increased because of sympathetic activation, or was slightly decreased as a result of overall hemodynamic improvement. Cardiac output and ejection fraction were increased by 10 to 30%. This hemodynamic improvement was evident at rest as well as during exercise.[5-7] In several studies, however, the hemodynamic improvement was greater during exercise or was evident only during exercise.[8-10] This phenomenon may result from inhibition of greater sympathetic tone during exercise. The hemodynamic response to prazosin varied widely among patients with congestive heart failure. Hemodynamic improvement was usually associated with clinical improvement.

A triphasic response to the effect of prazosin was described by Awan and colleagues, as follows: (1) acute hemodynamic response after initiation of treatment; (2) early attenuation of the effect after several doses; and (3) enhancement of the effect to the initial level in about two-thirds of patients and late development of tolerance to the hemodynamic and clinical effect in the remaining third.[11] The early attenuation of response results from activation of compensatory mechanisms common to all vasodilators. Late tolerance may result from inhibition of presynaptic alpha-2-adrenoreceptors and may increase the release of plasma norepinephrine. Another explanation is activation of the renin-angiotensin system.

Effects in Children. Dillon and associates reported five children with severe congestive heart failure who were treated with intravenous nitroprusside.[12] Four of these patients had a favorable initial response, and nitroprusside was replaced by orally administered prazosin. Another child with severe congestive heart failure who did not receive nitroprusside was also treated with prazosin. All five children also received digoxin and diuretics. During continued treatment, two of the children became entirely asymptomatic, one child showed marked symptomatic improvement, and another showed minimal symptomatic improvement. These authors concluded that "afterload reduction may be life-saving in children who are virtually moribund because of congestive heart failure."[12] In reaching this conclusion, however, these investigators failed to take into account that prazosin is a balanced vasodilator with an effect on the venous circulation. I believe that the beneficial effect of prazosin in children with congestive heart failure results from the drug's combined arteriolodilatory and venodilatory properties.

Vasodilators should not be used in patients with severe, fixed, left ventricular outflow obstruction. Therefore, I advise against administering prazosin to infants and children with congestive heart failure associated with severe valvar aortic stenosis or discrete subaortic stenosis.

Prazosin has an important advantage in children because it resembles nitroprusside in its hemodynamic effects, but unlike nitroprusside, prazosin may be administered orally. Nitroprusside is one of the most widely used vasodilators in cardiovascular medicine. The ability to initiate treatment with intravenous nitroprusside and to continue it with oral prazosin, which has the same effect, is an important advantage.

Comparison with Hydralazine. The effect of prazosin is comparable to that of hydralazine in patients with congestive heart failure.[13, 14] Because prazosin is a balanced vasodilator and hydralazine is mainly an arteriolar dilator, prazosin may be superior to hydralazine in patients with congestive heart failure whose predominant symptoms are of elevated left ventricular filling pressure. Hydralazine has been effective in some patients with congestive heart failure resistant to prazosin.[15]

Effects in Valvar Diseases

Prazosin has produced hemodynamic improvement in patients with aortic or mitral insufficiency and congestive heart failure. The results of hemodynamic studies are controversial, however. For example, Jebavy and co-workers reported that, in 17 patients with aortic insufficiency, prazosin reduced left ventricular filling pressure and regurgitant flow and did not produce significant changes in heart rate, cardiac output, and myocardial contractility.[16] These findings indicate that the predominant effect of prazosin in aortic insufficiency is preload reduction due to peripheral venodilation. On the other hand, Hockings and associates reported that, in 8 patients with aortic insufficiency and congestive heart failure, prazosin increased cardiac output and decreased systemic vascular resistance to a greater extent than it decreased left ventricular filling pressure.[17] These findings indicate that prazosin acts mainly by afterload reduction because of a decrease in peripheral vascular resistance. In patients with mitral insufficiency, prazosin decreases both afterload and preload.[18]

Effects on Hypertension

Prazosin effectively lowers elevated systemic arterial pressure. This effect results from peripheral arteriolar dilation (reduction in systemic vascular resistance) and possibly also from a decrease in cardiac output caused by venodilation.[19, 20] Because the increase in heart rate produced by prazosin in hypertensive patients is less than that produced by the classic, nonselective alpha-adrenoreceptor blocking agents, prazosin is clinically useful. Certain hypertensive patients may develop tachycardia during treatment with prazosin, however.[21] In most hypertensive patients in one study, prazosin did not alter cardiac output at rest, but increased it during exercise.[20]

Many clinical studies have confirmed the antihypertensive efficacy of prazosin, either alone or in combination with other antihypertensive agents.[22-25] Prazosin is usually combined with a diuretic or a beta-adrenoreceptor blocking agent. About 50% of the patients studied responded to prazosin monotherapy. The maximum effect was observed during the first week of treatment or was delayed for up to 8 weeks after the initiation of treatment. The antihypertensive effect was sustained throughout prolonged therapy in the majority of these patients.

No cases of hypertensive children treated with prazosin have been reported. My colleagues and I studied 2 male patients aged 17 years, in whom essential hypertension was found during a routine evaluation prior to military service. In one patient, prazosin was added to a regimen including a diuretic agent and methyldopa. In the other patient, prazosin was used alone, at a dose of 1 mg 3 times daily. Blood pressure was adequately controlled in both patients.

Prazosin is also effective and well tolerated in hypertensive patients with impaired renal function.[26, 27]

Effect on Pulmonary Function

Prazosin does not impair pulmonary function and may even cause bronchodilation, owing to blockade of alpha-adrenoreceptors in the pulmonary airways. Therefore, prazosin is safer than beta-blocking agents in hypertensive patients with bronchospastic diseases.

Effect on Plasma Lipid Levels

When young hypertensive patients are treated for many years to reduce the cardiovascular complications of hypertension, such treatment should not adversely affect other cardiovascular risk factors. Several beta-adrenoreceptor blockers and diuretic agents used to treat hypertension produce adverse changes in plasma lipids, including a decrease in the level of high-density lipoprotein (HDL) cholesterol or in the ratio of HDL to low-density lipoprotein (LDL) cholesterol and an increase in LDL cholesterol or plasma triglyceride levels. This lipid profile is associated with an increased risk for coronary atherosclerosis.

In several small studies, prazosin either did not produce these changes or brought about opposite changes in plasma lipids; the result was a more favorable lipid profile.[21, 28] It is yet to be confirmed whether these reported changes are also valid for children.

Discontinuance of the Drug

No rebound phenomena have been observed after discontinuance of prazosin in adults. We recommend, however, that if the drug must be discontinued, the process should be gradual.

Clinical Pharmacology

Prazosin is well, although not completely, absorbed from the gastrointestinal tract after oral administration. Maximal plasma levels are achieved within 1 to 3 hours.[29] Systemic bioavailability of prazosin is 43 to 83%, because of incomplete absorption as well as first-pass hepatic metabolism.[30, 31] Prazosin is rapidly distributed in the body, with maximal concentrations in the heart, blood vessels, and lungs.[32] Maximal plasma concentrations of prazosin range between 3 and 40 ng/ml.[31, 33] The volume of distribution of prazosin is 0.5 to 1.0 L/kg. More than 90% of prazosin in the plasma is protein-bound, mainly to alpha-1-acid glycoprotein.[31] Protein binding is decreased in patients with congestive heart failure, renal failure, or severe hepatic diseases.

Less than 10% of the absorbed amount of prazosin is excreted unchanged in the urine. The predominant route of elimination is hepatic metabolism.[30, 31] The metabolites of prazosin have some antihypertensive activity. The elimination half-life of prazosin is about 2 to 3 hours;[30, 31, 34] total clearance occurs at a rate of approximately 0.14 L/hour/kg.

Side Effects

The initiation of treatment with prazosin may be complicated in a few patients by syncope or hypotension, the "first-dose effect." Except for this serious side effect, prazosin is well tolerated.

Excessive decrease of arterial pressure may occur in up to 10% of hypertensive patients during initiation of treatment with prazosin. About 10% develop dizziness, the most common adverse effect of prazosin. The Veterans Administration Cooperative Study Group on Antihypertensive Agents reported that 48% of patients developed orthostatic dizziness.[35] Most of these patients were concomitantly receiving other antihypertensive agents, however.

Syncope may occur within 30 to 90 minutes of oral administration of the first dose of prazosin. Postural symptoms occur primarily in patients with sodium or volume depletion or in those concomitantly treated with beta-adrenoreceptor blockers.[36-38] To minimize the first-dose effect, one should start treatment while the patient is hospitalized and at low doses initially.

Other, less-common side effects include headache, nausea, palpitations, sedation and other central nervous system effects, blurred vision, dry mouth, constipation, diarrhea, and cutaneous and genitourinary symptoms.

Dosage and Administration

Dillon and colleagues used oral doses of 14 to 25 µg/kg every 6 hours in infants and children with congestive heart failure.[12] My colleagues and I administered doses of 1 mg 3 times daily to 17-year-old hypertensive patients.

References

1. Constantine, J.W.: Analysis of the hypotensive action of prazosin. In Prazosin: Evaluation of a New Antihypertensive Drug. Edited by D.W.K. Cotton. Amsterdam, Excerpta Medica, 1974, p. 16.
2. Chatterjee, K., et al.: Beneficial effects of vasodilator agents in severe mitral regurgitation due to dysfunction of subvalvar apparatus. Circulation, 48:684, 1973.
3. Hess, H.J.: Biochemistry and structure-activity studies with prazosin. In Prazosin: Evaluation of a New Antihypertensive Drug. Edited by D.W.K. Cotton. Amsterdam, Excerpta Medica, 1974, p. 4.
4. Schapel, G.J., and Betts, W.H.: The effect of a single oral dose of prazosin on venous reflex response, blood pressure and pulse rate in normal volunteers. Br. J. Clin. Pharmacol., 12:873, 1981.
5. Awan, N.A., et al.: Prazosin—an oral nitroprusside: demonstration of similar peripheral circulatory actions on systemic resistance and capacitance beds with marked hemodynamic improvement in severe chronic congestive heart failure patients. (Abstract.) Circulation, 56 (Suppl. 2):865, 1977.
6. Awan, N.A., Miller, R.R., and DeMaria, A.N.: Efficacy of ambulatory systemic vasodilator therapy with oral prazosin in chronic refractory heart failure. Circulation, 56:346, 1977.
7. Awan, N.A., et al.: Clinical pharmacologic and therapeutic application of prazosin in acute and chronic refractory congestive heart failure. Am. J. Med., 65:146, 1978.
8. Parmley, W.W., et al.: Hemodynamic effects of prazosin in chronic heart failure. Am. Heart J., 102:622, 1981.
9. Chatterjee, K., et al.: Influence of oral prazosin therapy on exercise hemodynamics in patients with severe chronic heart failure. Am. J. Med., 71:140, 1981.
10. Goldman, S.A., et al.: Improved exercise ejection fraction with long-term prazosin therapy in patients with heart failure. Am. J. Med., 68:36, 1980.
11. Awan, N.A., et al.: Management of refractory congestive heart failure with prazosin. Am. Heart J., 102:626, 1981.
12. Dillon, T.R., et al.: Vasodilator therapy for congestive heart failure. J. Pediatr., 96:623, 1980.
13. Mehta, J., et al.: Comparison of haemodynamic effects of oral prazosin, oral hydralazine and intravenous nitroprusside in some patients with chronic heart failure. Br. Heart J., 42:664, 1979.

14. Magorien, R.D., et al.: Prazosin and hydralazine in congestive heart failure. Ann. Intern. Med., 95:5, 1981.
15. Packer, M., et al.: Hemodynamic and clinical tachyphylaxis to prazosin-mediated afterload reduction in severe chronic congestive heart failure. Circulation, 59:531, 1979.
16. Jebavy, P., Koudelkova, E., and Henzlova, M.: Unloading effects of prazosin in patients with chronic aortic regurgitation. Am. Heart J., 105:567, 1983.
17. Hockings, B.E.F., et al.: Comparison of vasodilator drug prazosin with digoxin in aortic regurgitation. Br. Heart J., 43:550, 1980.
18. Mehta, J., et al.: Acute haemodynamic effects of oral prazosin in severe mitral regurgitation. Br. Heart J., 43:556, 1980.
19. Mulvihill-Wilson, J., et al.: Hemodynamic and neuroendocrine responses to acute and chronic alpha-adrenergic blockade with prazosin and phenoxybenzamine. Circulation, 65:383, 1983.
20. Lund-Johansen, P.: Hemodynamic changes at rest and during exercise in longterm prazosin therapy for essential hypertension. Postgrad. Med. J., 45:31, 1975.
21. Rubin, P.C., and Baschke, T.F.: Studies on the clinical pharmacology of prazosin. I. Cardiovascular, catecholamine and endocrine changes following a single dose. Br. J. Clin. Pharmacol., 10:23, 1980.
22. Marshall, A.J., et al.: Evaluation of beta blockade, bendrofluazide, and prazosin in severe hypertension. Lancet, 1:271, 1977.
23. Fauchald, P., Helgeland, A., and Storm-Mathisen, H.: Behandling av hoyt blodtrykk med prazosin (Peripress). Tidsskr. Nor. Laegeforen., 98:1494, 1978.
24. Mroczek, W.J., et al.: Prazosin hypertension: a double-blind evaluation with methyldopa and placebo. Curr. Ther. Res., 16:769, 1974.
25. Brogden, R.N., et al.: Prazosin: a review of its pharmacological properties and therapeutic efficacy in hypertension. Drugs, 14:163, 1979.
26. Harter, H.R., Tindira, C., and Delmez, J.A.: Blood pressure control in hemodialysis patients: the long-term effects of prazosin. J. Cardiovasc. Med., (Suppl.):49, 1981.
27. Baciarello, G., et al.: Efficacy of prazosin in therapy of arterial hypertension of chronic uremic patients undergoing dialysis treatment: 6-month follow-up. Curr. Ther. Res., 28:326, 1980.
28. Velasco, M., et al.: Effect of prazosin on blood lipids and on thyroid function in hypertensive patients. J. Cardiovasc. Pharmacol., 4 (Suppl. 2):S225, 1982.
29. Letcher, R.L., Chien, S., and Laragh, J.H.: Changes in blood viscosity accompanying the response to prazosin in patients with essential hypertension. J. Cardiovasc. Pharmacol., 1 (Suppl.):S8, 1979.
30. Bateman, D.N., et al.: Prazosin, pharmacokinetics and concentration effect. Eur. J. Clin. Pharmacol., 16:177, 1979.
31. Graham, A., et al.: Prazosin kinetics in hypertension. Clin. Pharmacol. Ther., 30:439, 1981.
32. Taylor, A., et al.: Antagonism of cardiac chronotropic responses to endogenous and exogenous catecholamine agonists by prazosin in the dog. Clin. Res., 27:105, 1979.
33. Hobbs, D.C., Twomey, T.M., and Palmer, R.V.: Pharmacokinetics of prazosin in man. J. Clin. Pharmacol., 18:402, 1978.
34. Rubin, P.C., Scott, J.W., and Reid, J.L.: Prazosin disposition in young and elderly subjects. Br. J. Clin. Pharmacol., 12:401, 1981.
35. Veterans Administration Co-operative Study Group on Antihypertensive Agents: Comparison of prazosin with hydralazine in patients receiving hydrochlorothiazide: a randomized, double-blind clinical trial. Circulation, 64:772, 1981.
36. Graham, R.M., et al.: A controlled study in hypertensive patients of the first dose phenomenon observed with prazosin therapy. Aust. N. Z. J. Med., 7:211, 1977.
37. Brogden, R.N., et al.: Prazosin: a review of its pharmacological properties and therapeutic efficacy in hypertension. Drugs, 14:163, 1979.
38. Elliott, H.L., et al.: Immediate cardiovascular responses to oral prazosin effects of concurrent β-blockers. Clin. Pharmacol. Ther., 29:303, 1981.

Chapter 15

Tolazoline

Tolazoline is an alpha-adrenoreceptor blocking agent. Its only use in cardiovascular medicine today is for treatment of neonatal hypoxemia. Even for this indication, the role of tolazoline remains controversial.

Effects on Neonatal Hypoxemia

Severe neonatal hypoxemia with pulmonary vasoconstriction may impair cardiac function, even in the presence of a structurally normal heart. Neonates with this disease may be thought to have a cyanotic congenital heart disease. Tolazoline has been tried in patients with this disease, in an attempt to improve the condition by relief of pulmonary vasoconstriction and afterload reduction.

The efficacy and safety of this mode of treatment are controversial. For example, Sandor and co-workers reported that 79% of 29 hypoxic neonates studied showed marked improvement during tolazoline infusion.[1] Right ventricular function, which had been impaired, was improved by tolazoline, as evaluated by measurements of systolic time intervals. Left ventricular function was also improved, although to a lesser extent than right ventricular function. A favorable clinical response, defined as a rise in Pa_{O_2} of more than 20 mm Hg, was obtained in 23 of the patients. Twenty of these patients were weaned from the respirator, and 3 died. Six patients did not respond initially, and 4 of them died. Failure to respond to tolazoline or to be weaned from the respirator was usually associated with additional pathologic features. In the neonates with oliguria before treatment, urine output improved during treatment.[1]

Side Effects and Complications

In contrast to these findings several other investigators reported less favorable results or serious complications, including systemic arterial hypotension, impairment of renal function, and hemorrhagic problems.[2-5] Even in the study reported by Sandor and associates, which showed good results, a fall in blood pressure was observed in 19 of 29 patients during tolazoline treatment.[1] True hypotension occurred in 4 of these patients.

Dosage and Administration

Tolazoline is given as an initial intravenous bolus of 1 mg/kg. If no response is noted a greater dose of up to 4 mg/kg may be used. If the response is favorable, repeated bolus injections or a continuous infusion may be given for up to about a week.

References

1. Sandor, G.G.S., et al.: Clinical and echocardiographic evidence suggesting afterload reduction as a mechanism of action of tolazoline in neonatal hypoxemia. Pediatr. Cardiol., 5:93, 1984.
2. Goetzman, B.W., et al.: Neonatal hypoxia and pulmonary vasospasm: response to tolazoline. J. Pediatr., 89:617, 1976.
3. Johnson, G.L., et al.: Echocardiography in hypoxemia neonatal pulmonary disease. J. Pediatr., 96:617, 1980.
4. Levin, D.L., et al.: Persistent pulmonary hypertension of the newborn infant. J. Pediatr., 89:626, 1976.
5. Stevenson, D.K., et al.: Refractory hypoxemia associated with neonatal pulmonary disease: the use and limitations of tolazoline. J. Pediatr., 95:595, 1979.

AGENTS AFFECTING THE RENIN-ANGIOTENSIN SYSTEM

The renin-angiotensin system is one of the homeostatic mechanisms regulating vascular tone and electrolyte balance. In adults, agents affecting this system at various points are used for treatment of systemic hypertension and congestive heart failure. Such agents include angiotensin II competitive antagonists (saralasin), angiotensin-converting-enzyme inhibitors (captopril, enalapril, MK-521), renin inhibitors of the substrate analogue type, and aldosterone antagonists (spironolactone).

Captopril is the most important member of this group that has been studied in children. It is used in infants and children for treatment of severe refractory congestive heart failure, hypertension, or both, and for treatment of refractory pulmonary hypertension. The use of captopril in young age groups is still investigational. Spironolactone has also been used to treat congestive heart failure in infancy and childhood.

Chapter 16

Captopril

Captopril (SQ 14225) is a synthetic, reversible inhibitor of angiotensin-converting enzyme. It may be given intravenously or orally, and it is used in adults mainly for the treatment of congestive heart failure and hypertension. This drug has an important advantage over other vasodilators in that the development of tolerance during long-term treatment is either minimal or absent. Captopril has also been used for treatment of pulmonary hypertension, with limited success. The therapeutic effect of this agent results mainly from peripheral vasodilation, which is balanced; that is, the drug acts similarly on arteries and veins.

The experience with captopril in infants and children is limited to treatment of a small number of hypertensive infants and children and a few infants with severe coarctation of the aorta associated with refractory congestive heart failure and hypertension. The drug has also been evaluated in children with primary pulmonary hypertension.

Structure

Captopril is D-3-mercapto-2-methylpropanoyl-L-proline. It contains a sulfhydryl group that contributes to the affinity of the molecule for the enzyme. Five different interactions are possible between the molecule of captopril and the active site of the converting enzyme.

Unlike the peptide-converting-enzyme inhibitors obtained from snake venom, captopril is not cleared by the enzyme.

Pharmacologic Effects

Captopril inhibits the enzyme that converts angiotensin I to angiotensin II. This enzyme is located mainly in the lungs. As a result of this inhibition, the plasma angiotensin II and aldosterone levels are reduced, and the angiotensin I levels are elevated. To block the renin-angiotensin system effectively, the converting enzyme's activity should be reduced to 10 to 20% of control values. The effect of captopril on plasma prorenin levels is inconsistent. In a study of patients with essential hypertension, it increased the plasma prorenin levels.[1] In a study of patients with renovascular hypertension, captopril initially lowered prorenin levels 30 minutes after oral administration; 4 hours later, however, peripheral prorenin levels rose.[2] This sequence may result from differences in rates of secretion of prorenin and renin from the kidney with renal artery stenosis.

Plasma electrolyte changes occur because of the inhibition of aldosterone release. The plasma sodium level is reduced, whereas the potassium level is elevated. Captopril has also been reported to increase the production of vasodilator prostaglandins and bradykinin, either systemically or locally.[3,4] This phenomenon is further discussed in the section of this chapter on mechanisms of captopril's antihypertensive effect.

The effects of captopril on the renin-angiotensin system were studied by Friedman and Chesney in nine hypertensive children.[5] In all patients, captopril reduced the elevated blood pressure. After treatment with captopril, these patients showed an increase in plasma renin activity and plasma angiotensin I levels, with a concomitant fall in plasma angiotensin II and plasma aldosterone concentrations. Thus, the effects of captopril on the renin-angiotensin system in children are similar to those observed in adults.

Hemodynamic Effects

Effects in Hypertension

The role of captopril in the treatment of severe or refractory hypertension has been established by numerous studies.[6-10] Captopril lowers elevated blood pressure at rest and during exercise in the supine and standing positions. The drug is effective in patients with essential and renovascular hypertension, as well as in those with hypertension associated with coarctation of the aorta, the accurate mechanism of which is not clear. Captopril lowers both systolic and diastolic blood pressures.

Captopril acts directly on the arterial vascular bed and lowers the elevated peripheral vascular resistance. Thus, captopril directly affects the abnormal hemodynamic parameter. Captopril also dilates the venous vascular bed. In hypertensive patients, the alterations in heart rate and cardiac output are not significant.[11-14]

The antihypertensive effect of captopril is sustained throughout long periods of treatment. In a study of adults with severe and refractory essential or renovascular hypertension, the effect of captopril persisted for more than 2 years.[7] In large series of patients with drug-resistant hypertension, captopril controlled blood pressure adequately in about a third of the patients and partially controlled it in another third.[15]

Treatment with captopril has been associated with an increase in plasma creatinine levels in patients with renovascular hypertension.[16] Therefore, renal function should be continuously monitored in patients treated with captopril who have renal artery stenosis. In patients with hypertension of undetermined cause and elevated plasma creatinine levels, renal artery stenosis should be suspected.

During prolonged antihypertensive treatment with captopril, the dose may be reduced without diminishing the initial effect. Several mechanisms may account for this phenomenon, as follows: (1) control of hypertension resulting in a decrease of the arteriolar wall-to-lumen ratio and peripheral resistance;[17] (2) inhibition of converting enzymes in tissues that persists with lower doses of the drug; and (3) accumulation of vasodilating substance such as prostaglandins and bradykinin. The relationship between the effect of captopril and the pretreatment level of plasma renin activity is inconsistent. Several investigators have found a direct correlation between the antihypertensive effect of short-term administration of captopril and the pretreatment level of plasma renin activity.[16,18-20] This correlation has not been observed during long-term administration of the drug.[21]

In several hypertensive patients studied, the following triphasic response to captopril was observed: (1) a favorable initial response; (2) a partial transient attenuation of the initial response during the first week of therapy; and (3) late restoration of the effect by administering higher doses of the drug.[18,22]

Caucasian patients in several studies responded better to captopril than black patients.[10,23] This difference has also been observed with other antihypertensive drugs and has been attributed to impairments of the renin-angiotensin or kallikrein-kinin systems in black patients.

Mechanisms of the Antihypertensive Effect. The most probable mechanism of the antihypertensive effect of captopril is inhibition of the renin-angiotensin system. Inhibition of the formation of angiotensin II prevents the vasoconstricting activity of this agent and the production of aldosterone, which causes salt and fluid retention. This theory is supported by the finding that captopril and other converting-enzyme inhibitors lower elevated blood pressure in patients with high plasma renin activity.[6,16,18] In low or absent renin stages, captopril does not lower blood pressure, and the angiotensin II antagonist saralasin even has a pressor effect. In a group of six children, the reduction of elevated blood pressure was associated with an increase in angiotensin I levels and a decrease in angiotensin II levels.[24] This theory is opposed by the weak correlation between the plasma renin activity and the reduction in blood pressure observed in several studies, however.[25,26]

In ten hypertensive children, no correlation was found between the pretreatment level of plasma renin activity and the magnitude of the blood pressure reduction by captopril.[27] It was also shown that captopril controls blood pressure at doses that do not adequately block circulating angiotensin-converting-enzyme activity.[17] The disparity in intensity and kinetics between plasma-converting-enzyme inhibition and the antihypertensive effect of captopril does not exclude an effect mediated by converting-enzyme inhibition in tissues.

Another mechanism of the antihypertensive effect of captopril is the drug's effect on the kallikrein-kinin system. This local hormonal system participates in the regional regulation of blood flow. Angiotensin-converting enzyme is also kininase II, an enzyme responsible for elimination of the vasodilator agent bradykinin.[3] Accumulation of bradykinin, perhaps not in the plasma but in certain tissues, may play a role in the mechanism of the antihypertensive effect of captopril.

Other possible mechanisms are increased production of vasodilator prostaglandins,[3] impairment of vasoconstriction mediated by the sympathetic nervous system, increased parasympathetic activity, potentiation of the baroreflex, and inhibition of vasopressin.[16, 28-31]

Combination with Other Antihypertensive Drugs. The antihypertensive effect of captopril is enhanced by combination with other drugs. The effect of captopril is especially pronounced in hypertensive patients with high levels of plasma renin activity. Because diuretic agents elevate the levels of plasma renin activity, it is rational to use a combination of captopril and diuretics. The efficacy of this combination has been demonstrated in large series and with various diuretic agents. For example, a Veterans Administration co-operative study revealed that, in a series of 475 patients with mild-to-moderate hypertension, the addition of hydrochlorothiazide enhanced the effect of captopril.[10] The addition of diuretics may be essential to control blood pressure adequately in patients with severe hypertension.

Captopril causes elevation of plasma renin activity. The addition of beta-adrenoreceptor blocking agents can suppress the elevated plasma renin activity and may enhance the antihypertensive effect of captopril.[15] One report notes an additive effect of captopril and prazosin combined. In several children studied, other antihypertensive drugs were required during the first week of treatment with captopril, until the antihypertensive effect of captopril became sustained.[24]

Treatment of Childhood Hypertension. In the past several years, several cases of hypertensive children successfully treated with captopril have been reported. The first case of treatment of malignant hypertension with captopril was reported by Oberfield and co-workers in 1979.[32] This 10-year-old child had blood pressure of 230/170 mm Hg that was resistant to diazoxide, reserpine, and spironolactone. Intravenous nitroprusside lowered the patient's blood pressure to 160/110 mm Hg. The renal arteries were normal, and plasma renin activity was elevated. The child was dependent on intravenous infusion of nitroprusside for control of blood pressure. After a single oral dose of captopril, 12.5 mg, the patient's blood pressure decreased from 160/130 to 140/105 mm Hg. The dose of captopril was increased to 225 mg daily, combined with chlothalidone. This treatment lowered blood pressure to 96/64 mm Hg. This child had a triphasic response to captopril, as seen in adults: an initial response, transient attenuation of the response, and late increase in response. It is possible that the transient attenuation of response results from activation of baroreceptor mechanisms.

Friedman and colleagues reported the cases of 6 children with severe hypertension, resistant to several antihypertensive agents, who responded favorably to captopril.[24] Three of these patients showed the classic triphasic response to captopril, consisting of an immediate response in the first day, followed by a transient attenuation of the effect, and finally an almost complete restoration of the initial effect in 10 to 30 days. The remaining 3 patients did not show an immediate improvement in blood pressure after administration of captopril and required coadministration of diazoxide or hydralazine for the first month. Treatment with captopril was effectively continued for 3 to 16 months. The blood pressure of all these patients was reduced without a change in weight. In 2 of the 6 children in this group, treatment was discontinued for up to a month before reinstitution of therapy became necessary.

Sinaiko and associates studied the efficacy and safety of captopril in 10 young hypertensive patients aged 3.5 to 20 years.[27] The hypertension was secondary in all 10 patients; 4 had renal parenchymal disease, 4 had renal transplant rejection, and 2 had renal artery stenosis. The patients received oral doses of 0.5, 1.0, and 2.0 g captopril. Blood pressure began to fall within 15 minutes of oral administration. No correlation was found between the dose of captopril and the magnitude of the blood pressure reduction. A significant reduction in both systolic and diastolic blood pressure was observed in all patients after a week of treatment, and this reduction was maintained during continuous therapy in 9 of the 10 patients. In 5 of the patients, adequate control was achieved when captopril was combined with hydrochlorothiazide, whereas the other 4 patients required a combination of captopril and other antihypertensive drugs. The pretreatment level of plasma renin activity did not predict the patient's response to captopril.

In conclusion, captopril is an effective agent in hypertensive children. It should usually be combined with diuretic agents and, occasionally, with other antihypertensive agents. The antihypertensive effect of captopril is maintained throughout long periods of treatment.

Treatment of Neonatal Hypertension. The successful use of captopril for treatment of hypertension in newborn infants without coarctation of the aorta was first reported in 1982 by Bifano and co-workers.[33] They reported the cases of three patients, as described in the following paragraphs.

A 1770-g newborn girl with a patent ductus arteriosus and congestive heart failure had intimal aortic dissection involving the left renal artery that was probably caused by an umbilical artery catheter. No blood flow to the left kidney was seen on a nuclear scan. The infant developed hypertension resistant to furosemide, hydralazine, methyldopa, nitroprusside, and propranolol, alone and in combination. The patient's blood pressure was controlled only when captopril, 1.2 mg daily in divided doses over 24 hours, was added to a regimen of hydralazine and furosemide. Following a left nephrectomy on the thirteenth day of hospitalization, the doses of antihypertensive drugs were reduced.[33]

A 3600-g infant girl with cyanotic congenital heart disease developed bilateral renal artery thrombosis and hypertension following the use of an umbilical artery catheter. Captopril therapy was initiated on the sixteenth day of hospitalization. With captopril as the sole antihypertensive agent, at a dose of 1.2 mg every 6 hours, the patient's systolic blood pressure fell from 110 to 90 mm Hg.[33]

A 3020-g infant boy developed right renal artery thrombosis following the use of an umbilical artery catheter. Furosemide, hydralazine, and nitroprusside did not adequately control blood pressure, and propranolol produced excessive bradycardia. An infusion of saralasin showed that the elevated blood pressure was sensitive to converting-enzyme inhibition. Captopril, 2 mg 4 times daily, was initiated and effectively controlled the blood pressure. All these neonates had elevated plasma renin activity ranging from 20 to 39 ng/ml/hour.

An interesting problem has been observed in three other neonates who developed hypertension resistant to several drugs including nitroprusside, diuretics, propranolol, and hydralazine (L.C. Blieden: personal communication). In these neonates, the cause of hypertension was renal artery thrombosis after insertion of an umbilical artery catheter. Captopril effectively controlled the elevated blood pressure. Serial echocardiograms showed a decrease in left ventricular volume, but also progressive left ventricular hypertrophy, which advanced despite the fall in blood pressure.[33] The mechanism and significance of this phenomenon are unknown. The mechanisms of the beneficial effect of captopril in congestive heart failure are probably similar to those of its antihypertensive effect. They are discussed in a previous section of this chapter.

Although captopril is effective and safe in infants, one should restrict its use to short periods because the drug-metabolizing systems of infants are immature, and side effects may occur.

In summary, captopril is effective in infants with severe, refractory hypertension. At present I recommend that the drug be used only in patients whose hypertension is resistant to conventional agents.

Treatment of Refractory Hypertension in Patients with Chronic Renal Failure and Renal Transplantation. Hamilton and Maidment reported the case of a 13-year-old boy with atrial septal defect and severe, crescentic glomerulonephritis who developed malignant hypertension refractory to several antihypertensive agents.[34] Captopril, 100 mg 3 times daily, lowered his blood pressure from 170/125 to 150/95 mm Hg. He died several months later, because of a large left-to-right shunt and congestive heart failure.

These authors also reported the case of a 14-year-old girl who received a renal transplant because of hemolytic uremic syndrome. One year later, she developed blood pressure of 240/180 mm Hg, which was poorly controlled by conventional therapy. Captopril, 50 mg 3 times daily, as the sole antihypertensive therapy, effectively controlled the patient's elevated blood pressure.[34]

Other patients with this condition are included in the series reported by Sinaiko and colleagues,[27] which was discussed earlier in this chapter.

Effects in Pulmonary Hypertension

Pulmonary hypertension in children may be either primary or secondary to various congenital heart diseases. In infants, persistence of the fetal circulation causes pulmonary hypertension.

Because the angiotensin-converting enzyme is present mainly in the endothelial cells of the pulmonary capillaries, and because the conversion of angiotensin I to angiotensin II occurs largely in the lungs, it was initially expected that captopril would be effective in patients with pulmonary hypertension. Captopril was ineffective in lowering elevated pulmonary arterial resistance and pressure, however.[12, 35, 36] In only one case, that of a young male patient with primary pulmonary hypertension, captopril lowered pulmonary arterial resistance and pressure.[37] At present, it is not recommended to administer captopril to children with pulmonary hypertension.

Effects in Congestive Heart Failure

Captopril produces hemodynamic and clinical improvement in patients with congestive heart failure. Captopril may be especially beneficial among the vasodilators in this respect because most patients do not develop tolerance to its effect during treatment for up to several years.[38-46]

The short-term administration of captopril to patients with congestive heart failure causes either no change or a decrease in heart rate, decreases in arterial pressure, systemic vascular resistance, left ventricular end-diastolic pressure, left ventricular volumes, and right atrial pressure, an increase in cardiac output and either an increase or no change in stroke work index. Because systemic resistance, cardiac output, and left ventricular filling pressure are almost comparably altered by up to 40%, captopril may be considered a balanced vasodilator. The reduction in heart rate is observed in adult patients with congestive heart failure, but not in those with hypertension. It is not known whether this difference would be observed in children, whose resting heart rate is higher than that of adults.

The negative inotropic and chronotropic effects of captopril limit the increase in cardiac output evoked by peripheral vasodilation. In one report, captopril reduced the pulmonary vascular resistance in patients with congestive heart failure, but to a lesser extent than it reduced systemic resistance.[47] The hemodynamic improvement was evident both at rest and during exercise. Captopril has also prolonged the exercise duration in patients with congestive heart failure.

Several investigators consider captopril to be free of tolerance. Packer and associates have classified the response to captopril in their experience as follows: (1) an initial hemodynamic improvement observed after the first dose and sustained during prolonged administration in about half the patients; (2) minimal effect initially, with either a slight or no further effect during the next weeks in about 20% of the patients; (3) a triphasic effect, with a marked initial effect, early tolerance after 48 hours, and spontaneous restoration of the effect after several weeks in about 15% of the patients; and (4) a marked initial effect followed by early tolerance that was not reversed during continued therapy in about 15% of the patients.[48] Thus, favorable results were obtained in the majority of adults and were sustained for long periods.

The findings in infants and children have been less satisfactory than in adults. In the experience of my colleagues and myself and in a study of Liebau and colleagues,[38] children with complex congenital heart diseases such as single ventricle and tetralogy of Fallot developed severe hypotension after administration of captopril. Patients of all ages who developed this complication had normal left ventricular function, but high left atrial pressure was needed to supply a sufficient volume load to the left ventricle to maintain cardiac output.[38] Captopril, which lowers left atrial pressure, should not be given to children with this unique hemodynamic condition.

Serum aldosterone levels are higher in infants with congestive heart failure (151 ± 38 mg/dl) than in normal infants (29 ± 7 mg/dl). In one study, increasing serum aldosterone levels were related to increasing plasma renin activity.[49] The response to furosemide was inversely related to the serum aldosterone concentration. Four of the infants in this study improved when treated with the aldosterone-antagonist spironolactone.[49] It is reasonable to assume that captopril may be especially beneficial in infants with congestive heart failure, high plasma renin activity, and high serum aldosterone levels.

Effects in Coarctation of the Aorta

Infants with severe coarctation of the aorta often have combined cardiovascular disease in the first days or week of life. They have rapidly deteriorating left and right congestive heart failure and severe hypertension. The definitive treatment is, of course, surgical resection of the coarctation. The rapid deterioration of the patient's condition, however, may lead to death prior to the surgical procedure and is responsible for high surgical mortality rates. It is preferable to treat congestive heart failure and hypertension preoperatively.

Hypertensive patients with coarctation of the aorta often have high plasma renin activity because hypertension in these patients is probably due to decreased blood flow to the kidneys, with resulting hyperactivity of the renin-angiotensin system. Captopril is theoretically an ideal drug in these patients with combined congestive heart failure and high-renin hypertension.

My colleagues and I have recently studied 2 such infants, resistant to various drugs, who responded favorably to captopril. The first infant developed severe congestive heart failure on the second day of life. He was digitalized and underwent cardiac catheterization at the age of 10 days. Severe coarctation of the aorta distal to the origin of the left subclavian artery was seen. Left ventricular ejection fraction was 0.32; blood pressure after catheterization was 160/80 mm Hg. Treatment with captopril was initiated, at 1 mg/kg/day in 3 divided doses. The patient's blood pressure was lowered to 110/70 mm Hg after the second dose. Repeated cardiac catheterization showed left ventricular ejection fraction of 0.45. Captopril treatment was continued for 5 days, and the clinical signs of congestive heart failure disappeared. The child then successfully underwent surgical treatment.

The second infant in our study was a 5000-g boy who developed congestive heart failure and blood pressure of 160/90 mm Hg. Cardiac catheterization showed severe coarctation of the aorta, ventricular septal defect with left-to-right shunt, and pulmonary hypertension. Captopril administration reduced the elevated blood pressure and alleviated the signs of congestive heart failure within 4 days of treatment.

As a result of the foregoing experience, I conclude that captopril is especially suitable for short-term treatment of combined high-renin hypertension and congestive heart failure in infants with coarctation of the aorta prior to surgical correction.

Severe systemic hypertension may complicate the postoperative course of patients undergoing surgical repair of coarctation of the aorta. This paradoxic phenomenon results from activation of the sympathetic and renin-angiotensin systems. Casta and associates reported that captopril effectively controlled severe hypertension that developed in a 15-year-old boy after successful surgical repair of coarctation of the aorta.[50] The elevated blood pressure in this patient was inadequately controlled by nitroprusside, methyldopa, and propranolol.

Effects in Takayasu's Disease

Takayasu's disease is a complex disorder consisting of characteristic eye changes and arterial lesions, mainly in the aorta and its primary branches. These arterial lesions include narrowing and loss of elasticity that may lead to dilatation. Renovascular hypertension due to acquired coarctation of the aorta or renal artery stenosis is a well-known complication of this disease. Takayasu's disease occurs most commonly in Asian-born, usually young, women. It accounts for about 25% of the cases of renovascular hypertension in Japan.[51] Takayasu's disease may cause also congestive heart failure because lesions of the aortic origin and the aortic valve may result in aortic regurgitation. This disease may also occur in children.

Theoretically, captopril is the ideal agent for treatment of complex Takayasu's disease associated with renovascular hypertension, aortic regurgitation, and congestive heart failure.

In the Sheba Medical Center, Tel Aviv, Israel, four patients with Takayasu's disease and renovascular hypertension, two of them children, were treated with captopril. Three of these cases have previously been reported by Grossman and co-workers.[52]

A 31-year-old woman with normal renal function, hypertension, aortic regurgitation, and right renal artery stenosis developed episodes of pulmonary edema. Captopril, 50 mg daily, controlled both congestive heart failure and hypertension and elevated the patient's plasma renin activity from 43 to 82 ng/ml/hour.

A 23-year-old woman was diagnosed as having hypertension. The patient's blood pressure had been well controlled by various antihypertensive agents for 10 years, but then it became refractory to treatment with hydralazine, diuretics, propranolol, methyldopa, and prazosin. Aortographic examination showed stenosis of the left subclavian artery and occlusion of the right renal artery. Captopril, 300 mg daily, normalized blood pressure for many months of follow-up and increased the plasma renin activity from 4.4 to 10.7 ng/ml/hour.

A 6-year-old male patient with blood pressure of 140/80 mm Hg underwent aortography because his right radial and both femoral pulses were not palpable. Aortographic study showed an aneurysm of the innominate artery and retrograde filling of the right subclavian artery from the right vertebral artery. Narrowing and aneurysmatic dilatation of 2 segments of the descending aorta were also observed. At the age of 11 years, the patient's condition deteriorated, and his blood pressure rose to 230/120 mm Hg. His renal function was normal. Repeated aortographic study showed that the disorder had spread and included bilateral renal artery stenosis. Antihypertensive treatment with propranolol, hydralazine, and diuretics was ineffective. The addition of captopril, 40 mg daily, to this combined regimen resulted in an immediate and sustained normalization of blood pressure. The patient's renal function did not deteriorate. Despite these favorable results, my associates and I failed to control hypertension with captopril in a 10-year-old female patient with Takayasu's disease and left renal artery stenosis. The patient responded only to high doses of minoxidil and propranolol. Nevertheless, it may be concluded from these data that captopril treatment should be tried in hypertensive children and young adults with Takayasu's disease.

Effects on the Coronary Circulation and Myocardial Energetics

Captopril reduces preload and afterload and, as a result, myocardial oxygen consumption. In a study of patients with coronary artery disease, captopril did not alter coronary vascular resistance and slightly decreased coronary blood flow.[53] Of course, excessive reduction of arterial pressure decreases coronary perfusion. Captopril may therefore be used in infants with anomalous origin of the left coronary artery from pulmonary artery and congestive heart failure, provided arterial pressure is not lowered excessively. I am not aware of any such report.

Effect on Renal Function

Captopril consistently increases renal blood flow and sodium excretion and, occasionally, the glomerular filtration rate in patients with congestive heart failure and hypertension.[54-56] In patients with renal artery stenosis, captopril elevates serum creatinine levels.

Effects in Ventricular Septal Defect

Vasodilators may be beneficial in patients with ventricular septal defect. Captopril may be especially helpful because not only is it a vasodilator, but also it has a specific effect on the renin-angiotensin system. Boucek and co-workers studied the role of the renin-angiotensin system and the effect of captopril in lambs with surgically created ventricular septal defect.[56a] In this study, the fasting plasma renin activity was determined prior to and 10 days after the creation of the ventricular septal defect. This activity increased from 2.2 ± 1.0 to 3.9 ± 1.5 ng/ml/hour following creation of the ventricular septal defect. In 7 lambs with a pulmonary-to-systemic flow ratio greater than 3:1, the plasma renin activity increased from 1.8 ± 0.7 to 4.4 ± 1.6 ng/ml/hour. The pulmonary-to-systemic flow ratio correlated with the change in plasma renin activity.[56a]

After administration of captopril, 5 mg/kg, to the foregoing lambs the systemic vascular resistance decreased by 30% and the pulmonary-to-systemic flow ratio decreased by 34%, from 3:5 to 2:3. Captopril, by decreasing pulmonary flow by 19%, was unique among vasodilators. The left atrial pressure fell from 18.8 to 10.6 mm Hg. Boucek and colleagues concluded that plasma renin activity is increased in cases of congestive heart failure associated with ventricular septal defect.[56a] This increase may contribute to the pathophysiologic features of hemodynamic disturbances associated with ventricular septal defect. Inhibition of the renin-angiotensin system by captopril causes partial reversal of hemodynamic abnormalities.

Studies of captopril in human patients with ventricular septal defect have yet to be performed.

Discontinuance of the Drug

Studies of the discontinuance of captopril were made in adults with congestive heart failure; no hemodynamic deterioration was observed for 9 days after discontinuing the drug, but mean arterial pressure was elevated by 10 mm Hg. Discontinuance of captopril for longer periods produced hemodynamic and clinical deterioration.[44] The question whether and when captopril should be discontinued in infants and children undergoing surgical procedures has not yet been answered. Because captopril attenuates the sympathetic activation resulting from hypotension induced by anesthesia, however, excessive hypotension may be an expected effect of anesthesia in children treated with captopril. The effect of discontinuance of captopril before surgical correction of coarctation of the aorta on the development of postoperative paradoxic hypertension is not known.

Clinical Pharmacology

Almost all pharmacokinetic studies of captopril have been performed in adults, usually either healthy volunteers or hypertensive patients. The experience in patients with congestive heart failure is limited.

Captopril may be given intravenously or orally. About 75% of the oral dose is absorbed, and the rate of absorption is rapid. Maximal plasma concentration is achieved within 1 to 1.5 hours of oral administration. A hypotensive effect may be evident within 15 min of oral administration and may become maximal in 1.5 hours.[37, 57-59] Food may interfere with the absorption of captopril.[59] In adults, the drug should be given at least 2 hours after or an hour before a meal. In a study of children, the antihypertensive effect of captopril was evident within 15 min of oral administration and reached a peak within 1.5 hours.[27] Captopril undergoes some first-pass hepatic elimination, and its absolute oral bioavailability is about 60%.

In adults, the drug is widely distributed in almost all body tissues, except the brain. Animal experiments have shown that such may not be the case in infants, however. In fetuses of rats, captopril crossed the blood-brain barrier at the age of 7 days and was found in the brain; this phenomenon results from immaturity of the blood-brain barrier.[60] Captopril may be transferred by breast milk. About 30% of the captopril in the plasma is bound to proteins.[61]

Captopril is rapidly excreted by the kidneys; up to 90% is recovered in the urine within 24 hours. About half the amount in the urine is in the form of the unchanged drug, whereas the remainder is excreted as metabolites.[57] About 25% of the dose is excreted in the feces.[62] The elimination half-life of captopril is 1 to 2 hours.[62, 63] Captopril and its metabolite accumulate in patients with severe renal dysfunction. The drug can be eliminated by hemodialysis.[64]

In a study of hypertensive children with renal dysfunction, the antihypertensive effect of captopril was maintained for up to 10 hours. In 5 children with creatinine clearance between 10 and 21 ml/min/1.73 m^2, the clearance of captopril ranged from 14.1 to 18.8 ml/min/kg.[27] As previously mentioned, captopril is partially metabolized by the liver. The main metabolite is captopril disulfide with glutathione and cysteine.

Side Effects

Treatment with captopril is associated with some serious side effects. These effects were especially evident during the early years of experience with this drug, when high doses were given for treatment of hypertension. Because lower doses are now administered for hypertension and even lower doses are given for congestive heart failure, the incidence of side effects has declined.

Cardiovascular Effects

Severe bradycardia may result from the negative chronotropic effect of captopril, but this reaction is uncommon. The combination of captopril with a beta-blocking agent may be especially deleterious.

Hypotension occurred during dialysis in 2 children treated with captopril; this side effect required a reduction in dosage.[24] Hypotension is especially prevalent in patients with volume depletion because of treatment with diuretics. Severe hypotension may develop in patients with congestive heart failure and serum sodium levels of less than 130 meq/L.[65]

Hematopoietic Depression

Captopril may cause agranulocytosis or neutropenia,[26, 66, 67] although this side effect is rare. Cooper reviewed the world literature and found 38 reports of patients who developed leukopenia, usually neutropenia, during treatment with captopril and no other drug known to cause neutropenia.[67a] The effect almost always occurred during the first 3 months of treatment and was more common in patients with connective tissue diseases or impariment of renal function than in other patients.

Renal Damage

Hypertensive patients, especially those with renovascular hypertension, often have elevated serum creatinine levels during treatment with captopril. An important, but rare, side effect is nephrotic syndrome. About 50 patients who developed proteinuria or in whom proteinuria worsened during treatment with captopril have been reported in the literature; pretreatment renal damage increased the likelihood of proteinuria in these patients.[68-72] No pathognomonic histopathologic renal changes have been observed as a result of treatment with captopril.

Hyperkalemia

Hyperkalemia, a well-known adverse effect of captopril in adults,[15, 72] is uncommon in children. For example, only one of six children reported by Friedman and associates had hyperkalemia during treatment with captopril, and that patient had also had hyperkalemia prior to treatment.[24]

Dysgeusia

Dysgeusia, or loss of taste perception, occurred in about 70% of adults studied who were treated with captopril.[73] It is not known whether this side effect occurs in children as well, but the possibility of feeding difficulties due to captopril-induced dysgeusia should be kept in mind.

Other Side Effects

A rash appears in up to 10% of patients receiving captopril. Angioedema, ulceration of the tongue, abdominal pain, nausea, vomiting, constipation, dry mouth, and dyspnea are uncommon. Eosinophilia and antinuclear antibodies may develop.[73-75]

Drug Interactions

Indomethacin

An interaction of captopril with indomethacin may be important in children. One of the suggested mechanisms for the antihypertensive effect of captopril is impairment of catabolism of bradykinin, a compound that releases vasodilating prostaglandins from various tissues. Indomethacin is an inhibitor of prostaglandin synthesis and may thereby reduce the effect of captopril.[76]

Ibuprofen

Ibuprofen can inhibit the acute hypotensive effect of captopril, probably by a mechanism similar to that of indomethacin.[77]

Dosage and Administration

Doses of 0.1 to 0.4 mg/kg, given 1 to 4 times daily, were used by Bifano and co-workers.[33] My colleagues and I have used 0.3 mg/kg intravenously, 3 times daily, in infants with coarctation.

In children, one should start with 1 mg, increase the dose to 2.5 mg and then to 5 mg at 2-hour intervals, and increase the dose further by 12.5 mg every 8 to 24 hours, until the patient's diastolic blood pressure falls below 105 mm Hg.[24] The final single dose should not exceed 2 mg/kg.

References

1. Glorioso, N., et al.: Active and inactive renin after a single dose of captopril in hypertensive subjects. Am. J. Cardiol., 49:1552, 1982.
2. Derkx, F.H.M., et al.: Asynchronous changes in prorenin and renin secretion after captopril in patients with renal artery stenosis. Hypertension, 5:244, 1983.
3. Swartz, S.L., and Williams, G.H.: Angiotensin-converting enzyme inhibition and prostaglandins. Am. J. Cardiol., 49:1405, 1982.
4. Mookherjee, S., et al.: Acute effects of captopril on cardiopulmonary function, hemodynamics and renin-angiotensin-aldosterone-bradykinin profile in hypertension. Am. Heart. J., 106:106, 1983.
5. Friedman, A.L., and Chesney, R.W.: Effect of captopril on the renin-angiotensin system in hypertensive children. J. Pediatr., 103:806, 1983.
6. Gavras, H., et al.: Antihypertensive effect of oral angiotensin converting-enzyme inhibitor SQ 14225 in man. N. Engl. J. Med., 298:991, 1978.
7. Case, D.B., et al.: Long-term efficacy of captopril in renovascular and essential hypertension. Am. J. Cardiol., 49:1440, 1982.
8. Case, D.B., et al.: Successful acute and chronic treatment of severe and malignant hypertension with oral converting enzyme inhibitor captopril. (Abstract.) Circulation, 59, 60 (Suppl. II):II-130, 1979.
9. Campbell, B.C., Shepher, A.N., and Reid, J.L.: Effects of the angiotensin converting enzyme inhibitor, captopril, in essential hypertension. Br. J. Clin. Pharmacol., 13:213, 1982.

10. Veterans Administration Co-operative Study Group on Antihypertensive Agents: Racial differences in response to low-dose captopril are abolished by the addition of hydrochlorothiazide. Br. J. Clin. Pharmacol., 14:97S, 1982.
11. Fouad, F.M., et al.: Contrasts and similarities of acute hemodynamic responses to specific antagonism of angiotensin II (Sar, Thr, A II) and to inhibition of converting enzyme (captopril). Circulation, 61:163, 1980.
12. Fagard, R., et al.: Response of the systemic and pulmonary circulation to converting-enzyme inhibition (captopril) at rest and during exercise in hypertensive patients. Circulation, 65:33, 1982.
13. Muirhead, E.E., et al.: Anti-hypertensive action of the orally active converting enzyme inhibitor (SQ 14225) in spontaneously hypertensive rats. Circ. Res., 43 (Suppl. 1):1-53, 1978.
14. Cody, R.J., et al.: Hemodynamics of orally active converting enzyme inhibitors (SQ 14225) in hypertensive patients. Clin. Sci. Mol. Med., 55:453, 1978.
15. Raine, A.E.G., and Ledingham, J.G.G.: Clinical experience with captopril in the treatment of severe drug-resistant hypertension. Am. J. Cardiol., 49:1475, 1982.
16. Aldigier, J.C., et al.: Comparison of the hormonal and renal effects of captopril in severe essential and renovascular hypertension. Am. J. Cardiol., 49:1447, 1982.
17. Mimran, A., and Jover, B.: Maintenance of the antihypertensive efficacy of captopril despite consistent reduction in daily dosage. Br. J. Clin. Pharmacol., 14:818, 1982.
18. Case, D.B., et al.: Clinical experience with blockade of the renin-angiotensin-aldosterone system by an oral converting-enzyme inhibitor (SQ 14225, captropril) in hypertensive patients. Prog. Cardiovasc. Dis., 21:195, 1978.
19. DeCarvalho, J.G.R., et al.: Hemodynamic correlates of saralasin-induced arterial pressure changes. Circulation, 57:373, 1978.
20. Brunner, H.R., et al.: Angiotensin II—blockade in man by Sar-1-Ala 8 angiotensin II for understanding and treatment of high blood pressure. Lancet, 2:1045, 1973.
21. Sen, S., Tarari, R.C., and Bumpus, F.M.: Cardiac effects of angiotensin antagonists in normotensive rats. Clin. Sci. Mol. Med., 56:494, 1979.
22. Case, D.B., et al.: Use of the first dose response on plasma renin activity to predict long-term effect of captopril: identification of triphasic pattern of blood pressure response. J. Cardiovasc. Pharmacol., 2:339, 1980.
23. Moser, M., and Lunn, J.: Responses to captopril and hydrochlorothiazide in black patients with hypertension. Clin. Pharmacol. Ther., 32:307, 1982.
24. Friedman, A., et al.: Effective use of captopril (angiotensin I-converting enzyme inhibitor) in severe childhood hypertension. J. Pediatr., 97:664, 1980.
25. Wenting, G.J., et al.: Hemodynamic effects of captopril in essential hypertension, renovascular hypertension and cardiac failure: correlations with short and long term effects on plasma renin. Am. J. Cardiol., 49:1453, 1982.
26. Havelka, J., et al.: Acute and chronic effects of the angiotensin-converting enzyme inhibitor captopril in severe hypertension. Am. J. Cardiol., 49:1467, 1982.
27. Sinaiko, A.R., et al.: Antihypertensive effect and elimination kinetics of captopril in hypertensive children with renal disease. J. Pediatr., 103:799, 1983.
28. Antonaccio, M.J., and Korwin, L.: Pre- and postjunctional inhibition of vascular sympathetic function by captopril in SHR. Implication of vascular angiotensin II in hypertension and antihypertensive actions of captopril. Hypertension, 3 (Suppl. I):54, 1981.
29. Okuno, T., et al.: Sq 14,225 attenuates the vascular response to norepinephrine in the rat mesenteric arteries. Life Sci., 25:1343, 1979.
30. Mancia, G., et al., Modification of arterial baroreflexes by captopril in essential hypertension. Am. J. Cardiol., 49:1415, 1982.
31. Bravo, E.L., and Tarazi, R.C.: Hemodynamics of an angiotensin II antagonist in normal unanesthetized dogs. Circ. Res., 43 (Suppl.):1-27, 1978.
32. Oberfield, S.E., et al.: Use of the oral angiotensin I-converting enzyme inhibitor (captopril) in childhood malignant hypertension. J. Pediatr., 95:641, 1979.
33. Bifano, H., et al.: Treatment of neonatal hypertension with captopril, J. Pediatr., 100:145, 1982.

34. Hamilton, D.V., and Maidment, G.: Captopril for refractory hypertension in patients with chronic renal failure and renal transplantation. J. R. Soc. Med., *74*:357, 1981.
35. Leier, C.V., et al.: Captopril in primary pulmonary hypertension. Circulation, *67*:155, 1983.
36. Rich, S., et al.: Captopril as treatment for patients with pulmonary hypertension. Br. Heart J., *48*:272, 1982.
37. Horowitz, J.D., et al.: Effects of captopril (SQ 14,225) in a patient with primary pulmonary hypertension. Postgrad. Med. J., *57*:115, 1981.
38. Leibau, G., et al.: Captopril in congestive heart failure. Br. J. Clin. Pharmacol., *14*:193S, 1982.
39. Davis, R., et al.: Treatment of chronic congestive heart failure with captopril, an oral inhibitor of angiotensin-converting enzyme. N. Engl. J. Med., *301*:117, 1979.
40. Tarazi, R., et al.: Renin, aldosterone and cardiac decompensation: studies with an oral converting enzyme inhibitor in heart failure. Am. J. Cardiol., *44*:1013, 1979.
41. Levine, T.B., Franciosa, J.A., and Cohn, J.N.: Acute and long-term response to an oral converting-enzyme inhibitor, captopril, in congestive heart failure. Circulation, *62*:35, 1980.
42. Ader, R., et al.: Immediate and sustained haemodynamic and clinical improvement in chronic heart failure by oral angiotensin-converting enzyme inhibitor. Circulation, *81*:931, 1980.
43. Awan, N.A., et al.: Efficacy of oral angiotensin-converting enzyme inhibition with captopril therapy in severe chronic heart failure. Am. Heart J., *101*:22, 1981.
44. Dzau, V.J., et al.: Sustained effectiveness of converting-enzyme inhibition in patients with severe congestive heart failure. N. Engl. J. Med., *302*:1373, 1980.
45. Faxon, D.P., Halperin, J.L., and Schick, E.C.: Angiotensin inhibition in severe heart failure: acute central and limb haemodynamic effects of captopril with observations on sustained oral therapy. Am. Heart J., *101*:548, 1981.
46. Awan, N.A., et al.: Long-term haemodynamic and clinical efficacy of captopril therapy in ambulatory management of severe chronic congestive heart failure. Am. Heart J., *103*:474, 1982.
47. Packer, M., et al.: Quantitative differences in the hemodynamic effects of captopril and nitroprusside in severe chronic heart failure. Am. J. Cardiol., *51*:184, 1983.
48. Packer, M., Medina, N., and Yushak, M.: Identification of four different hemodynamic patterns of response to captopril therapy in severe heart failure. ACC 1983.
49. Baylen, B.G., et al.: The occurrence of hyperaldosteronism in infants with congestive heart failure. Am. J. Cardiol., *45*:305, 1980.
50. Casta, A., et al.: Effective use of captopril in postoperative paradoxical hypertension of coarctation of the aorta. Clin. Cardiol., *5*:551, 1982.
51. Kimoto, S.: The history and present status of aortic surgery in Japan, particularly for aortitis syndrome. J. Cardiovasc. Surg., *20*:107, 1979.
52. Grossman, E., et al.: Clinical use of captopril in Takayasu's disease. Arch. Intern. Med., *144*:95, 1984.
53. Halperin, J.L., et al.: Coronary hemodynamic effects of angiotensin inhibition by captopril and teprotide in patients with congestive heart failure. Am. J. Cardiol., *50*:967, 1982.
54. Zimmerman, B.G., Gomer, S.K., and Liao, J.C.: Action of angiotensin on vascular adrenergic nerve ending; facilitation of norepinephrine release. Fed. Proc., *31*:1344, 1972.
55. Creager, M.A., et al.: Acute regional circulatory and renal hemodynamic effects of converting-enzyme inhibition in patients with congestive heart failure. Circulation, *64*:483, 1981.
56. Hollenberg, N.K., and Passan, D.R.: Specificity of the renal vascular response to captopril: studies during saralasin infusion in the DOCA-treated, salt-loaded rabbit. In press.
56a. Boucek, M.M., et al.: Elevated plasma renin in lambs with ventricular septal defect and hemodynamic improvement following captopril. AHA 1984.
57. Kripalani, K.J., et al.: Disposition of captopril in normal subjects. Clin. Pharmacol. Ther., *27*:636, 1980.

58. Kramer, B., Massie, B., and Topie, N.: Controlled trial of captopril for heart failure: effects on hemodynamics, scintigraphy and exercise tolerance. Am. J. Cardiol., *49*:925, 1982.
59. Singhvi, S.M., et al.: Effect of food on the bioavailability of captopril in healthy subjects. J. Clin. Pharmacol., *22*:135, 1982.
60. Ita, C.E., et al.: Distribution of captopril to feuses and milk of rats. Xenobiotica. In press.
61. Macda, T., et al.: Studies on the metabolism of a new antihypertensive agent, SQ 14,225 (captopril). I. In vitro studies on the binding to plasma protein and behaviour in blood. *In* Proceedings of the Ninety-Ninth Annual Meeting of the Pharmaceutical Society of Japan, Sapporo, August 28-30, 1979.
62. Duchin, K.L., et al.: Captopril kinetics. Clin. Pharmacol. Ther., *31*:452, 1982.
63. Romankiewicz, J.A., et al.: Captopril: an update review of its pharmacological properties and therapeutic efficacy in congestive heart failure. Drugs, *25*:6, 1983.
64. Pierides, A.M., et al.: Captopril elimination during hemodialysis and in chronic renal failure. Trans. Am. Soc. Artif. Intern. Organs, *9*:59A, 1980.
65. Packer, M., Medina, N., and Yushak, M.: Identification of patients at high risk of symptomatic hypotension during captopril therapy for severe heart failure. AHA 1983.
66. Heel, R.C., et al.: Captopril: a preliminary review of its pharmacological properties and therapeutic efficacy. Drugs, *20*:409, 1980.
67. Forslund, T., Borgmasters, H., and Fyhrquist, F.: Captopril-associated leucopenia confirmed by rechallenge in patient with renal failure. Lancet, *1*:166, 1981.
67a. Cooper, R.A.: Captopril-associated neutropenia: who is at risk? Arch. Intern. Med., in press.
68. Tarazi, R.C., et al.: The role of captopril in the treatment of hypertension. Br. J. Clin. Pharmacol., *14*:241S, 1982.
69. Prins, E.J.L., et al.: Nephrotic syndrome in patient on captopril. Lancet, *2*:306, 1979.
70. Rosendorff, C., et al.: Nephrotic syndrome during captopril therapy. S. Afr. Med. J., *58*:172, 1980.
71. Seedat, Y.K.: Nephrotic syndrome from captopril. S. Afr. Med. J., *57*:390, 1980.
72. Woodhouse, K., Farrow, P.R., and Wilkinson, R.: Reversible renal failure during treatment with captopril. Br. Med. J., *2*:1146, 1979.
73. Nicholls, M.G., et al.: Ulceration of the tongue: a complication of captopril therapy. Ann. Intern. Med., *94*:659, 1981.
74. Kayanakis, J.G., et al.: Eosinophilia during captopril treatment. Lancet, *2*:923, 1980.
75. Kallenberg, C.G.M., et al.: Antinuclear and antinative DNA antibodies during captopril treatment. Acta Med. Scand., *211*:297, 1982.
76. Silberbauer, K., Stanek, B., and Templ, H.: Acute hypotensive effect of captopril in man modified by prostaglandin synthesis inhibition. Br. J. Clin. Pharmacol., *14*:87S, 1982.
77. Goldstone, R., et al.: Captopril vasodepressor action is mediated both by converting enzyme inhibition (CEI) and prostaglandins. Clin. Res., *29*:525A, 1981.

Chapter 17

Saralasin

Saralasin, an antagonist of angiotensin II, was first described in 1971.[1] This agent reduces blood pressure in normotensive and hypertensive patients by reducing the peripheral vascular resistance. Occasionally, it increases peripheral resistance ("pressor response"). Saralasin also has a direct negative inotropic effect or an inhibitory effect on the positive inotropic effect of angiotensin II. This action is responsible for a decrease in cardiac output. Because saralasin causes marked reductions in blood pressure in patients with renovascular hypertension and high plasma renin activity, it has been used as a screening test for renovascular hypertension. The sensitivity of this test is low, however.[2] An intravenous infusion of saralasin may be used to predict a patient's response to oral captopril.

Antihypertensive Effect

Bifano and associates reported the case of an infant who developed hypertension and congestive heart failure due to right renal artery stenosis.[3] Infusion of saralasin, 0.05 µg/kg/min reduced blood pressure within 30 min from 145/78 to 96/60 mm Hg. Hypertension recurred when saralasin was discontinued.

Ruley and co-workers reported the cases of 2 hypertensive children, aged 51 days and 8 years, respectively, who became refractory to conventional parenterally administered antihypertensive medications and had an ileus that precluded oral administration of drugs.[4] Both patients had a reduction of 30% in blood pressure during infusion of saralasin, at a rate up to 15 µg/kg/min. The elevated blood pressure was controlled during continuous infusion of saralasin for 8 and 13 days, respectively. In an 8-month old infant with hypertension due to coarctation of the aorta, blood pressure was adequately controlled by an infusion of saralasin. The infusion was continued for 20 hours, throughout surgical correction, without recognized adverse effects.[4]

Side Effects

Adverse effects associated with the administration of saralasin include excessive reduction or elevation of blood pressure during initiation of infusion, premature ventricular beats, nausea, sweating, anxiety, and flushing of the skin.

I suggest that saralasin be used for short periods only in hypertensive children who are resistant to or are unable to tolerate conventional antihypertensive agents.

References

1. Pals, D.T., et al.: Specific competitive antagonist of the vascular action of angiotensin II. Circ. Res., 29:664, 1971.
2. Krakoff, L.R., et al.: Saralasin infusion in screening patients for renovascular hypertension. Am. J. Cardiol., 45:609, 1980.
3. Bifano, H., et al.: Treatment of neonatal hypertension with captopril. J. Pediatr., 100:145, 1982.
4. Ruley, E.J., Bock, G.H., and Smith, D.S.: Use of continuous saralasin infusion to control hypertension. J. Pediatr., 101:1013, 1982.

Section IV

BETA-ADRENORECEPTOR BLOCKING AGENTS

Beta-adrenoreceptor blocking agents produce a reversible and competitive inhibition of beta-adrenergic stimulation in various tissues. Their introduction to clinical use 30 years ago was one of the greatest advances in cardiovascular therapy. After initial failures, some of which ended tragically, such as the experience with practolol, several lines of development were determined. This development resulted in the synthesis of numerous beta-adrenoreceptor blocking agents. About 20 of these agents are in routine clinical use in adult patients for the treatment of systemic hypertension, angina pectoris, myocardial infarction, arrhythmias, hypertrophic and, occasionally, congestive cardiomyopathies, thyrotoxicosis, portal hypertension, migraine, various neurologic and psychiatric disturbances, glaucoma, and other diseases.

Most of the diseases for which beta-blocking agents are prescribed in adults also occur in the pediatric age groups. Further indications for these drugs in infancy and childhood are tetralogy of Fallot and other conditions associated with dynamic infundibular obstruction.

Modern research has made available a large group of beta-adrenoreceptor blocking drugs from which appropriate agents can be selected for each clinical condition. This selection is restricted to treatment of adults, however, because pediatric cardiologists limit themselves almost exclusively to propranolol. This conservative approach to the use of beta-blocking agents in infants and children may be less effective and less safe than other approaches. For example, it is well known that beta-blocking drugs can aggravate bronchospasm. In adults, various attempts have been made to limit this adverse effect in patients with bronchospastic diseases. These attempts include the use of selective beta-blockers, beta-blockers with intrinsic sympathomimetic activity, or beta-blockers with both these properties. Few of these advances have been incorporated into the daily practice of pediatric cardiology.

This introduction describes the classification of beta-blocking agents according to their ancillary properties, the practical implications of this classification, and the effects of beta-blocking drugs as a group. In Chapters 18 and 19, the experience with specific beta-blocking agents in children is described, and the potential use of new beta-blocking drugs in children is discussed.

Structure

All beta-adrenoreceptors are analogues of the beta-stimulator isoproterenol. The molecule of beta-blocking agents consists of an aromatic ring and a side chain, both of which carry various substituents. The structure of the aromatic ring determines the potency of beta-adrenoreceptor blockade, the potency of intrinsic sympathomimetic activity, and lipid solubility. The substituents on the aromatic ring of beta-blocking agents are less potent in stimulating beta-adrenoreceptors than those present on the ring of beta-agonists, such as the two hydroxyl groups on the aromatic ring of isoproterenol.

The alkyl side chain determines the affinity of beta-blocking agents to the receptors. Most beta-blocking drugs, including propranolol, atenolol, metoprolol, oxprenolol, acebutolol, pindolol, sotalol, and labetalol, have an isopropylaminopropoxy side chain, with or without some substitutions. An asymmetric beta-carbon atom on the side chain determines the pharmacologic activity of these agents.

Classification

Beta-blocking agents may be classified according to their ancillary and certain pharmacokinetic properties. The most important characteristics are potency of beta-blockade, selectivity, intrinsic sympathomimetic activity, membrane-stabilizing activity, associated class 3 antiarrhythmic properties, associated vasodilatory properties, and lipid solubility.

Potency

Beta-blocking agents differ in their potency on a weight-to-weight basis. Potency may be determined by the dose of isoproterenol required to overcome the blockade. Pindolol and timolol, the most potent beta-blockers, are six times more potent than propranolol and atenolol. Absolute potency is only one of the determinants of clinical dosage and has little value in practice.

Selectivity

Beta-adrenoreceptors may be divided into beta-1-receptors, which are present mainly in the heart, and beta-2-receptors, which are present in many other organs and tissues, including blood vessels and pulmonary airways. Some of the cardiac beta-adrenoreceptors are of the beta-2 type. For most clinical indications of beta-blocking agents, the important effect is blockade of beta-1-receptors.

Selective beta-blocking agents may produce fewer adverse effects than nonselective drugs. For example, nonselective beta-blockers also block the beta-2-adrenoreceptors, which mediate relaxation in the peripheral circulation and in pulmonary airways; this process leaves unopposed the constricting adrenergic stimuli mediated by alpha-adrenoreceptors. Therefore, nonselective beta-blocking agents aggravate the symptoms of bronchospasm and peripheral vascular disease. With selective beta-blocking drugs, such side effects are less common.[1,2] These side effects are not completely absent with selective beta-blocking agents because (1) selectivity is relative, and at high doses, beta-1 "selective" blocking agents also block beta-2-receptors; and (2) in all organs, mixed beta-adrenoreceptors of both types are found. Nonselective beta-blocking drugs may prolong insulin-induced hypoglycemia, whereas with selective blockers, this effect is absent or minimal.[3]

Thus, in patients with bronchospasm, peripheral vascular disease, or severe diabetes mellitus, selective beta-blocking agents are potentially superior to nonselective beta-blocking drugs. On the other hand, nonselective beta-blockers are superior in the treatment of tremor and migraine. The most widely used nonselective beta-blocking agent is propranolol, and the most widely used selective beta-blocking drug is atenolol.

Intrinsic Sympathomimetic Activity

In addition to inhibition of the effect of pure beta-adrenoreceptor agonists, beta-blocking agents may partially activate the beta-adrenoreceptors. This partial agonist activity is called intrinsic sympathomimetic activity. A certain compound may be both a potent beta-blocker and a potent partial agonist because, while the agent attaches to the receptor and partially activates it, the access of pure potent agonists to the receptor is inhibited.

Beta-blocking agents with intrinsic sympathomimetic activity theoretically have several advantages or disadvantages over beta-blockers devoid of this property. For example, at a certain degree of beta-blockade, these agents produce less bradycardia. This feature is important mainly in elderly patients and is of little relevance in the pediatric age group. By activation of beta-2-receptors, these beta-blocking drugs may produce less bronchospasm and less constriction of peripheral blood vessels than beta-blockers devoid of intrinsic sympathomimetic activity. Such potential advantages are yet to be confirmed. Intrinsic sympathomimetic activity partially protects patients against prolongation of atrioventricular conduction time.

Although some investigators have suggested that intrinsic sympathomimetic activity may help to prevent aggravation of congestive heart failure by beta-blocking agents, other reports have indicated that congestive heart failure may be aggravated even by beta-blockers with intrinsic sympathomimetic activity.[4-6] Intrinsic sympathomimetic activity modifies the effects of beta-blockade on myocardial contractility at rest, but not during exercise.[7] If intrinsic sympathomimetic activity is too potent, adverse effects such as arrhythmias, palpitations, and tremor may occur. The most clinically important beta-blocking agents with intrinsic sympathomimetic activity are pindolol, oxprenolol, and alprenolol.

Membrane-Stabilizing Activity

Membrane-stabilizing activity or local anesthetic activity is the property of inhibition of the fast sodium current across cell membranes. It is common to all Class I antiarrhythmic agents and to several beta-blocking drugs. All these agents reduce the rate of rise of phase 0 depolarization.[8,9] The concentration of beta-blocking agents required to produce this effect is much higher than that required for beta-blockade. Membrane-stabilizing activity may contribute to the antiarrhythmic effect of beta-blockers, but it usually plays no role in their cardiovascular effects. For example, D-propranolol, which has a membrane-stabilizing activity similar to that of L-propranolol or racemic propranolol, has a much weaker cardiodepressant effect than racemic or L-propranolol.

Vasodilatory Activity

Beta-blocking agents usually produce vasoconstriction as a result of a compensatory effect because of the decrease in cardiac output and as a result of adrenergic stimulation of peripheral alpha-adrenoreceptors in the presence of beta-blockade. Several beta-blockers do have vasodilatory properties, however. These drugs are of two types: (1) agents that combine beta- and alpha-adrenoreceptor blocking activity, such as labetalol; and (2) agents with a direct vasodilatory effect, such as prizidilol.

Effect on Oxyhemoglobin Dissociation

Propranolol alters the oxyhemoglobin dissociation curve and thereby increases oxygen delivery to the tissues. Other beta-blocking agents do not have this property, which may contribute to the therapeutic effect of propranolol in ischemic heart disease. In children, the effect on the oxyhemoglobin dissociation curve is of special importance in cases of tetralogy of Fallot, in which this effect may be one of the mechanisms of action of the drug.

Pharmacokinetic Differences

Beta-blocking agents differ from one another by several pharmacokinetic parameters. Many of these differences result from variations in lipid solubility of these agents. The long-acting beta-blocking drugs, such as atenolol, are given once daily; the short-acting beta-blockers, such as propranolol, are given 3 to 4 times daily; and the ultrashort-acting beta-blockers, such as esmolol, are effective only for a few minutes. Beta-blocking agents differ in the extent and rate of absorption, bioavailability, route of elimination, protein binding, and other pharmacokinetic factors.

Hemodynamic Effects

The hemodynamic effects common to all beta-blocking agents are slowing of heart rate, decreases in myocardial contractility, cardiac output, and systemic arterial pressure, and for most beta-blockers, an increase in systemic vascular resistance. Most of these effects result directly from beta-blockade. The increase in peripheral vascular resistance is compensatory to the decrease in cardiac output, but it also results from unopposed stimulation of alpha-adrenoreceptors in blood vessels. The initial increase in systemic vascular resistance may be partially attenuated by continued treatment.

Most beta-blocking agents reduce renal plasma flow, both because of reduction in cardiac output and because of local renal effects. This change is accompanied by a decrease in glomerular filtration rate and is more prominent with nonselective beta-blockers. Nadolol may increase renal plasma flow.

Beta-blocking drugs usually reduce plasma renin activity and are considered to be more effective in patients with high-renin than low-renin hypertension.

Pulmonary Effects

Because relaxation of bronchial smooth muscles is mediated by beta-2-adrenoreceptors, beta-blocking agents may precipitate or may aggravate bronchoconstriction. Therefore, beta-blockers, especially nonselective agents, may cause deterioration of pulmonary function in patients with pulmonary obstructive diseases.[10] The increased release of histamine from mast cells may contribute to the adverse pulmonary effect of beta-blockers.[11]

Effect on Peripheral Circulation

Beta-blocking drugs decrease cardiac output and increase systemic vascular resistance. Therefore, they reduce peripheral blood flow. In patients with peripheral vascular diseases, these drugs may aggravate symptoms.

Therapeutic Indications

The therapeutic indications for beta-blocking agents are discussed in detail in Chapter 18. In general, they include angina pectoris, myocardial infarction, systemic hypertension, cardiomyopathies, arrhythmias, tetralogy of Fallot, thyrotoxicosis, and various neurologic and psychiatric disorders.

Side Effects

Beta-blocking agents have side effects specific to each agent, as well as side effects common to the whole group. The most famous and hazardous side effect is the oculomucocutaneous syndrome produced by practolol, which was the cause of withdrawal of this important cardioselective blocker from clinical use. Side effects common to the whole group result directly from beta-blockade. They include bradycardia, myocardial depression, hypotension, fatigue, bronchoconstriction, central nervous system effects (which are less common with the hydrophilic beta-blockers), aggravation of symptoms of peripheral vascular disease, hypoglycemia, constipation, diarrhea, nausea, and various skin lesions. Nonselective beta-blocking agents may cause coronary spasm due to unopposed alpha-adrenergic stimulation in the coronary arteries.

Drug Discontinuance

Rebound aggravation of angina pectoris or hypertension has been reported in several patients in whom beta-blocking agents were abruptly withdrawn. This reaction is further discussed in Chapter 18.

References

1. Perks, W.H., et al.: Comparison of atenolol and oxprenolol in patients with angina or hypertension and co-existent chronic airways obstruction. Br. J. Clin. Pharmacol., 5:101, 1978.
2. Benson, M.K., et al.: Cardioselective and non-cardioselective beta-blockers in reversible obstructive airways disease. Postgrad. Med. J. 53(Suppl. 3):143, 1977.
3. Waal-Manning, H.J.: Metabolic effects of beta-adrenoceptor blockers. Drugs, 11 (Suppl. 1):121, 1976.
4. Lyon, L.J. and Nevins, M.A.: Alprenolol treatment of angina pectoris. JAMA, 215:1669, 1971.
5. Bianchi, C., et al.: Beta blockade and angina pectoris: a controlled multi-centre clinical trial. Pharmacol. Clin., 1:161, 1969.
6. Apthorp, G.H., et al.: The effects of sympathectomy on the electro-cardiogram and effort tolerance in angina pectoris. Br. Heart J., 26:218, 1964.
7. Choong, C.Y.P., et al.: Hemodynamic effects of beta blockade with and without intrinsic sympathomimetic activity (ISA) in patients with stable exertional angina. AHA 1982.

8. Connolly, M.E., et al.: The clinical pharmacology of beta-adrenoceptor blocking drugs. Prog. Cardiovasc. Dis., *19*:203, 1976.
9. Waal-Manning, H.J.: Can β-blockers be used in diabetic patients? Drugs, *17*:157, 1979.
10. McDevitt, D.G.: Beta-adrenoceptor antagonists and respiratory function. Br. J. Clin. Pharmacol., *5*:97, 1978.
11. Micolaesau, V., et al.: Beta-adrenergic blockade with practolol in acetylcholine sensitive asthma patients. Respiration, *29*:139, 1972.

Chapter 18

Propranolol

Propranolol is a non-selective beta-adrenoreceptor blocking agent without intrinsic sympathomimetic activity, but with membrane-stabilizing activity. It is the most widely used beta-adrenoreceptor blocking drug in adults. In pediatric cardiovascular therapy, propranolol is the only beta-adrenoreceptor blocking agent in routine clinical use. The drug is used also for a variety of noncardiovascular indications, most of them of little relevance to pediatric therapy.

The main indications for propranolol in infants and children are hypertension, tetralogy of Fallot, hypertrophic obstructive cardiomyopathy, arrhythmias, and thyrotoxicosis. In adults, propranolol is used mainly for prevention of anginal episodes in patients with coronary artery disease and angina pectoris and for treatment of hypertension. The drug also reduces mortality rates in patients who have had acute myocardial infarction.

Pharmacologic Properties

Propranolol is a nonselective beta-adrenoreceptor blocking agent that affects both beta-1 and beta-2-adrenoreceptors. It is commercially available as a racemate; however, the beta-blocking effect of L-propranolol is up to 50 times higher than that of D-propranolol. Although propranolol has no partial sympathomimetic activity, it has a membrane-stabilizing activity (local-anesthetic or quinidine-like effect). This effect is independent of the beta-adrenoreceptor blocking action and is equal for both optical isomers of propranolol.[1-3] These features are discussed in the introduction to Section IV.

Hemodynamic Effects

The most important effects of propranolol are decreases in heart rate, myocardial contractility, and systemic arterial pressure, resulting from blockade of cardiac beta-adrenoreceptors. The primary effects, the decreases in heart rate and contractility, probably lead to the third important effect, the decrease in arterial pressure.

Propranolol decreases heart rate at rest and during exercise, after short-term as well as prolonged administration. Propranolol inhibits, but does not prevent, the exercise-induced increase in heart rate, owing to a combined effect of sympathetic blockade and withdrawal of parasympathetic activity. The decrease ranges between 10% in healthy persons to up to about 50% in patients with hypertension or ischemic heart disease.[4–7] Several investigators have suggested that the other hemodynamic effects of propranolol are completely or partially dependent on the decrease in heart rate.[8–11] The depressant effect on myocardial contractility is probably primary, however, because it has persisted during atrial pacing at a constant rate.[12]

The negative inotropic effect of propranolol has been shown in animal and human studies, both in normal and failing hearts. This effect was demonstrated by several indices of contractility, including RD/dt_{max}, mean ejection rate, maximum blood flow velocity and acceleration, and various other noninvasively and invasively measured indices.[12–14] Results of several studies in healthy men or in patients without myocardial dysfunction showed no change in myocardial contractility after propranolol administration, especially when the drug was given orally, however.[15–17] Conflicting data on the effect of propranolol on ejection fraction in healthy subjects were reported. Marshall and co-workers reported that propranolol did not alter global and regional ejection fraction at rest, but decreased it during exercise in healthy human subjects,[10] whereas Port and colleagues reported that propranolol decreased ejection fraction at rest by up to 21% in 8 of 12 healthy human subjects.[8] During exercise, the drug decreased ejection fraction, as compared with the control exercise value of this parameter. This change resulted mainly from the decrease in control resting ejection fraction in the treated subjects, but also from inhibition of the exercise-induced increase in ejection fraction. Erhardt and associates reported that propranolol decreased left ventricular ejection fraction at rest by 4% and during exercise by 12%.[11]

In patients with coronary artery disease, propranolol may decrease, may not change, or may increase ejection fraction and its response to exercise. The effect depends on pretreatment myocardial function and on the effect of propranolol on the ischemic state.

This subject is of little or no value in pediatric cardiologic practice. In studies of normotensive subjects, propranolol either increased or failed to alter the systemic vascular resistance; the increase in this parameter probably resulted from unopposed peripheral alpha-adrenergic stimulation in the presence of beta-adrenergic blockade.[18, 19]

Propranolol decreased cardiac output at rest and during exercise in normotensive and hypertensive patients.[8, 20] This effect resulted mainly from the decrease in cardiac rate and contractility. This subject is further discussed in the section of this chapter on the mechanism of the antihypertensive effect of propranolol.

In patients with cardiovascular disease other than hypertrophic cardiomyopathy, propranolol has little or no effect on the diastolic properties of the heart.[21] In patients with hypertrophic obstructive cardiomyopathy, propranolol may improve diastolic left ventricular filling.[22]

Propranolol reduces myocardial oxygen uptake because of decreases in heart rate, contractility, and arterial pressure. In several studies, the drug reduced blood flow in the normal myocardium and reduced, failed to alter, or even increased blood flow in the ischemic myocardium.[23–26] The reduction in blood flow may result from decreased demand or from coronary vasoconstriction due to unopposed coronary alpha-adrenergic stimulation.

Propranolol may impair renal function, as evident by reductions in renal blood flow, glomerular filtration rate, and creatinine clearance observed in several studies.[19, 22, 27, 28] This effect was attributed to the propranolol-induced decrease in cardiac output, and possibly also to renal vasoconstriction produced by a direct effect of propranolol.

Effects in Hypertension

Propranolol is effective in treatment of systemic hypertension in all age groups. The drug lowers both systolic and diastolic blood pressures, at rest and during exercise. It is effective in patients with essential hypertension as well as in those with renovascular hypertension and hypertension associated with parenchymal renal diseases. The antihypertensive effect of propranolol is dose-dependent.[29] The drug's effect is greater on systolic pressure than on diastolic pressure.

In patients with mild hypertension, propranolol may be given as the sole antihypertensive therapeutic agent. The results with propranolol when used alone have been poor, although many cases of mild essential hypertension can be controlled thus.[30, 31] Propranolol is now considered to be the standard beta-blocking agent used in hypertension, and all other beta-blockers are compared to it. In patients with severe hypertension, propranolol is rarely used alone. Although the drug may be used alone, especially in patients with high-renin hypertension,[32] it is not recommended.

The antihypertensive effect of propranolol was correlated with the pretreatment level of plasma renin activity. Patients with high-renin hypertension showed the greatest effect, whereas in patients with low-renin hypertension, propranolol was ineffective.[32] Moreover, patients with high-renin hypertension required lower doses of propranolol to control the elevated blood pressure than patients with low-renin hypertension.[33] This feature is important for infants and children with coarctation of the aorta and high-renin hypertension. The antihypertensive efficacy of propranolol was comparable to that of diuretics and reserpine.[30]

The combination of propranolol and diuretic agents is more effective than the use of either drug alone in the control of hypertension.[30] Diuretic agents increase the plasma renin activity, and the addition of propranolol suppresses it. This phenomenon is one of the explanations for the additive effect, which has been confirmed by several clinical studies. For example, Zacharias and co-workers reported that, in 107 hypertensive patients treated with diuretic agents, blood pressure was 201/116 mm Hg; during treatment with propranolol in addition to diuretics, the mean blood pressure of these patients fell to 150/88 mm Hg.[34]

The combination of propranolol with vasodilators such as hydralazine and minoxidil also exerts an additive antihypertensive effect. These vasodilators cause adrenergic activation, leading to compensatory increases in heart rate and contractility. Propranolol inhibits this compensatory mechanism. The combination of propranolol, a diuretic agent, and hydralazine or, less commonly, minoxidil, has been effective in children with severe hypertension. Occasionally, an intravenously administered vasodilator such as nitroprusside may be required in children with hypertensive emergencies during treatment with propranolol.

Mechanism of the Antihypertensive Effect. Several mechanisms have been suggested to account for the antihypertensive effect of propranolol. First is the decrease in cardiac output. The cardiac beta-adrenoreceptor blockade by propranolol causes negative chronotropic and inotropic responses. This process leads to a decrease in cardiac output. If the decrease in cardiac output is not associated with an equal compensatory increase in peripheral vascular resistance, blood pressure will be lowered.[35-37] This mechanism is considered to be primarily responsible for the antihypertensive effect of propranolol. The concept is contrasted by several findings, however. Blood pressure is not always reduced despite significant reduction in cardiac output. Prolonged treatment with propranolol is associated with a sustained antihypertensive effect, even though cardiac output may return to its pretreatment level. Moreover, administration of propranolol rapidly causes beta-blockade, as evident by a decrease in heart rate, whereas the antihypertensive effect may appear only after several days of treatment and may peak only after several weeks.[36]

Decrease of plasma renin activity is a possible mechanism. Propranolol is more effective in high-renin hypertension than in low-renin hypertension, and a correlation exists between the decrease in blood pressure and the suppression of plasma renin activity. These findings indicate that suppression of the renin-angiotensin system plays a role in the mechanism of the antihypertensive effect of propranolol.[32] This concept is opposed by the findings that, despite an early decrease in plasma renin activity, the antihypertensive effect of propranolol may be delayed,[36,38] and doses required to control hypertension are higher than those required to decrease the plasma renin activity.[39,40] Moreover, the correlation between reduction in blood pressure and reduction in plasma renin activity has not occurred in all patients studied.[41] To resolve this controversy, a dual mechanism has been suggested: (1) a renin-dependent effect produced by low doses of propranolol and (2) a renin-independent effect produced by high doses.[33]

Resetting of baroreceptors has been suggested as a possible mechanism,[42] but this theory is yet to be confirmed.

Reduction of sympathetic outflow from the central nervous system, another possible mechanism, has been suggested for several beta-blocking agents, but it is especially valid for propranolol, which has a high liposolubility and easily penetrates the central nervous system.[29] The decrease in sympathetic outflow causes a decrease in cardiac output and, consequently, in arterial pressure. As mentioned earlier, treatment with propranolol is associated with an increase in peripheral vascular resistance. Despite this effect, propranolol is a potent antihypertensive agent.

Effects in Hypertrophic Obstructive Cardiomyopathy

The introduction of propranolol is one of the most important achievements in the treatment of hypertrophic obstructive cardiomyopathy. In children, propranolol is the preferred drug for treatment of hemodynamic abnormalities and rhythm disturbances associated with this disease.

About 18 years ago, it was reported that propranolol produces significant symptomatic improvement in patients of all ages with hypertropic obstructive cardiomyopathy.[43-45] Hemodynamic improvement in systole and diastole is considered to be the mechanism of the beneficial clinical effect. In the early days of propranolol treatment in patients with this disease, the suppression of myocardial contractility, leading to a reduction in the systolic pressure gradient over the left ventricular outflow, was considered to be the main hemodynamic effect of propranolol. Later, it was accepted that the main hemodynamic abnormality in this condition may be impairment of left ventricular diastolic filling. The primary impairment probably occurs in early diastolic rapid filling. Propranolol may improve left ventricular compliance and filling in these patients. This improvement has been observed in more than half the patients studied.[46-49] The improved diastolic filling was shown to be independent of age, of dose of propranolol, and of the degree of hypertrophy.[49] It was also shown to be at least partially independent of the slowing of heart rate by propranolol.[49]

Despite the potentially favorable profile of propranolol in hypertrophic cardiomyopathy, the success of treatment largely depends on the appropriate selection of patients. Patients with mild symptoms and a small or latent gradient have been reported to derive greater benefit from propranolol than those with severe symptoms, mainly dyspnea, and a high pressure gradient.[50, 51] These findings are from studies in adults, however, and may not be valid in children, as evident from improvement of two neonates with hypertrophic cardiomyopathy and congestive heart failure who were treated with propranolol.[52]

Data on the effect of propranolol on arrhythmias and sudden death in patients with hypertrophic cardiomyopathy have been controversial. Several investigators have reported that propranolol prevented sudden death and arrhythmias,[53, 54, 66] whereas others have noted no effect on mortality rates and even no significant suppression of ventricular and supraventricular arrhythmias.[44, 55, 56] In one study, propranolol alone suppressed arrhythmias in only 4 of 11 patients with hypertrophic cardiomyopathy.[66]

Gillette and associates studied the effects of propranolol in 6 infants and children with hypertrophic obstructive cardiomyopathy.[52] Indications for treatment were congestive heart failure in 2 newborn infants, syncope in 1 child, and chest pain in 4 children. Symptoms and abnormal signs were abolished by propranolol in all 6 patients. None of them required surgical intervention, and none died. Echocardiographic study showed regression of septal hypertrophy. In the 2 neonates with congestive heart failure, propranolol was discontinued after 2 years and 9 months, respectively, and they remained clinically well. The 4 remaining patients were treated with propranolol for 2.5 to 6.0 years and were still receiving the drug when the paper was written. In 3 of these patients, propranolol abolished premature ventricular beats.[52]

My colleagues and I studied a child with discrete subaortic stenosis associated with progressive cardiomyopathy and dynamic left ventricular outflow obstruction, as shown by repeated catheterization. After initiation of propranolol, a repeat echocardiographic study did not reveal progression of the hypertrophy over a period of 2.5 years.

Propranolol may also be effective in tiny infants with hypertrophic obstructive cardiomyopathy. Shand and co-workers studied an 8-week-old infant with this disease. This patient had a pressure gradient of 120 mm Hg across the left ventricular outflow tract and right ventricular gradient with marked hypertrophy of both ventricles and the interventricular septum.[57] In view of the age of the patient, a trial of propranolol was preferred to operation. Propranolol was given at doses that maintained a plasma level of 40 to 90 ng/ml. The patient showed clinical improvement. During a repeat cardiac catheterization at the age of 22 months, performed 24 hours after discontinuance of propranolol, no left ventricular outflow pressure gradient was noted, and the right ventricular outflow pressure gradient was reduced. Isoproterenol produced a small left ventricular outflow gradient of 20 mm Hg. At the age of 3 years, the child was clinically well; however, cardiac enlargement was visible on a thoracic roentgenogram, and biventricular hypertrophy was evident on an electrocardiogram.[57]

At a certain stage in its natural course, hypertrophic cardiomyopathy may be converted to congestive cardiomyopathy. The continued administration of propranolol beyond this point may result in hemodynamic deterioration. Therefore, children with hypertrophic cardiomyopathy should be carefully followed, and follow-up should include serial echocardiograms.

Effects in Tetralogy of Fallot

The introduction of propranolol in the treatment of patients with tetralogy of Fallot is the most important achievement in the nonsurgical management of this anomaly. The definitive treatment of this anomaly is complete surgical correction. If infants or small children develop complications such as hypoxemic spells, and if they are too small to undergo complete surgical correction, a palliative aortopulmonary shunt is created, and complete correction is delayed for several years. This procedure exposes the patient to the risks of a second operation however. Moreover, in some small children a shunt is difficult to create. In such patients, administration of propranolol may produce symptomatic relief, may eliminate the need for a shunt, and may allow complete surgical correction to be delayed. Propranolol produces hemodynamic and clinical improvement in patients with tetralogy of Fallot. It prevents the appearance of paroxysmal hypoxemic spells for at least several months in the majority of the patients.

Garson and colleagues reported that the responders to propranolol were older and received higher doses of propranolol than the nonresponders.[58] High doses may improve the effect of propranolol in younger children.

Ponce and associates studied 22 patients with tetralogy of Fallot who were treated with oral propranolol, 1 mg/kg every 6 hours.[59] In 13 infants, aged 3 to 20 months, the drug was used in an effort to postpone surgical correction. In 9 children, 2 to 11 years of age, the drug was used while awaiting the operation or when the patients' parents refused to allow surgical correction. Eight of the patients received propranolol intravenously during cardiac catheterization. The drug increased resting oxygen saturation by 4%. Blood pressure and heart rate decreased by 8 mm Hg and 11 beats/min, respectively. Heart murmurs increased in intensity, indicating an increased flow across the pulmonary valve and right ventricular infundibulum. Eighteen of the patients had hypoxic spells before therapy. Prolonged oral administration of propranolol abolished or lessened these episodes in all but a single patient. Five of the 22 patients were refractory to treatment with propranolol. Surgical correction was performed 3 to 27 months after initiation of therapy. Postoperative complications attributable to propranolol were not observed.[59]

Garson and co-workers studied 35 infants who received propranolol as palliative treatment for hypoxemic spells associated with tetralogy of Fallot.[58] Propranolol effectively abolished spells for at least 3 months in 80% of the patients. The dose of propranolol was considered to be the main determinant of response. In the infants in whom propranolol was effective, surgical treatment was postponed by 13.1 months. The only significant adverse effect was congestive heart failure, which developed in 1 patient. Surgical repair was performed in 16 patients. Propranolol was administered until the morning of the operation. Of the 2 operative deaths, neither was related to the use of propranolol. Garson and colleagues concluded that propranolol is the preferred palliation for tetralogy of Fallot.

In tetralogy of Fallot, the right ventricular outflow obstruction may occur at various levels. In addition to dynamic obstructions in the right ventricle and the infundibulum, fixed pulmonic valvar or supravalvar stenosis may be present. Because propranolol affects mainly myocardial contractility, some investigators have suggested that the drug may be especially effective in patients who have only dynamic obstructions.[60, 61] Such is not always the case, however. I have observed a favorable response to propranolol in patients with combined infundibular and moderate-to-severe valvar pulmonic stenosis. Garson and associates reported good results in two infants with severe, fixed obstructions; one of these patients had pulmonary valvar atresia, and the other had atresia of the left pulmonary artery.[58] These investigators found no specific anatomic pattern associated with responsiveness or unresponsiveness in patients with tetralogy of Fallot.

The following mechanisms may account for the beneficial effect of propranolol in tetralogy of Fallot. First, the negative inotropic effect of propranolol causes a decrease in ventricular contractility and in the extent of the dynamic right ventricular obstruction, mainly at the infundibular level. This change causes a decrease in right ventricular pressure and in right-to-left shunting and results in improved peripheral oxygenation.[62] Second, rapid heart rate is associated with a higher degree of right-to-left shunting.[63] Propranolol slows the heart rate, and this effect contributes to the decrease of the shunting. Third, propranolol can increase peripheral vascular resistance because, in the presence of nonselective peripheral vascular beta-blockade, the vasoconstricting alpha-adrenoreceptor stimulation is left unopposed. This increase results in an increase in left ventricular systolic pressure and a decrease in cardiac output, causing a reduction in the magnitude of right-to-left shunting.[64] Finally, propranolol shifts the oxyhemoglobin dissociation curve to the right and thus improves the delivery of oxygen to tissues.

In summary, propranolol effectively and safely provides hemodynamic and clinical improvement in patients with tetralogy of Fallot. It allows one to delay complete surgical repair and obviates the need for palliative shunting.

Effect on Pulmonary Function

Like other nonselective beta-adrenoreceptor blocking agents, propranolol may cause bronchospasm in patients with pulmonary obstructive disease and even in healthy subjects. This phenomenon is due to blockade of the bronchial beta-2-adrenoreceptors that mediate bronchodilation. This effect of propranolol may impair pulmonary function.[65, 66] Several patients have developed bronchial asthma during prolonged treatment with propranolol.[67] This subject is further discussed in the section of this chapter on the side effects of propranolol.

Effect on Platelet Function

Propranolol reduces platelet aggregation.[68–70] In studies of patients with various cardiovascular diseases, propranolol also reduced the production of thromboxane A_2, a vasoconstricting prostaglandin derivative, by the platelets.[71, 72] This antiplatelet activity is not related to beta-blockade. It may result from the membrane-stabilizing effect of propranolol or from a direct effect on prostaglandin metabolism.[73] The antiplatelet activity may contribute to the beneficial effect of propranolol in hypertension and angina pectoris.

Effect on Oxyhemoglobin dissociation

Propranolol can shift the oxyhemoglobin dissociation curve to the right in healthy human subjects and in patients with coronary artery disease. The drug thereby decreases the affinity of hemoglobin to oxygen; the result is improved oxygen supply to the tissues. This effect may play a role in the beneficial effect of propranolol in angina pectoris and possibly also in tetralogy of Fallot.

Effects in Angina Pectoris

Propranolol is effective in patients with coronary artery disease and stable angina pectoris. It reduces the number of spontaneous anginal episodes, nitroglycerin consumption, and electrocardiographic evidence of ischemia and it increases exercise tolerance. These effects have been observed after both intravenous and oral therapy.[76-79] The beneficial effect of propranolol is usually associated with decreases in heart rate, systemic arterial pressure, and the rate-pressure product. These findings suggest that reduction in myocardial oxygen demand is the most important mechanism of the antianginal effect of propranolol. Other mechanisms are shift of the oxyhemoglobin dissociation curve to the right, improvement in the oxygen supply to the ischemic myocardium, and antiplatelet activity.

The antianginal effect is sustained for at least several years, unless the coronary disease deteriorates. For example, Warren and co-workers reported that, in a group of 63 patients treated for 8 years, 84% experienced at least a 50% reduction in the frequency of anginal attacks.[67] Propranolol may be given alone or in combination with other antianginal agents such as nitrates and calcium antagonists. It is also effective in unstable angina unassociated with coronary spasm.

The use of propranolol in variant angina resulting from coronary spasm is controversial. Propranolol may aggravate coronary spasm due to unopposed alpha-adrenergic stimulation in the coronary arteries.[80, 81] Clinical studies have shown an improvement,[82, 83] minimal beneficial effect,[84, 85] or even a detrimental effect.[86]

Electrophysiologic Effects

The electrophysiologic effects of propranolol result from its beta-adrenoreceptor blocking action and, to some extent, also from its quinidine-like (local anesthetic) effect.

Effect on the Sinus Node

In adults, propranolol prolongs the sinus node cycle length and the sinoatrial conduction time. It may prolong or may shorten the sinus node recovery time. The most consistent change is prolongation of the cycle length, which may range between 10 and 30% in healthy human subjects.[87, 88] The effect on other parameters is inconsistent. In a study of patients with sinus nodal dysfunction, propranolol prolonged the sinus node cycle length and sinus recovery time, but not the sinoatrial conduction time.[89] In another group of patients with sinus nodal dysfunction, propranolol increased the sinus cycle length by 17% and the sinoatrial conduction time by 18%. Limited data have been reported on the effect of propranolol on sinus nodal function in children. Yabek and colleagues evaluated the effect of propranolol, 0.1 mg/kg intravenously, in 10 children without clinical evidence of sinus nodal dysfunction.[90] The drug increased the spontaneous sinus cycle length in all patients. The mean increase was 13.4%, from 635 ± 200 msec to 720 ± 202 msec. The maximum corrected sinus node recovery time increased in 9 patients after propranolol administration. The mean corrected sinus node recovery time increased by 63%, from 203 ± 61 msec to 330 ± 190 msec. An inconsistent effect on sinoatrial conduction time was observed, and the mean sinoatrial conduction time changed little. Therefore, the effects of propranolol on the sinus node in children appear to be similar to those observed in adults, that is, suppression of the sinus node's automaticity with an inconsistent effect on sinoatrial conduction time.[90] Unlike in adults, in whom about 50% may show shortening of the corrected sinus node recovery time, almost all children studied showed prolongation of this parameter.

Effect on the Atrioventricular Node

It is generally accepted that propranolol increases anterograde atrioventricular conduction time in the atrioventricular node.[87, 91] Some controversy exists, however, concerning the effect of propranolol on the anterograde atrioventricular nodal effective refractory period. Several investigators have reported that propranolol prolongs this period,[87] whereas others have found no significant change.[92] The effect of propranolol on the atrioventricular node results from beta-adrenoreceptor blockade and accounts for the beneficial effect of this drug on patients with re-entrant arrhythmias. The depressant effect on the atrioventricular node prolongs the P-R and A-H intervals. For example, in 2 patients, both 16 years old, propranolol increased anterograde atrioventricular nodal conduction time from 95 to 110 and 135 msec, respectively.[93] In a 17-year-old patient, propranolol prolonged the A-H interval from 90 to 105 msec.[87] Propranolol prolongs retrograde conduction across the atrioventricular node.[93]

Effect on Accessory Atrioventricular Pathways

Propranolol has no significant effect on the anterograde or retrograde effective refractory periods of accessory atrioventricular pathways in adults.[94] Results of electrophysiologic studies have been reported for only a few children with Wolff-Parkinson-White syndrome. Barrett and co-workers reported that, in a 16-year-old patient, propranolol prolonged the conduction time in the accessory pathway from 100 to 115 msec and the effective refractory period of the accessory pathway from 185 to 230 msec.[93] In another 16-year-old patient, propranolol shortened the conduction time in the accessory pathway from 120 to

110 msec and prolonged the effective refractory period from 225 to 240 msec.

Effect on the Ventricles

Propranolol does not usually alter conduction or refractoriness in the His-Purkinje system and the ventricular myocardium.

Propranolol shortens the QTc interval in the majority of patients, but this effect is not uniform. For example, in the study reported by Seides and colleagues, propranolol shortened the QTc interval in 9 of 16 patients.[87] This effect is beneficial in the treatment of children with congenitally prolonged QT syndrome.

Effects in Arrhythmias

Supraventricular Tachycardia

Propranolol has been effective in termination and prevention of supraventricular tachycardia.[95, 96] Some controversy exists concerning the efficacy of propranolol in supraventricular tachycardia associated with Wolff-Parkinson-White syndrome. In my experience as well as in several reported studies, propranolol was effective in suppressing this arrhythmia in patients with Wolff-Parkinson-White syndrome.[96, 97] Results of one study showed, however, that intravenous propranolol did not prevent the initiation of re-entrant tachycardia in a group of 14 patients with Wolff-Parkinson-White syndrome.[93]

Supraventricular tachycardia is the most common sustained cardiac tachyarrhythmia in infancy and childhood. Tingelstad and associates were the first to report, in 1968, that propranolol, administered concomitantly with digoxin, was particularly helpful in the treatment of persistent supraventricular tachycardia in childhood.[98] Since then, propranolol has been successfully used, alone or in combination with other drugs, in infants and children with this arrhythmia.

Gillette and colleagues studied 41 infants and children with cardiac arrhythmias who were treated with propranolol.[52] Thirty of them had supraventricular tachycardia. Propranolol was effective in treatment of this arrhythmia in 6 of 8 patients with Wolff-Parkinson-White syndrome, in 7 of 9 patients with concealed anomalous pathway, in 6 of 8 patients with automatic ectopic focus, and in 3 of 5 patients with undetermined mechanism. In the patients without Wolff-Parkinson-White syndrome, propranolol was usually effective only when co-administered with digoxin. In 3 of the patients with Wolff-Parkinson-White syndrome, propranolol diminished, but did not abolish, the supraventricular tachycardia.

My colleagues and I have followed, for a period of 2 to 5 years, 5 patients with corrected transposition of the great arteries or Ebstein's anomaly and Wolff-Parkinson-White syndrome with supraventricular tachyarrhythmias. Propranolol, given orally, effectively prevented the recurrences of arrhythmias in all these patients throughout the follow-up period. One patient died suddenly after 3 years of treatment.

Pickoff and co-workers studied 5 infants and children, aged 3 weeks to 11 years, with supraventricular tachycardia resistant to digitalis.[99] In 3 of them, electrophysiologic studies showed concealed Wolff-Parkinson-White syndrome and in 1 patient, atrioventricular nodal pathways were noted. Propranolol was added to the medical treatment at oral doses of 7 to 14 µg/kg/day. Four of the children remained free of the arrhythmia, and the remaining child had supraventricular tachycardia during febrile illnesses.

Treatment of Fetal Tachycardia. Only a few cases of administration of propranolol during pregnancy have been reported. In most of these cases, the drug was used for treatment of diseases of the mother. Propranolol, which crosses the placenta, may be used for treatment of fetal tachycardia during pregnancy, however.

Sustained fetal supraventricular tachycardia is a well-recognized cause of heart failure in utero and of nonimmune hydrops fetalis. For example, in a series of 13 cases of nonimmune hydrops fetalis, 3 were caused by this arrhythmia alone. Propranolol may be tried in fetal supraventricular tachycardia, especially when it is resistant to digoxin.

Teuscher and colleagues reported a case of fetal tachycardia with heart rate of 200 beats/min.[100] Propranolol was given to the mother in the last 20 days of pregnancy and lowered heart rate to 120 to 160 beats/min. After birth, the propranolol level in the neonatal blood was 20% of the level in the maternal blood. The newborn infant had paroxysmal supraventricular tachycardia, and propranolol was again required for maintenance of a normal heart rate. The cause of the arrhythmia in this case was unknown, but it was probably related to Wolff-Parkinson-White syndrome. Combined maternal treatment with propranolol and digoxin may be tried.

Atrial Flutter

Propranolol is uncommonly used in patients of any age with atrial flutter. Atrial flutter is rare in childhood, and treatment can be difficult, especially in infants. Martin and Hernandez reviewed their experience with 10 infants with congenital and paroxysmal forms of this arrhythmia.[101] In 2 of the infants, D.C. cardioversion was the initial therapeutic technique. In both patients, the arrhythmia converted to sinus rhythm but reverted to atrial flutter, immediately or after several hours. These 2 patients were treated with digoxin and propranolol and eventually regained sinus rhythm. Another patient was first seen at 9 weeks of age with atrial flutter and congestive heart failure. D.C. cardioversion was attempted several times. It converted the patient's heart rhythm to normal sinus rhythm, but the rhythm immediately reverted to atrial flutter. The infant was treated with digoxin and propranolol, improved clinically, and was discharged from hospital. Ambulatory monitoring showed a decrease in frequency of episodes of flutter and an increase in periods of normal sinus rhythm. At 6 months, the patient's electrocardiogram showed a normal sinus rhythm, and propranolol was discontinued. The child died suddenly at home 2 weeks later. Endocardial fibroelastosis was found at autopsy.

My colleagues and I have studied a similar case. A 6-month-old infant with endocardial fibroelastosis had congestive heart failure. The diagnosis was confirmed during cardiac catheterization, and treatment with digoxin was initiated. Within the next few months, the child had recurrent episodes of atrial flutter. Propranolol was added to digoxin and controlled the arrhythmia. Because of progressive congestive heart failure, propranolol had to be discontinued. The child died at the age of 15 months of severe congestive heart failure. This case, and our experience with other patients with endocardial fibroelastosis, showed that atrial flutter associated with endocardial fibroelastosis is one of the most difficult arrhythmias to treat. Even if the condition responds to propranolol, hemodynamic deterioration may require discontinuance of this drug.

Gillette and associates studied three children with atrial flutter. Underlying diseases were not specified.[52] Propranolol was effective in only one of the children.

After Mustard's operation for complete transposition of the great arteries, atrial flutter is the most frequent arrhythmia in patients who had tachycardia as the dominant rhythm. In one study, 64% of 29 such patients had atrial flutter.[102] Treatment with available antiarrhythmic agents, including propranolol, did not reduce the risk of sudden death in these patients.

In summary, propranolol, alone or in combination with digoxin, is moderately effective in infants and children with atrial flutter. The limited effect of propranolol should be interpreted in view of the well-known resistance of atrial flutter in these age groups to all forms of treatment.

Atrial Fibrillation

In patients of any age, propranolol is rarely used in treatment of atrial fibrillation. It is occasionally given together with quinidine when treatment with quinidine is initiated, to prevent the early acceleration of ventricular rate resulting from the vagolytic effect of quinidine.

Atrial fibrillation is rare in childhood. My colleagues and I studied a child with hypertrophic cardiomyopathy and atrial fibrillation in whom the arrhythmia was controlled by the combination of propranolol and amiodarone. Gillette and co-workers reported that propranolol was effective in a child with atrial fibrillation.[52]

Ventricular Arrhythmias

Propranolol has been effective in suppressing chronic ventricular arrhythmias. For example, Gibson and Sowton reported that propranolol suppressed ventricular arrhythmias in 44% of 125 patients.[2] Woosley and associates reported that propranolol totally suppressed ventricular arrhythmias in 25% of 32 patients and produced a greater-than-70% suppression in another 50% of the patients.[103] Propranolol also suppressed ventricular arrhythmias in patients after acute myocardial infarction.[104] The increased survival rates of patients treated with propranolol after acute myocardial infarction are partially attributed to suppression of ventricular arrhythmias.

The experience in children with ventricular arrhythmias is limited. In a child with a congenitally prolonged QT interval, propranolol effectively suppressed ventricular tachycardia. Milne and associates studied a 6-year-old child with a congenitally prolonged QT interval and palpitations precipitated by exercise.[105] Propranolol shortened the QTc interval and the QT interval during atrial and ventricular pacing. Based on their experience in adults, Milne and co-workers concluded that propranolol shortens the QT interval in patients with congenital, but not acquired, idiopathic QT prolongation.[105] The mechanism of action is not clear, but it may resemble that of stellectomy.

Wennevold and Sandol reported their experience with 3 children with paroxysmal ventricular tachycardia and fibrillation treated with propranolol for 6 to 14 years.[105a] The first patient was a girl whose recurrent syncopal episodes had begun at the age of 6 years. For 2 years, she had been misdiagnosed and had been treated for epilepsy. At the age of 8 years, an exercise electrocardiogram had confirmed the diagnosis of malignant ventricular tachycardia. Propranolol had been initiated, and the patient had been asymptomatic for 2 years. Throughout the next 14 years, she had only a few episodes of arrhythmia, which were attributed to failure to take the drug or to her outgrowing of the dose. This patient had an uncomplicated pregnancy and delivery during continued beta-blockade at the age of 21 years and is doing well at the age of 22 years.

The second patient was a girl who had started to have episodes of fainting at the age of 8 years. The electrocardiogram had shown sinus bradycardia. At the age of 12 years, the diagnosis of brief malignant ventricular tachycardia had been confirmed by exercise electrocardiogram. Treatment with propranolol partially abolished the fainting spells. These spells stopped at the age of 18, but she died suddenly 4 years later.

The third patient was a 3-year-old boy with cardiomyopathy. At the age of 6 years, syncopal episodes had appeared, the patient's heart had been enlarged, and an electrocardiogram had shown ischemic changes. Ventricular fibrillation had been recorded during syncope when the patient was 10 years old. He was treated with propranolol and practolol with partial response and died suddenly at 16 years of age, 4 years after his last episode of syncope.[105a] It is possible that death could have been prevented in this patient by the implantation of a pacemaker.

In summary, propranolol can abolish syncope associated with malignant ventricular arrhythmias, but sudden death may nevertheless occur.

Effects in Thyrotoxicosis

Propranolol is effective in the treatment of thyrotoxicosis. It abolishes cardiovascular and other symptoms and reduces the plasma level of the active thyroid hormone T_3. These effects may result from reduction of peripheral activation of T_4 and its conversion to the active hormone T_3.[106] As a result, the serum level of T_4 is increased, that of T_3 is decreased, and that of reversed T_3 is increased. When propranolol is abruptly discontinued, a rebound increase in free T_3 in the serum occurs. Because of these effects, propranolol had been used in the past 20 years for treatment of thyrotoxicosis. Propranolol may be given alone, but it is usually combined with antithyroid drugs or radioiodine. Propranolol is also used in preparation for thyroidectomy.[107]

Several investigators have reported that propranolol is useful for treatment of thyrotoxicosis in neonates, infants, and children.[108–111] Feld (personal communication) treated two children with thyrotoxicosis and a hyperkinetic circulatory state with propranolol, given alone as initial therapy. The patients' symptoms improved.

Lawrence and colleagues reported the cases of 2 children with acute excessive ingestion of thyroid hormones who were treated with propranolol.[112] A 3-year-old boy ingested 80 tablets of 0.15 mg levothyroxine. He was treated by gastric lavage, activated charcoal, magnesium citrate, propranolol 10 mg every 6 hours, prednisone, propylthiouracil, and cholestyramine. In 48 hours, the child's heart rate was accelerated, and the dose of propranolol was increased to 20 mg every 6 hours. The child remained asymptomatic during hospitalization and at follow-up clinic visits. A 2-year-old girl ingested 40 tablets of 0.1 mg levothyroxine. She was treated with charcoal and propranolol, 20 mg every 6 hours. This dose of propranolol controlled the patient's heart rate.[112]

In cases of acute ingestion of thyroid hormones in infants and children, propranolol is effective as part of combined therapy including the following: (1) gastric lavage and activated charcoal, to decrease absorption of the hormones; (2) cholestyramine, to bind thyroid hormones and to decrease enterohepatic accumulation; (3) prednisone or propylthiouracil, to decrease peripheral conversion of T_4 to T_3; and (4) propranolol, to block the hemodynamic and metabolic effects of thyroid hormones.[112]

Neonatal thyrotoxicosis is a rare, transient disease related to the presence of long-acting thyroid stimulator in the neonate's blood. Fewer than 50 cases have been reported. Since this disease is self-limiting, symptomatic control in the early postnatal phase is sufficient. Such control may be achieved with propranolol.

In 1973, Smith and Howard reported the case of a patient with neonatal thyrotoxicosis in whom the disease was controlled by the combination of propranolol, digoxin, phenobarbitone, propylthiouracil, and Lugol's iodine.[113] Pemberton and associates reported on another patient with neonatal thyrotoxicosis in whom propranolol, 0.5 to 8 mg 4 times daily as sole therapy, effectively controlled the disease.[108] Propranolol reduced activity of the child, heart rate, and cutaneous blood flow. When the patient's protein-bound iodine level had returned to normal, propranolol was discontinued, and the symptoms did not return.

In summary, propranolol, whether alone or in combined therapy, is effective in controlling thyrotoxicosis of various causes in neonates, infants, and children.

Effect on Plasma Lipids

Long-term administration of propranolol may be complicated by an adverse effect on a patient's plasma lipid profile. This feature has been seen in adults and may pose a special problem in children with hypertension or hypertrophic cardiomyopathy who require treatment for many years. The most important effect of propranolol on lipids is an increase in serum triglycerides.

Total cholesterol levels are not usually altered, but the distribution of cholesterol may be unfavorably altered, with a decrease in high-density lipoprotein (HDL) cholesterol and an increase in very low-density and low-density lipoprotein (VLDL and LDL) cholesterol when compared to untreated patients.[114-117]

This lipid profile is associated with a higher incidence of coronary artery disease. It is not known, however, whether the slight-to-moderate changes produced by propranolol are also associated with increased incidence of coronary artery disease in young age groups. Most of the studies on the effect of propranolol on lipids have been performed in adults with hypertension or coronary artery disease.

Effect on Glucose Metabolism

Propranolol inhibits hepatic glycogenolysis and thereby lowers plasma glucose levels. By this mechanism, propranolol may potentiate insulin-induced hypoglycemia or may prolong its duration.[118] The effect of propranolol on glucose metabolism in children has been evaluated by several investigators. In a series of 64 children treated with propranolol for long periods, no signs of hypoglycemia were observed.[52] On the other hand, several children developed hypoglycemia after short-term ingestion of high doses of propranolol.[119, 120] A 4-year-old child developed hypoglycemic seizures after 3 days of refusal of solid food because of an oral wound. The possibility of propranolol-induced hypoglycemia should be considered in children treated with propranolol during changes in diet or febrile diseases. Hypoglycemia may occur in neonates whose mothers had been treated with propranolol during pregnancy. Habib and McCarthy found hypoglycemia in 4 neonates with good Apgar scores whose mothers had received propranolol during pregnancy.[121] Cottrill and associates also reported hypoglycemia in a neonate whose mother had received 160 mg propranolol daily.[122] Although the potential risk of hypoglycemia in neonates of mothers treated with propranolol has been questioned,[123] it should still be considered.

Effect on Anterior Pituitary and Sex Hormones

In healthy human subjects, propranolol has reduced the plasma levels of follicle-stimulating hormone and testosterone, has elevated plasma levels of cortisol and has not altered the levels of growth hormone, luteinizing hormone, and prolactin. These effects have varied among patients.[124] The presence and significance of these changes in children have not been defined.

Drug Discontinuance

Studies in adults have shown that abrupt discontinuance of the long-term administration of propranolol may result in serious withdrawal symptoms. The propranolol withdrawal syndrome has been reported mainly in patients with coronary artery disease or hypertension. The extreme presentations of this syndrome are sudden death and acute myocardial infarction. Other presentations are deterioration of angina pectoris, rebound hypertension, provocation or worsening of cardiac arrhythmias, palpitations, headache and sweating. The withdrawal syndrome usually appears within 3 to 10 days of discontinuance of the drug. Although it is difficult to evaluate the incidence of this syndrome, 5 to 10% of patients with cardiovascular disease may develop it.[69, 125, 126]

The incidence of propranolol withdrawal syndrome in infants and children has not been evaluated, but isolated cases have been reported. Martin and Hernandez reported the case of a child with endocardial fibroelastosis and atrial flutter who died suddenly 2 weeks after discontinuance of propranolol.[101] Because propranolol effectively suppressed the arrhythmia in this patient, recurrence of the arrhythmia may have been the cause of death.

I have studied an infant with tetralogy of Fallot and hypoxemic spells responsive to propranolol. Ten days after his parents discontinued treatment at home, the spells increased in frequency. No controlled trials of propranolol withdrawal have been performed in infants and children.

The propranolol withdrawal syndrome may result from several mechanisms, as follows: (1) increased sensitivity to beta-adrenoreceptor stimulation, possibly because of increased density of beta-adrenoreceptors in target organs during treatment with propranolol; (2) elevation of levels of thyroid hormones; (3) enhanced platelet aggregation; (4) increased levels of plasma catecholamines and increased plasma renin activity; (5) progression of underlying cardiovascular diseases; and (6) continuance of high levels of physical activity after discontinuance of the protective beta-blocking agent.

Clinical Pharmacology

Propranolol may be given orally or intravenously. The commercially available drug for both routes of administration is racemic propranolol. More than 90% of an oral dose is absorbed from the gastrointestinal tract.[127] The rate of absorption is rapid, and the maximal plasma concentration is reached within 2 hours of administration of a single oral dose.[128] The rate and extent of absorption of propranolol may be increased in patients with celiac disease.

After absorption, propranolol undergoes extensive first-pass hepatic metabolism, by oxidation, N-dealkylation, deamination, and glucuronidation. This process results in systemic bioavailability of 30 to 40%, with a wide variation among patients.[129] During prolonged oral administration of propranolol, the plasma concentrations of the metabolites are much higher than those of the parent drug. Most metabolites are pharmacologically inactive, but one of them, 4-hydroxy propranolol, exerts some beta-adrenoreceptor blocking effect. The systemic bioavailability of L-propranolol is lower than that of D-propranolol.[130]

Plasma levels of propranolol were reported to range between 20 and 580 nmol/L after short-term administration and between 20 and 84 ng/ml during long-term administration.[131, 132] The variability in plasma concentrations results from variability in first-pass hepatic metabolism of the drug. During prolonged administration of racemic propranolol, the plasma levels of L-propranolol were reported to be higher than those of D-propranolol.[133]

A significant level of beta-blockade is achieved in more than half the patients at plasma levels of 0.5 to 5 ng/ml and in almost all patients at plasma levels of up to 30 ng/ml.[134] At the lower concentration range, a positive correlation between plasma concentration and beta-blockade has been found. An antianginal effect has been reported at plasma levels of about 20 to 40 ng/ml.[16] A weaker correlation between the antianginal effect and the log of plasma level of propranolol has been observed.[135] These findings are controversial because several investigators found no correlation between plasma levels and clinical effects of propranolol.[128]

In studies of children with tetralogy of Fallot, a correlation between the effect and the dose was found. The responders received about twice the dose of the nonresponders. The plasma level required for suppression of ventricular arrhythmias in at least half the patients was reported to range between 40 and 320 ng/ml, although much higher plasma levels were required on rare occasions.[136, 137] These levels are higher than those required to achieve beta-blockade. The level of free propranolol may correlate better with the therapeutic effects than with the level of total propranolol.[138]

Propranolol is bound by about 90% to plasma proteins, including alpha-1-acid glycoprotein, albumin, and lipoprotein.[139] The plasma levels of these proteins are increased in several diseases and result in a decrease in free propranolol.[140, 141] Excessive protein binding was the cause of resistance to propranolol in 4 of 6 patients.[142]

Propranolol is eliminated by hepatic metabolism and renal excretion of the metabolites, as well as small amounts of the unchanged drug.[127] The systemic clearance of the metabolites correlates with hepatic blood flow. In patients with renal or hepatic failure, the metabolites of propranolol may accumulate. In patients with normal hepatic and renal function, the elimination half-life of propranolol ranges between 3 and 6 hours.[143, 144] The pharmacodynamic half-life of propranolol is longer than the elimination half-life.[145]

Children with Down's syndrome have an impaired metabolism of propranolol.[59] In 2 infants with tetralogy of Fallot and Down's syndrome, plasma levels of 211 and 467 ng/ml, respectively, were found 2 hours following an oral dose of propranolol, as compared with 20 to

115 ng/ml in children with tetralogy of Fallot but without Down's syndrome.

Side Effects

The side effects of propranolol are usually predictable because most are related to beta-adrenoreceptor blockade. The most important side effects of propranolol are cardiovascular.

Bradycardia

Almost all patients treated with propranolol show some slowing of heart rate because of beta-adrenoreceptor blockade. Bradycardia was observed, however, in only 0.56% of 1435 patients treated with propranolol. Two of 22 infants and children with tetralogy of Fallot reported by Ponce and co-workers, developed marked bradycardia during treatment with propranolol.[59] In my experience, propranolol had to be discontinued in 2 of 31 infants and children with tetralogy of Fallot because of severe bradycardia. This side effect is dose-dependent and usually responds to reduction in dose. Patients with sick sinus syndrome are more prone to develop sinus bradycardia during treatment with propranolol.

Complete Atrioventricular Block

Complete atrioventricular block is an unusual complication of propranolol therapy and is rare in children. Seis and colleagues reported on a 9-year-old boy receiving maintenance hemodialysis who had an emergency admission to a pediatric ward because of severe hypertension, congestive heart failure, and pulmonary edema.[146] The patient's chest roentgenogram revealed an enlarged heart with bilateral pulmonary congestion. The electrocardiogram showed left ventricular hypertrophy. The patient received intravenous diazoxide. Digitalization and hemodialysis were initiated immediately. Oral antihypertensive treatment consisted of propranolol, 10 mg 3 times daily, and hydralazine, 25 mg 4 times daily. Digoxin was discontinued when the patient's condition improved after 7 days. Thirteen days later, the patient developed complete atrioventricular block, with a ventricular rate of 50 beats/min. Propranolol was discontinued, and 48 hours later, the electrocardiogram was normal. When propranolol was readministered, first-degree atrioventricular block developed.

I have studied a child with tetralogy of Fallot who developed complete atrioventricular block after accidental ingestion of eight times his therapeutic dose of propranolol. The possibility of atrioventricular nodal conduction disturbances due to propranolol in children is rare, but it should be kept in mind.

Congestive Heart Failure

The negative inotropic and chronotropic effects of propranolol may result in provocation or aggravation of congestive heart failure. This effect was found in 0.48% of 1435 patients treated with propranolol, although a much higher incidence was found in patients with coronary artery disease who were treated for long periods with propranolol.[67] In my experience, 2 of 31 children with tetralogy of Fallot developed congestive heart failure during treatment with propranolol. One of them improved after a reduction in dose, whereas the other required discontinuance of the drug. Ponce and associates reported that 1 of 22 infants and children with tetralogy of Fallot developed congestive heart failure.[59]

Peripheral Vascular Effects

Propranolol elevates peripheral vascular resistance because it blocks the vascular beta-adrenoreceptors through which peripheral vasodilation is mediated and leaves the vasoconstricting alpha-adrenoreceptor stimulation unopposed. It also decreases cardiac output. These effects result in a decrease in blood flow to the extremities that may cause a cold feeling in the extremities or even claudication. These adverse peripheral vascular effects are usually observed in adults with peripheral vascular disease and rarely present a problem in infants and children.

Pulmonary Effects

Because propranolol blocks the bronchodilatory beta-adrenoreceptors in the lungs and leaves the alpha-adrenoreceptors unopposed, bronchospasm may be caused or may be aggravated, especially in patients with pulmonary obstructive diseases. Propranolol is contraindicated in children with active bronchial asthma.

Effects on the Central Nervous System

Propranolol causes vivid dreams, depression, dizziness, hallucinations, somnolence, headache, paresthesias, anxiety, and other effects related to the central nervous system, each in less than 1% of the patients. Central-nervous-system-related side effects of propranolol in children may be more common than previously thought.

Arrhythmogenic Effect

Beta-adrenoreceptor blocking agents rarely have an arrhythmogenic effect. In contrast, Class I antiarrhythmic agents may provoke or may aggravate arrhythmias in a few patients. Even though amiodarone has also a membrane-stabilizing activity similar to that of Class I antiarrhythmic agents, it is rarely associated with an arrhythmogenic effect. Pioselli and co-workers reported on a 7-year-old child with mitral valve prolapse who had more than 190 bouts of ventricular tachycardia daily.[147] Several antiarrhythmic agents were tried, with good results. Propranolol was the only drug that increased the number of premature ventricular beats in this patient.

Growth Retardation

Some concern exists about whether prolonged treatment with beta-blocking agents from infancy may cause growth retardation. Long-term oral propranolol administration to growing rats reduced both their growth rate and the absolute weight of most organs; this effect was entirely reversible on discontinuance of treatment and occurred independently of changes in growth hormone and hypothalamic somatostatin concentration.[148]

Drug Interactions

Cimetidine

Cimetidine increases the steady-state plasma concentration of propranolol.[149,150] This change results from reduced hepatic clearance of propranolol, both because of a decrease in hepatic blood flow and a direct effect of cimetidine on hepatic enzymes.[149,151]

Lidocaine

Propranolol reduces the clearance of lidocaine because of a decrease in hepatic blood flow.[152]

Quinidine

Co-administration of quinidine can increase the systemic bioavailability of propranolol.[153]

Dosage and Administration

Oral Administration

Doses of 1 to 3 mg/kg/day have been used in infants and children. The total daily dose is given as 3 to 4 divided doses, at 6 to 8 hour intervals. Occasionally, oral doses as low as 0.5 mg/kg/day or as high as 4.0 mg/kg/day have been used.[52] Pickoff and colleagues used even higher doses of 7 to 14 mg/kg/day for management of supraventricular tachycardia in infants and children.[99] Children with tetralogy of Fallot who responded to propranolol received a mean dose of 2.6 mg/kg/day.[58]

Intravenous Administration

Doses of 0.1 to 0.2 mg/kg were given intravenously during hemodynamic studies in children with tetralogy of Fallot and during electrophysiologic studies in children with arrhythmias.

References

1. Gettes, L.S.: Beta-adrenergic blocking drugs in the treatment of cardiac arrhythmias. Cardiovasc. Clin., 2:211, 1970.
2. Gibson, D., and Sowton, E.: The use of beta-adrenergic receptor-blocking drugs in dysrhythmias. Prog. Cardiovasc. Dis., 12:16, 1969.
3. Howitt, G., et al.: The effect of the dextro isomer of propranolol in sinus rate and cardiac arrhythmias, Am. Heart J., 76:736, 1968.
4. Thadani, U., et al.: Comparison of adrenergic beta-receptor antagonists in angina pectoris. Br. Med. J., 1:138, 1973.
5. Davidson, C., et al.: Comparison of antihypertensive activity of beta-blocking drugs during chronic treatment. Br. Med. J., 2:7, 1976.
6. Epstein, S.E., et al.: Effects of beta adrenergic blockade on the cardiac response to maximal and submaximal exercise in man. J. Clin. Invest., 44:1745, 1965.
7. Milne, J.R., et al.: Effect of intravenous propranolol on QT interval. A new method of assessment. Br. Heart J., 43:1, 1980.
8. Port, S., Cobb, F.R., and Jones, R.H.: Effects of propranolol on left ventricular function in normal men. Circulation, 61:358, 1980.
9. Friedman, M.J., et al.: Effects of propranolol on resting and postextrasystolic potentiated left ventricular function in patients with coronary artery disease. Am. Heart J., 81, 1983.
10. Marshall, R.C., et al.: Effect of oral propranolol on rest, exercise and postexercise left ventricular performance in normal subjects and patients with coronary artery disease. Circulation, 63:572, 1981.
11. Erhardt, J.C., Verani, M.S., and Marcus, M.L.: Exercise isotope ventriculogram: use in assessing changes in left ventricular function. (Abstract.) Circulation, 56 (Suppl. II):II-61, 1978.
12. Klinke, W.P., et al.: Use of catheter-tip velocity pressure transducer to evaluate left ventricular function in man: effects of intravenous propranolol. Circulation, 61:946, 1981.
13. Dwyer, E.M., Jr., Wiener, L., and Cox, W.J.: Effects of beta-adrenergic blockade on left ventricular hemodynamics and the electrocardiogram during exercise induced angina pectoris. Circulation, 38:250, 1968.
14. Wiener, L., Dwyer, E.M., Jr., and Cox, J.W.: Hemodynamic effects of nitroglycerin, propranolol and their combination in coronary heart disease. Circulation, 39:623, 1969.
15. Sapru, R.P., et al.: Effect of isoprenaline and propranolol on left ventricular function as determined by nuclear angiography. Br. Heart J., 44:75, 1980.
16. Pine, M., et al.: Correlation of plasma propranolol concentration with therapeutic response in patients with angina pectoris. Circulation, 52:886, 1975.
17. Crawford, M.H., Lindenfeld, J., and O'Rourke, R.A.: Effects of oral propranolol on left ventricular size and performance during exercise and acute pressure loading. Circulation, 61:549, 1980.
18. Robin, E., et al.: A comparative study of nitroglycerin and propranolol. Circulation, 36:175, 1967.
19. Fenyvesi, T., and Kallay, K: The presence of beta-adrenergic receptors in the renal vascular bed. Acta Physiol. Acad. Sci. Hung., 38:159, 1970.
20. Franciosa, J.A., Johnson, S.M., and Tobian, L.J.: Hemodynamic effects of oxprenolol and propranolol in hypertension. Clin. Pharmacol. Ther., 26:676, 1979.

21. Bonow, R.O., et al.: Effects of verapamil and propranolol on left ventricular systolic function and diastolic filling in patients with coronary artery disease. Circulation, 64:787, 1981.
22. Nies, A.S., McNeil, J.S., and Schrier, R.W.: Mechanism of increased sodium reabsorption during propranolol administration. Circulation, 44:596, 1971.
23. Vatner, S.F., et al.: Effects of propranolol on regional myocardial function, electrograms and blood flow in conscious dogs with myocardial ischemia. J. Clin. Invest., 60:353, 1977.
24. Vatner, S.F., et al.: Effects of a cardiac glycoside in combination with propranolol on the ischemic heart of conscious dogs. Circulation, 57:568, 1978.
25. Pitt, B., and Craven, P.: Effect of propranolol on regional myocardial blood flow in acute ischemia. Cardiovasc. Res., 4:176, 1970.
26. Pearle, D.L., Williford, D., and Gillis, R.A.: Superiority of practolol versus propranolol in protection against ventricular fibrillation induced by coronary occlusion. Am. J. Cardiol., 42:960, 1978.
27. Carriere, S.: Effect of norepinephrine, isoproterenol, and adrenergic blockers upon the intrarenal distribution of blood flow. Can. J. Physiol. Pharmacol., 47:199, 1969.
28. Krauss, X.H., et al.: Effects of chronic beta-adrenergic blockade on systemic and renal hemodynamic responses to hyperosmotic saline in hypertensive patients. Clin. Sci., 43:385, 1972.
29. Van Hooff, M.E.J., et al.: Time course of blood pressure changes after intravenous administration of propranolol or furosemide in hypertensive patients. J. Cardiovasc. Pharmacol., 5:773, 1983.
30. Jackson, M., et al.: Propranolol in the treatment of essential hypertension. JAMA, 237:2303, 1977.
31. Galloway, D.B., et al.: Propranolol in hypertension: a dose-response study. Br. Med. J., 2:140, 1976.
32. Buhler, F.R., et al.: Propranolol inhibition of renin secretion: a specific approach to diagnosis and treatment of renin-dependent hypertensive diseases. N. Engl. J. Med., 287:1209, 1972.
33. Hollifield, J.W., et al.: Proposed mechanisms of propranolol's antihypertensive effect in essential hypertension. N. Engl. J. Med., 68, 1976.
34. Zacharias, F.J., et al.: Propranolol in hypertension: a study of long term therapy, 1964–1970. Am. Heart J., 83:755, 1972.
35. Davies, R., et al.: Blockade of cardiac and renal beta-receptors by low dose propranolol in normal subjects: clues to its antihypertensive effect. Br. Heart J., 41:331, 1979.
36. Pritchard, B.N.C.: Propranolol as an antihypertensive agent. Am. Heart J., 79:128, 1970.
37. Ulrych, M., et al.: Immediate hemodynamic effects of beta-adrenergic blockade with propranolol in normotensive and hypertensive man. Circulation, 37:411, 1968.
38. Frohlich, E.D., et al.: The paradox of beta-adrenergic blockade in hypertension. Circulation, 37:417, 1968.
39. Michelakis, A.M., and McAllister, R.G.: The effect of chronic adrenergic blockade on plasma renin activity in man. J. Clin. Endocrinol. Metab., 34:386, 1972.
40. Zweifler, A., and Esler, M.: Blood pressure, renin activity and heart rate changes during propranolol therapy of hypertension. Am. J. Cardiol., 40:105, 1977.
41. Bravo, E.L., et al.: Beta-adrenergic blockade in diuretic-treated patients with essential hypertension. N. Engl. J. Med., 292:66, 1975.
42. Pritchard, B.N.C., and Gillam, P.M.S.: Treatment of hypertension with propranolol. Br. Med. J., 1:7, 1969.
43. Thompson, D.S., et al.: Effects of propranolol on myocardial oxygen consumption, substrate extraction, and haemodynamics in hypertrophic obstructive cardiomyopathy. Br. Heart J., 44:488, 1980.
44. Sloman, G.: Propranolol in management of muscular subaortic stenosis. Br. Heart J., 29:783, 1967.
45. Swan, D.A., et al.: Analysis of symptomatic course and prognosis and treatment of hypertrophic obstructive cardiomyopathy. Br. Heart J., 33:671, 1971.

46. Tabatznik, B.: Ambulatory monitoring in the late post myocardial infarction period. Postgrad. Med. J., 52(Suppl. 7):56, 1976.
47. Goodwin, J.F., and Kirkler, D.M.: Sudden death in cardiomyopathy. Adv. Cardiol., 25:96, 1978.
48. Pichard, A.D., et al.: Septal perforator compression (narrowing) in idiopathic hypertrophic subaortic stenosis. Am. J. Cardiol., 40:310, 1977.
49. Alvares, R.F., and Goodwin, J.F.: Non-invasive assessment of diastolic function in hypertrophic cardiomyopathy on and off beta adrenergic blocking drugs. Br. Heart J., 48:204, 1982.
50. Wigle, E.D., Adelman, A.G., and Felderhof, C.H.: Medical and surgical treatment of the cardiomyopathies. Circ. Res., 34,35(Suppl. II):II-196, 1974.
51. Goodwin, J.F.: Prospects and predictions for the cardiomyopathies. Circulation, 50:210, 1974.
52. Gillette, P.C., et al.: Oral propranolol treatment in infants and children. J. Pediatr., 92:141, 1978.
53. Harris, A.: Long term treatment of paroxysmal cardiac arrhythmias with propranolol. Am. J. Cardiol., 18:431, 1966.
54. Cherian, G., et al.: Beta adrenergic blockade in patients with hypertrophic obstructive cardiomyopathy. Am. Heart J., 73:140, 1967.
55. Hardarson, T., et al.: Prognosis and mortality of hypertrophic obstructive cardiomyopathy. Lancet, 2:1462, 1973.
56. McKenna, W.J., et al.: Arrhythmia in hypertrophic cardiomyopathy: exercise and 48 hour ambulatory electrocardiographic assessment with and without beta adrenergic blocking therapy. Am. J. Cardiol., 45:1, 1980.
57. Shand, D.G., Sell, C.G., and Oates, J.A.: Hypertrophic obstructive cardiomyopathy in an infant—propranolol therapy for three years. N. Engl. J. Med., 285:843, 1971.
58. Garson, A., Gillette, P.C., and McNamara, D.G.: Propranolol: the preferred palliation for tetralogy of Fallot. Am. J. Cardiol., 47:1098, 1981.
59. Ponce, F.E., et al.: Propranolol palliation of tetralogy of Fallot: experience with long-term drug treatment in pediatric patients. Pediatrics, 52:100, 1973.
60. Keck, E.W., and Brode, P.: Beta receptor block in Fallot's tetralogy. Germ. Med. Month., 15:139, 1970.
61. Eriksson, B.O., Thoren, C., and Zetterqvist, P.: Long term treatment with propranolol in selected cases of Fallot's tetralogy. Br. Heart J., 31:37, 1969.
62. Nayler, W.G., Chipperfield, D., and Lowe, T.E.: The negative inotropic effect of adrenergic beta-receptor blocking drugs on human heart muscle. Cardiovasc. Res., 3:30, 1969.
63. King, S.B., and Franch, R.H.: Production of increased right-to-left shunting by rapid heart rates in patients with tetralogy of Fallot. Circulation, 44:265, 1971.
64. Honey, M., Chamberlain, D.A., and Howard, J.: The effect of beta sympathetic blockade on arterial oxygen saturation in Fallot's tetralogy. Circulation, 30:501, 1964.
65. Macdonald, I.A., et al.: The acute effects of metoprolol or propranolol on metabolic and cardiorespiratory responses to exercise in hypertensive patients. Proceedings of the S.P.S. and the B.P.S., 1982, p. 583P.
66. Frank, M.J., et al.: Long term medical management of hypertrophic obstructive cardiomyopathy. Am. J. Cardiol., 42:993, 1978.
67. Warren, S.G. Brewer, D.L., and Orgain, E.S.: Long term propranolol therapy for angina pectoris. Am. J. Cardiol., 37:420, 1976.
68. Keber, I., et al.: The influence of combined treatment with propranolol and acetyl salicylic acid on platelet aggregation in coronary heart disease. Br. J. Clin. Pharmacol., 7:287, 1979.
69. Frishman, W.H., et al.: Reversal of abnormal platelet aggregability and change in exercise tolerance in patients with angina pectoris following oral propranolol. Circulation, 50:887, 1974.
70. Thomas, D.: Effect of catecholamine on platelet aggregation caused by thrombin. Nature, 215:298, 1967.

71. Mehta, J., and Mehta, P.: Effects of propranolol therapy on platelet release and prostaglandin generation in patients with coronary heart disease. Circulation, 66:1294, 1982.
72. Vlachakis, N.D., and Aledort, L.: Hypertension and propranolol therapy: effect on blood pressure, plasma catecholamines and platelet aggregation. Am. J. Cardiol., 45:321, 1980.
73. Dray, F., Charbonnel, B., and Maclouf, J.: Radioimmunoassay of prostaglandins F_α, E_1 and E_2 in human plasma. Eur. J. Clin. Invest., 5:311, 1975.
74. Manchester, J., et al.: Relationship of antianginal agents to hemoglobin-oxygen affinity. (Abstract.) Circulation, 45,46 (Suppl. II):II-28, 1972.
75. Schrumpf, J.D., et al.: Altered hemoglobin-oxygen affinity with long-term propranolol therapy in patients with coronary artery disease. Am. J. Cardiol., 40:76, 1977.
76. Hamer, J., et al.: Effect of propranolol (Inderal) in angina pectoris: preliminary report. Br. Med. J., 2:720, 1964.
77. Prichard, B.N.C., Aellig, W.H., and Richardson, G.A.: The action of intravenous administration of oxprenolol, practolol, propranolol and sotalol on acute exercise tolerance in angina pectoris, the effect on pulse rate and the electrocardiogram. Postgrad. Med. J., 46 (Suppl.):77, 1970.
78. Zeft, H.J., Patterson, S., and Orgain, E.S.: The effect of propranolol in the longterm treatment of angina pectoris. Arch. Intern. Med., 124:578, 1969.
79. Wolfson, S., et al.: Propranolol and angina pectoris. Am. J. Cardiol., 18:345, 1966.
80. Nissri, J.: Variant angina and propranolol. N. Engl. J. Med., 294:1007, 1976.
81. Yasue, H., et al.: Prinzmetal's variant form of angina as a manifestation of alphaadrenergic receptor-mediated coronary artery spasm: documentation by coronary arteriography. Am. Heart J., 91:148, 1976.
82. Hernandez-Casas, G., Dear, W., and Leachman, R.D.: Prinzmetal's variant angina pectoris with normal coronary arteriograms: effect of long-term reserpine treatment. Cardiovasc. Dis., 1:194, 1974.
83. Guazzi, M., et al.: Treatment of spontaneous angina pectoris with beta blocking agents: a clinical, electrocardiographic, and haemodynamic appraisal. Br. Heart J., 37:1235, 1975.
84. Robertson, R.M., Breinig, J.B., and Robertson, D.: Chronic recurrent variant angina. South. Med. J., 72:1297, 1979.
85. Bodenheimer, M., et al.: Prinzmetal's variant angina: a clinical and electrocardiographic study. Am. Heart J., 87:304, 1974.
86. Yasue, H., et al.: Pathogenesis and treatment of angina pectoris at rest as seen from its response to various drugs. Jpn. Circ. J., 42: 1, 1978.
87. Seides, S.F., Josephson, M.E., and Batsford, W.P.: The electrophysiology of propranolol in man. Am. Heart J., 88:733, 1974.
88. Stern, S., and Eisenberg, S.: The effect of propranolol (Inderal) in the electrocardiogram of normal subjects. Am. Heart J., 77:192, 1969.
89. Narula, O.S., et al.: Effect of propranolol on normal and abnormal sinus node function. In The Sinus Node. Edited by F.I.M. Bonke. The Hague, Martinus Nijhoff, 1978, p. 112.
90. Yabek, S.M., et al.: Electrophysiologic effects of propranolol on sinus node function in children. Am. Heart J., 104:612, 1982.
91. Berkowitz, W.D., Wit, A.L., and Lau, S.H.: The effects of propranolol on cardiac conduction. Circulation, 40:855, 1969.
92. Wu, D., Denes, P., and Dhingra, R.: The effects of propranolol on induction of AV nodal reentrant paroxysmal tachycardia. Circulation, 50:665, 1974.
93. Barrett, P.A., et al.: The electrophysiologic effects of intravenous propranolol in the Wolff-Parkinson-White syndrome. Am. Heart J., 98:213, 1979.
94. Denes, P., Wu, D., and Amat-y-Leon, F.: The effect of propranolol on anomalous pathway refractoriness and circus movement tachycardia in patients with preexcitation. Am. J. Cardiol., 39:319, 1977.

95. Gettes, L.S., and Yoshonis, K.F.: Rapidly recurring supraventricular tachycardia: a manifestation of reciprocating tachycardia and an indication for propranolol therapy. Circulation, 41:689, 1970.
96. Chung, E.K.: Tachyarrhythmias in Wolff-Parkinson-White syndrome: antiarrhythmic drug therapy. JAMA, 237:376, 1977.
97. Gallagher, J.J., et al.: The Wolff-Parkinson-White syndrome and the pre-excitation dysrhythmias. Med. Clin. North Am., 60:101, 1976.
98. Tingelstad, J.B., et al.: Propranolol in the management of children with paroxysmal supraventricular tachycardia. Circulation, 38(Suppl. VI):194, 1968.
99. Pickoff, A.S., et al.: High-dose propranolol therapy in the management of supraventricular tachycardia. J. Pediatr., 94:144, 1979.
100. Teuscher, A., et al.: Effect of propranolol on fetal tachycardia in diabetic pregnancy. Am. J. Cardiol., 42:304, 1978.
101. Martin, T.C, and Hernandez, A.: Atrial flutter in infancy. J. Pediatr., 100:239, 1982.
102. Flinn, C.J., et al.: Cardiac rhythm after the Mustard operation for complete transposition of the great arteries. N. Engl. J. Med., 310:1635, 1984.
103. Woosley, R.L., et al.: Suppression of chronic ventricular arrhythmias with propranolol. Circulation, 60:819, 1979.
104. Koppes, G.M., Beckmann, C.H., and Jones, F.G.: Propranolol therapy or ventricular arrhythmias 2 months after acute myocardial infarction. Am. J. Cardiol., 46:322, 1980.
105. Milne, J.R., et al.: The long QT syndrome: effects of drugs and left stellate ganglion block. Am. Heart J., 104:194, 1982.
105a. Wennevold, A., and Sandøe, E.: 6–14 years; beta-blockade in three children with paroxysmal ventricular fibrillation. In Management of Ventricular Tachycardia— Role of Mexiletine: Proceedings of a Symposium, Copenhagen, 25–27, May, 1978. Edited by E. Sandøe, et al. Amsterdam, Excerpta Medica, 1978, p. 429.
106. Kristensen, B.O., Steiness, E., and Weeke, J.: Propranolol withdrawal and thyroid hormones in patients with essential hypertension. Clin. Pharmacol. Ther., 23:624, 1978.
107. Toft, A.D., Irvine, W.J., and Campbell, R.W.F.: Assessment by continuous cardiac monitoring of minimum duration of preoperative propranolol treatment in thyrotoxic patients. Clin. Endocrinol., (Oxf.) 5:195, 1976.
108. Pemberton, P.J., McConnell, B., and Shanks, R.G.: Neonatal thyrotoxicosis treated with propranolol. Arch. Dis. Child. 49:813, 1974.
109. Bullock, J.L., Harris, R.E., and Young, R.: Treatment of thyrotoxicosis during pregnancy with propranolol. Am. J. Obstet. Gynecol., 121:242,1975.
110. Buckle, R.M., Treatment of thyroid crisis by beta-adrenergic blockade. Acta Endocrinol. (Copenh.), 57:168, 1968.
111. Galaburda, M., Rosman, N.P., and Haddow, J.E. Thyroid storm in an 11-year old boy managed by propranolol. Pediatrics, 53:920, 1974.
112. Lawrence, M.A.J., et al.: Acute ingestions of thyroid hormones. Pediatrics, 73:313, 1984.
113. Smith, J., and Howard, S.: Propranolol in neonatal thyrotoxicosis. Arch. Dis. Child., 47:813, 1973.
114. Tanaka, N., et al.: Effect of chronic administration of propranolol on lipoprotein composition. Metabolism, 25:1071, 1976.
115. Wright, A.D., et al.: Beta-adrenoceptor blocking drugs and blood sugar control in diabetes mellitus. Br. Med. J., 1:159, 1979.
116. Leren, P., et al.: Effect of propranolol and prazosin on blood lipids: the Oslo Study. Lancet, 2:4, 1980.
117. Johnson, B.F.: The emerging problem of plasma lipid changes during antihypertensive therapy. J. Cardiovasc. Pharmacol. 4(Suppl. 2):S213, 1982.
118. Deacon, S.P., and Barnett, D.: Comparison of atenolol and propranolol during insulin-induced hypoglycaemia. Br. Med. J., 2:272, 1976.
119. Hesse, B., and Pedersen, J.T.: Hypoglycemia after propranolol on the humoral and metabolic responses to insulin-induced hypoglycemia. Lancet, 2:1386, 1966.
120. MacKintosh, T.F.: Propranolol and hypoglycemia. Lancet, 1:102, 1967.

121. Habib, A., and McCarthy, J.S.: Effects on the neonate of propranolol administered during pregnancy. J. Pediatr., *91*:808, 1977.
122. Cottrill, C.M., et al.: Propranolol therapy during pregnancy, labor and delivery: evidence for transplacental drug transfer and impaired neonatal drug disposition. J. Pediatr., *91*:812, 1977.
123. Rubin, P.C.: Beta blockers in pregnancy. N. Engl. J. Med., *305*:1323, 1981.
124. Lewis, M.J., et al.: The effects of propranolol and acebutolol on the overnight plasma levels of anterior pituitary and related hormones. Br. J. Clin. Pharmacol., *12*:737, 1981.
125. Shand, D.G., and Wood, A.J.J.: Propranolol withdrawal syndrome—why? Clin. Pharmacol. Ther., *23*:202, 1978.
126. Frishman, W.H., et al.: Comparative effects of abrupt withdrawal of propranolol and verapamil in angina pectoris. Am. J. Cardiol., *50*:1191, 1982.
127. Paterson, J.W., et al.: The pharmacodynamics and metabolism of propranolol in man. Pharmacol. Clin., *2*:127, 1970.
128. Thadani, U., and Parker, J.O.: Propranolol in the treatment of angina pectoris: comparison of duration of action in acute and sustained oral therapy. Circulation, *59*:571, 1979.
129. Dvornik, D., et al: Comparative bioavailability of propranolol twice-daily versus four-times-daily administration. J. Clin. Pharmacol., *21*:472, 1982.
130. Kawashima, K., Levy, A., and Spector, S.: Stereospecific radioimmunoassay for propranolol isomers. J. Pharmac. Exp. Ther., *196*:517, 1976.
131. Shand, D.G., Nuckolls, E.M., and Oates, J.A. Plasma propranolol levels in adults. Clin. Pharmacol. Ther., *11*:112, 1970.
132. Zacest, R., and Koch-Weser, J.: Relation of propranolol plasma level to beta-blockade during oral therapy. Pharmacology, *7*:178, 1972.
133. Jackman, G.P., et al.: No stereoselective first-pass hepatic extraction of propranolol. Clin. Pharmacol. Ther., *30*:291, 1981.
134. Mullane, J.F., et al.: Propranolol dosage, plasma concentration, and beta blockade. Clin. Pharmacol. Ther., *32*:692, 1982.
135. Prichard, B.N.C., and Gillam, P.M.S.: An assessment of propranolol in angina pectoris: a clinical dose response curve and the effect on the electrocardiogram at rest and on exercise. Br. Heart J., *33*:473, 1971.
136. Coltart, D.J., Gibson, D.G., and Shand, D.G.: Plasma propranolol levels associated with suppression of ventricular ectopic beats. Br. Med. J., *1*:490, 1971.
137. Nixon, J.V., et al.: Efficacy of propranolol in the control of exercise induced or augmented ventricular ectopic activity. Circulation, *57*:115, 1978.
138. McDevitt, D.G., et al.: Plasma binding and the affinity of propranolol for a beta receptor in man. Clin. Pharmacol. Ther., *20*:152, 1976.
139. Borga, Q., Piafsky, K.M., and Nielsen, O.G.: Plasma protein binding of basic drugs. I. Selective displacement from α-acid glycoprotein by tris (2-butosyethyl) phosphate. Clin. Pharmacol. Ther., *22*:539, 1977.
140. Sager, C., Nielsen, O.G., and Jacobsen, S.: Variable binding of propranolol in human serum. Biochem. Pharmacol., *28*:905, 1979.
141. Piafsky, K.M., et al.: Increased plasma protein binding of propranolol and chlorpromazine mediated by disease-induced elevations of plasma-acid glycoprotein. N. Engl. J. Med., *299*:1435, 1978.
142. Sager, G., et al.: Effect of heparin on serum binding of propranolol in the acute phase of myocardial infarction. Br. J. Clin. Pharmacol., *12*:613,1981.
143. Kornhauser, D.M., et al.: Biological determinant of propranolol disposition in man. Clin. Pharmacol. Ther., *23*:165, 1978.
144. Chidsey, C.A., et al.: Studies of the absorption and removal of propranolol in hypertensive patients during therapy. Circulation, *52*:313, 1975.
145. Berglund, G., et al.: Propranolol given twice daily in hypertension. Acta Med. Scand., *194*:513, 1973.
146. Seis, P.M., et al.: Complete atrioventricular block associated with propranolol therapy. J. Pediatr., *98*:326, 1981.

147. Pioselli, D., et al.: Management of paroxysmal ventricular tachycardia in patients with mitral valve prolapse. In Management of Ventricular Tachycarida—Role of Mexiletine: Proceedings of a Symposium, Copenhagen, 25-27 May, 1978. Edited by E. Sandøe, et al., Amsterdam, Excerpta Medica, 1978, p. 419.
148. Paraskevopoulos, J.A., et al.: Growth retardation following chronic administration of beta-blockers: the role of the hypothalamus-pituitary axis. Abstract submitted to the International Symposium on Cardiovascular Pharmacology, Geneva, 1985.
149. Feely, J., Wilkinson, G.R., and Wood, A.J.J.: Reduction of liver blood flow and propranolol metabolism by cimetidine. N. Engl. J. Med., *304*:692, 1981.
150. Reimann, I.W., et al.: Cimetidine increases steady state plasma levels of propranolol. Br. J. Clin. Pharmacol., *12*:785, 1981.
151. Rendic, S., et al.: Interaction of cimetidine with liver microsomes. Xenobiotica, *9*:555, 1979.
152. Ochs, H.R., Carstens, G., and Greenblatt, D.J.: Reduction in lidocaine clearance during continuous infusion and by coadministration of propranolol. N. Engl. J. Med., *303*:373, 1980.
153. Sakurai, T., et al.: Augmented effect of propranolol by pharmacokinetic interaction with quinidine. AHA 1983.

Chapter 19
Other Beta-Adrenoreceptor Blocking Agents

Atenolol

Atenolol is among the most promising of the beta-adrenoreceptor blocking agents introduced to cardiovascular medicine in the last decade. Although atenolol is one of the three most widely used beta-adrenoreceptor blockers in adults, pediatric cardiologists are not familiar with the drug. To the best of my knowledge, no study of the pediatric use of atenolol has been published. Therefore, the discussion focuses on a description of the properties of atenolol and on its potential advantage in children, as well as on the limited experience with this agent. Because atenolol crosses the placenta and appears in neonatal blood, and because it is an important agent of pregnancy-associated hypertension, the pediatric aspects of this treatment are also discussed.

Atenolol is a beta-1-selective adrenoreceptor blocking drug devoid of local anesthetic or intrinsic sympathomimetic activities. Its long elimination half-life allows once-daily administration. In adults, atenolol is routinely used for the treatment of hypertension, angina pectoris, and arrhythmias and has been investigated for use after myocardial infarction. In children, the experience is limited to a few patients with hypertension.

Structure

Atenolol is 4-(2-hydroxy-isopropylaminopropoxy)-phenylacetylamide.

Pharmacologic Properties

Atenolol is a beta-1-selective adrenoreceptor blocker with a beta-blocking potency resembling that of propranolol. Its selectivity is lost at high doses, and it may then block both beta-1 and beta-2-adrenoreceptors.[1] Atenolol also exerts a central effect, the reduction of the efferent sympathetic discharge from the central nervous system.[2]

Hemodynamic Effects

Like other beta-adrenoreceptor blocking agents, atenolol slows heart rate at rest and inhibits the increase in heart rate during exercise. In hypertensive patients who respond to atenolol, heart rate is reduced by 5 to 25%. The effect on systemic vascular resistance varies among patients. Short-term intravenous administration of atenolol increases systemic vascular resistance by about 25%[3,4] but prolonged oral administration often fails to alter this parameter. Propranolol, unlike atenolol, almost consistently increases systemic vascular resistance. This effect is disadvantageous in patients with coronary artery disease or hypertension, but it may be beneficial to patients with tetralogy of Fallot (see also Chap. 18). One of the suggested mechanisms for the favorable effect of propranolol in patients with tetralogy of Fallot is an increase in peripheral vascular resistance, resulting in a reduction in the magnitude of the right-to-left shunt. Therefore, a beta-blocking drug such as atenolol, which does not consistently increase peripheral vascular resistance, may not be useful in patients with this condition. This subject has not yet been studied hemodynamically or clinically.

The effect of atenolol on peripheral vascular resistance differs from that of propranolol because atenolol is a beta-1-selective adrenoreceptor blocker, which does not leave the vasoconstricting alpha-adrenoreceptors unopposed. Propranolol blocks the vascular beta-2-adrenoreceptors, which mediate vasodilation, and leaves the vasoconstricting alpha-adrenoreceptors unopposed.

Pediatric Aspects of Treatment During Pregnancy

Atenolol crosses the placenta and reaches high plasma levels in the neonate. Liedholm reported that, during long-term treatment, the plasma levels of atenolol in mothers and neonates were similar.[5] Therefore, atenolol given to pregnant women, usually for treatment of hypertension, may affect the fetus and the neonate. Rubin and co-workers compared the effects of atenolol and placebo in 120 women with pregnancy-associated hypertension.[6] No major birth malformations occurred in either group. Three of 55 children in the placebo group had developmental abnormalities, including a child with brain damage, during follow-up for a year. No developmental abnormalities were encountered in the atenolol group, which also included 55 children. Comparative data on neonatal heart rate were not given by these investigators. In an earlier report, these investigators had stated that the range of serious neonatal side effects in the atenolol group was the same as in the placebo group.

Liedholm reported that a perinatal mortality rate of 2.5% was found in newborns of 88 hypertensive mothers who had been treated with atenolol during pregnancy.[7] The report stated that this rate is acceptable in such a high-risk group.

Because of the long elimination half-life of atenolol and the possibility of impaired elimination in the neonate, I recommended that infants of mothers treated with atenolol during pregnancy should be followed for 10 days after birth for bradycardia or other signs of distress.

Effects in Hypertension

Atenolol effectively controls elevated systolic and diastolic blood pressure in the supine and standing positions, both at rest and during exercise.[8-12] The reduction in blood pressure is proportional to the patient's pretreatment blood pressure. The effect may be evident on the first day of treatment, although it usually takes a few days for the maximal effect to be noted. Occasionally, several weeks are required for the maximal effect to be achieved.[13]

Atenolol is probably more effective in patients with high-renin hypertension than in those with low-renin hypertension. Therefore, atenolol may be especially suitable for hypertensive children with coarctation of the aorta, who usually have high plasma renin activity. No correlation has been found between the extent of the antihypertensive effect and the decrease in plasma renin activity by atenolol. The antihypertensive effect of atenolol has been sustained during several years of treatment. No reports on the use of atenolol in hypertensive children have been published. My own experience and data gained by personal communications are limited to a few older children with essential or renovascular hypertension and to one child with hypertension after surgical correction of coarctation of the aorta. Atenolol, alone or in combination with other antihypertensive agents, appeared to be effective and safe in these patients.

I recommend that atenolol be considered, as an investigational agent, in pediatric patients in whom a beta-adrenoreceptor blocking drug is required to control hypertension.

Comparison with other Antihypertensive Drugs

Propranolol. Atenolol has several advantages over propranolol. Because propranolol is a nonselective beta-adrenoreceptor blocking agent, it also blocks the peripheral vascular beta-2-adrenoreceptors. The alpha-adrenoreceptors are left unopposed, and peripheral vasoconstriction occurs. Atenolol, which is a beta-1-selective adrenoreceptor blocking drug, does not, at least at low doses, affect the peripheral beta-adrenoreceptors and does not alter the systemic vascular resistance. Atenolol is potentially safer than propranolol in patients with bronchospastic disease and it also has a weaker metabolic effect than propranolol. Atenolol and propranolol have not been compared in children. In at least one study in hypertensive adults, however, atenolol was slightly more potent than propranolol.[14]

Methyldopa. The antihypertensive effect of atenolol is comparable to that of methyldopa.[15, 16]

Effect on Plasma Lipids

Controversial findings have been obtained in studies of the effect of atenolol on plasma lipids. One study showed that atenolol had no effect on plasma lipoproteins in hypertensive patients.[17] Other studies reported increases in plasma triglyceride and very low-density lipoprotein (VLDL) cholesterol levels without alterations of total cholesterol concentration.[18–20] We must reach a definite conclusion on this subject, especially in pediatric patients, because unfavorable changes in a plasma lipid profile in childhood may increase the risk of coronary atherosclerosis in early adulthood.

Clinical Pharmacology

Atenolol is the most hydrophilic beta-adrenoreceptor blocking agent in routine clinical use, and many of its pharmacologic properties result from this feature. About 50% of an oral dose of atenolol is absorbed from the gastrointestinal tract, at a rapid rate. Maximal plasma concentrations are achieved within 2 to 4 hours of oral administration. The pharmacodynamic effect is maximally evident at about the same time and is sustained for 24 hours. Therefore, atenolol is effective when given once a day.[13, 21]

Although the correlation between plasma levels of atenolol and the extent of beta-blockade is strong, the determination of these plasma levels is of little value in clinical practice, except to ascertain compliance of the patient. Atenolol is mainly eliminated by renal excretion of the unchanged drug, although some hepatic metabolism has been reported. The elimination half-life is 8 to 10 hours, but the pharmacodynamic half-life is longer.[22–24] Atenolol can be eliminated by hemodialysis.

Because atenolol is hydrophilic, it does not penetrate the central nervous system, and its concentration in the brain is much lower than in the plasma. Therefore, atenolol has many fewer adverse effects on the central nervous system than most other beta-adrenoreceptor blocking drugs.

Side Effects

The side effects of atenolol are usually related to the drug's beta-adrenoreceptor blocking effect and are thereby predictable. The incidence of side effects is low; especially notable is the low incidence of side effects related to the central nervous system. This feature makes atenolol safer than other beta-blocking agents in children.

Bradycardia is found in about 3% of patients treated with atenolol, and only in a small portion of them it is associated with dizziness.[25] Hemodynamic deterioration with congestive heart failure or shock may occur in patients with impaired left ventricular function. Hypertensive patients may develop hypotension after high doses of atenolol.

Postural hypotension may occur in up to 5% of the patients. Atenolol may aggravate bronchospasm, although theoretically, this drug is superior to nonselective beta-blockers in this respect. In patients with peripheral vascular disease, atenolol may cause a cold feeling in the extremities. Vertigo, fatigue, depression, lethargy, drowsiness, and other central-nervous-system side effects are rare. Diarrhea or nausea may occur. A single case of retroperitoneal fibrosis in a patient treated with atenolol has been reported.[26]

Dosage and Administration

An important advantage of atenolol is its flat dose-response curve, requiring only minimal dosage adjustments. The usual oral dose in adults is 100 mg once daily. About 20% of patients require a daily dose of 150 or 200 mg, and a few patients with severe hypertension receive 300 or 400 mg daily.

Dosage regimens for children are not available. I suggest that older children begin with 12.5 to 25 mg once daily. Adolescents may receive amounts in the lower dosage range recommended for adults.

Bucindolol

Bucindolol is a new beta-adrenoreceptor blocking agent with a peripheral vasodilatory effect. In adults, this drug has been effective in the treatment of systemic hypertension. Bucindolol may also be effective in the short-term management of congestive heart failure in children with congenital heart disease and left-to-right shunting. This beneficial effect has been attributed to pulmonary arteriolar vasoconstriction, resulting in a decrease in left-to-right shunting.

Structure

Bucindolol is 2-[2-hydroxy-3[C2-(3-indolyl)-1,1-dimethylethyl]-amino]propoxy]benzonitrile hydrochloride.

Pharmacologic Properties

Bucindolol is a potent selective beta-adrenoreceptor blocking drug.[27, 28] It also has weak intrinsic sympathomimetic activity, weak alpha-adrenoreceptor blocking activity, and a direct vasodilatory effect.[27, 29] Bucindolol has been reported to have a pulmonary vasoconstrictor effect.[30]

Hemodynamic Effect

Bucindolol usually slows heart rate,[29] owing to its beta-adrenoreceptor blocking effect, but it may accelerate heart rate, either because of intrinsic sympathomimetic activity or secondary to systemic vasodilation. Bucindolol lowers elevated systemic arterial pressure by means of its beta- and alpha-adrenoreceptor blocking activities and its direct vasodilatory effect.[27] Bucindolol may also exert a positive inotropic effect.

Leatherbury and colleagues evaluated the effect of bucindolol in 6 children, aged 1 to 21 months, with ventricular septal defect or endocardial cushion defect, congestive heart failure, left-to-right shunt of 10.4 L/min/m^2, pulmonary-to-systemic flow ratio of 3.9, and pulmonary vascular resistance of 3 "Wood" units.[30] The children received bucindolol, 0.05 mg/kg intravenously over 5 min. The drug decreased left-to-right shunt by 50%, pulmonary flow by 41%, and the ratio of pulmonary to systemic flow by 30%. Pulmonary resistance increased by 94%, whereas mean aortic pressure decreased. Mean pulmonary artery pressure, systemic flow, systemic vascular resistance, left ventricular end-diastolic pressure, peak left ventricular dP/dt, and shortening fraction were not much altered. This report concluded that bucindolol produces pulmonary arteriolar vasoconstriction, increases pulmonary vascular resistance, and thereby decreases pulmonary blood flow and left-to-right shunting. Bucindolol may be effective in the short-term management of congestive heart failure in children with congenital heart lesions and high pulmonary flow.[30]

Bucindolol has lowered elevated blood pressure in hypertensive patients. The antihypertensive effect of bucindolol is evident within 2 hours of oral administration. Bucindolol differs from other beta-blockers by its rapid onset of action, which probably results from the direct vasodilatory effects. Bucindolol increases plasma renin activity.

Electrophysiologic Effects

Bucindolol decreases or increases heart rate, decreases or does not alter the PR interval, increases or does not alter the atrial effective refractory period, and does not alter sinus node recovery time and the QRS and QTc intervals. When rapidly injected, bucindolol may cause transient narrowing of the P wave.[28, 29]

Clinical Pharmacology

Bucindolol may be given intravenously or orally. It is rapidly absorbed from the gastrointestinal tract after oral administration; maximal plasma levels are reached in under 2 hours. Bucindolol undergoes extensive first-pass hepatic metabolism, resulting in systemic bioavailability of about 20%. The drug is eliminated by hepatic metabolism, with an elimination half-life of 2.5 to 7.0 hours. The metabolites are excreted in the urine and bile. One of them, 5-hydroxybucindolol, is pharmacologically active.[29] Bucindolol is bound by 90% to plasma proteins.

Side Effects

Although bucindolol is usually well tolerated, it may cause dizziness, tiredness, and exercise-induced muscular weakness. Rarely, postural hypotension occurs.

Dosage and Administration

Oral Administration. In adults, doses of 20 to 300 mg are used. No dosage regimen has been established for children.

Intravenous Administration. In infants and children with a left-to-right shunt, doses of 0.05 mg/kg, given over 5 minutes, have been used.

Metoprolol

Metoprolol is a beta-1-selective adrenoreceptor blocker without intrinsic sympathomimetic activity and with mild membrane-stabilizing activity. Its potency is about one-third that of propranolol, but oral doses of both agents are about equal. In adults, metoprolol is used for treatment of hypertension, angina pectoris, arrhythmias, thyrotoxicosis, and tremor.[31-36] No well-controlled pediatric studies of metoprolol have been reported. Recently, however, this agent has been used for treatment of hypertension in pregnancy, and fetuses and neonates are exposed to its effect.

Metoprolol crosses the placenta and shows a varying distribution in the fetus, with a preference for the liver and the adrenal glands. The human fetus can metabolize metoprolol.[37]

In a placebo-controlled trial of treatment of hypertension during pregnancy with metoprolol in 52 women, no neonatal death occurred in the metoprolol-treated group, and no adverse neonatal effects were observed.[38] In another study, metoprolol decreased fetal heart rate, but this decrease did not adversely influence the condition of the fetus.[39]

Metoprolol may be given intravenously or orally. It undergoes extensive first-pass hepatic metabolism. Plasma protein binding is about 11%.[40] Metoprolol is eliminated by hepatic metabolism, at a genetically determined rate, and by urinary excretion of the metabolites. The elimination half-life is 2.5 to 7.5 hours. Maron and associates recently reported on a 10-year-old child with obstructive cardiomyopathy associated with only minimal left ventricular hypertrophy, who was successfully treated with metoprolol.[41] In this patient, a two-dimensional echocardiogram showed a region of minimal wall thickening confined to the anterior basal ventricular septum. No other portion of the left ventricle was hypertrophied. Moderately severe systolic anterior mitral motion (SAM) and midsystolic partial closure of the aortic valve were seen. The pressure gradient across the subaortic area was 120 mm Hg. This patient was treated with metoprolol, 100 mg twice daily, which abolished SAM on the M-mode echocardiogram and reduced the intensity of the systolic murmur, indicating a decrease in the pressure gradient.

Pindolol

Pindolol is a nonselective beta-adrenoreceptor blocking agent with potent intrinsic sympathomimetic activity and mild membrane-stabilizing activity. The beta-blocking effect of pindolol is about 20 to 40 times more potent than that of propranolol after oral administration and is 5 to 10 times more potent than that of propranolol after intravenous administration.[42-45] The intrinsic sympathomimetic activity of pindolol is the most potent of all the beta-blocking drugs in clinical use.

In patients with peripheral vascular disease or slow heart rate, the intrinsic sympathomimetic activity makes pindolol superior to beta-blocking agents devoid of this property. This feature is of little relevance in children; however, pindolol may be safer than beta-adrenoreceptor blockers devoid of intrinsic sympathomimetic activity in children with bronchial asthma.

In adults, pindolol is used for treatment of hypertension, angina pectoris, arrhythmias, and orthostatic hypertension due to neuropathies. The efficacy and safety of pindolol have not been determined in infants and children. Pindolol is secreted in human milk, and nursing mothers should not receive pindolol. Pindolol has recently been used to treat hypertension during pregnancy. Preliminary studies have shown no adverse fetal or neonatal effects.[46]

Labetalol

Labetalol is an agent with both beta- and alpha-adrenoreceptor blocking properties, and perhaps direct vasodilatory properties.[47-49] Labetalol is a nonselective beta-adrenoreceptor blocking agent. The potency of this effect is about 20% that of propranolol.[48] The beta-blocking effect is 4 to 16 times greater than the alpha-blocking effect. The alpha-blocking effect is selective for postsynaptic alpha-1-adrenoreceptors. Labetalol also has some beta-2-adrenoreceptor agonist activity.[50]

In adults, labetalol is used for treatment of hypertension and arrhythmias. In patients with these diseases and peripheral vascular disease, labetalol may be superior to other beta-blocking agents because of its vasodilatory effect. Such may be also be the case in patients with impairment of renal function.

No experience with labetalol in infants and children has been reported, but because labetalol has been used for treatment of hypertension during pregnancy, fetuses and neonates may be affected by this drug. In a study of 85 women treated with labetalol during pregnancy, a low perinatal mortality rate of 4.4% and no congenital malformations or severe neonatal adverse effects were observed.[51] In another study of 80 women treated with labetalol or bed rest alone, no short-term fetal effects were noted, even when high doses of labetalol were given intravenously. No problems during delivery were attributable to beta-blockade. The neonates' heart rate fell slightly after birth and for 6 hours thereafter. The umbilical cord blood levels of labetalol were equal to maternal blood levels.[52]

Thus, it appears that treatment with labetalol during pregnancy is not associated with an increase in fetal or neonatal adverse effects. At least one study has shown mild neonatal hypotension after maternal treatment with labetalol, however.[53] The effect of labetalol on preterm neonates has yet to be determined.

Timolol

Timolol is a nonselective beta-adrenoreceptor blocking agent devoid of intrinsic sympathomimetic or membrane-stabilizing activity. Its beta-adrenoreceptor blocking effect is eight times as potent as that of propranolol.[54–56] The reason for this high potency may be that timolol, unlike most other commercially available beta-adrenoreceptor blocking drugs, is prepared as the active levoisomer and not as the racemate; another reason may be the low protein binding of this drug.[57]

In adults, timolol is used for treatment of angina pectoris and hypertension, for secondary prevention of myocardial infarction, and uncommonly, for suppression of arrhythmias. It was the first beta-adrenoreceptor blocking agent clinically used for treatment of glaucoma. No pediatric experience with timolol in cardiovascular diseases has been reported, but young patients with glaucoma may be treated with this drug.

In 1967, it was reported that propranolol, administered systemically to hypertensive patients who also had glaucoma, reduced the elevated intraocular pressure.[58] Timolol is considered to be optimal for topical ocular application because of the absence of local anesthetic properties or intrinsic sympathomimetic activity. Clinical studies have shown that timolol effectively lowers the intraocular pressure by up to one-third in up to 90% of patients with open-angle glaucoma, but not closed-angle glaucoma. Timolol is reported to be at least as effective as epinephrine and pilocarpine.[59-60] When it is administered topically to the eyes, timolol may be systemically absorbed and may produce cardiovascular effects.

Sotalol

Sotalol is a nonselective beta-adrenoreceptor blocking agent devoid of intrinsic sympathomimetic or membrane-stabilizing activity. Its beta-adrenoreceptor blocking potency is about one-third that of propranolol.[61] Sotalol is the only beta-adrenoreceptor blocker that also has class III antiarrhythmic properties; that is, it prolongs repolarization. Thus, the features of sotalol resemble those of the combination of timolol and amiodarone. Because of this effect, sotalol is unique among beta-blocking agents in that it may prolong the QTc interval.[61, 62]

In adults, sotalol is used for treatment of arrhythmias, hypertension, and angina pectoris. It has been investigated for the secondary prevention of myocardial infarction. No experience exists with sotalol in infants and children; however, the worldwide use of propranolol and amiodarone for suppression of arrhythmias in children suggests that sotalol, which has properties of both these agents, will be used in the future in pediatric practice.

References

1. Aberg, H.: Plasma renin activity after the use of a new beta-adrenergic blocking agent (I.C.I. 66,082). Int. J. Clin. Pharmacol., 9:98, 1974.
2. Scott, E.M.: The effect of atenolol on the spontaneous and reflex activity of the sympathetic nerves in the cat: influence of cardiopulmonary receptors. Br. J. Pharmacol., 78:425, 1983.
3. Astrom, H., and Jonson, B.: Haemodynamic effects of different beta-blockers in angina pectoris. Scott. Med. J., 22:64, 1977.
4. Astrom, H., and Vallin, H.: Effect of a new beta-adrenergic blocking agent, I.C.I. 66,082, on exercise haemodynamics and airway resistance in angina pectoris. Br. Heart J., 36:1194, 1974.
5. Liedholm, H.: Transplacental passage and breast milk accumulation of atenolol in humans. Drugs, 25 (Suppl. 2):217, 1983.
6. Rubin, P.C., et al.: Atenolol in the management of pregnancy-associated hypertension: obstetric and paediatric aspects. Abstract presented at the International Symposium on Hypertension in Pregnancy, Milan, 1984.
7. Liedholm, H.: Atenolol in the treatment of hypertension of pregnancy. Drugs, 25 (Suppl. 2):206, 1983.
8. Myers, M.G., et al.: Atenolol in essential hypertension. Clin. Pharmacol. Ther., 19:502, 1976.
9. Douglas-Jones, A.P., and Cruickshank, J.M.: Once-daily dosing with atenolol in patients with mild or moderate hypertension. Br. Med. J., 1:990, 1976.
10. Marshall, A.J., et al.: Dose response and frequency of administration of atenolol in essential hypertension: once daily treatment with beta-blockade. Postgrad. Med. J., 53(Suppl 3):168, 1977.

11. Alicandri, C.L., et al.: Atenolol once daily in essential hypertension: a multicentre study. Drugs, 25(Suppl 2):70, 1983.
12. Floras, J.S. et al.: Ambulatory blood pressure and its variability during randomised double-blond administration of atenolol, metoprolol, pindolol, and long acting propranolol in subjects with mild to moderate hypertension. Drugs, 25(Suppl 2):19, 1983.
13. Heel, R.C., et al.: Atenolol: a review of its pharmacological properties and therapeutic efficacy in angina pectoris and hypertension. Drugs, 17:425, 1979.
14. Zacharias, F.J., and Cowen, K.J.: Comparison of propranolol and atenolol in hypertension. Postgrad. Med. J., 53(Suppl 3):111, 1977.
15. Basker, A.M., et al.: A double-blind comparison of atenolol ("Tenormin") and methyldopa in the treatment of moderate hypertension in general practice: a multicentre study. Curr. Med. Res. Opin., 4:618, 1977.
16. Wilson, C., et al.: Atenolol and methyldopa in the treatment of hypertension. Postgrad. Med. J., 53 (Suppl. 3):123, 1977.
17. Rossner, S., and Weiner, L.: A comparison of the effects of atenolol and metoprolol on serum lipoproteins. Drugs, 25 (Suppl. 2):322, 1983.
18. Eliasson, K., et al.: Serum lipoprotein changes during atenolol treatment of essential hypertension. Eur. J. Clin. Pharmacol., 20:335, 1981.
19. Shaw, J., et al.: Beta-blockers and plasma triglycerides. Br. Med. J., 1:986, 1978.
20. England, J.D.F., et al.: Beta-adrenoceptor-blocking agents and lipid metabolism. Clin. Sci. Mol. Med., 55 (Suppl. 4):323s, 1978.
21. Jackson, G., et al.: Atenolol: once-daily cardioselective beta blockade for angina pectoris. Circulation, 61:55, 1980.
22. Shanks, R.G., et al.: Correlation of reduction of exercise heart rate with blood levels of atenolol after oral and intravenous administration. Postgrad. Med. J., 53 (Suppl. 3):70, 1977.
23. McDevitt, D.G., et al.: Investigation of chronic dosing regimens of atenolol. Postgrad. Med. J., 53 (Suppl. 3):79, 1977.
24. McAinsh, J.: Clinical pharmacokinetics of atenolol. Postgrad. Med. J., 53(Suppl. 3):74, 1977.
25. Cruickshank, J.M.: Beta-blockers, bradycardia and adverse effects. Acta Ther., 7:309, 1981.
26. Doherty, C.C., et al.: Retroperitoneal fibrosis after treatment with atenolol. Br. Med. J., 2:1786, 1978.
27. Deitchman, D., et al.: β-Adrenoceptor and cardiovascular effects of MJ 13105 (bucindolol) in anesthetized dogs and rats. Eur. J. Pharmacol., 61:263, 1980.
28. Deitchman, D., et al.: Cardiovascular effects of bucindolol (MJ 13105) in conscious dogs. Arch. Int. Pharmacodyn., 274:76, 1980.
29. Deitchman, D., et al.: Bucindolol. In New Drugs Annual: Cardiovascular Drugs. Edited by Alexander Scriabine. New York, Raven Press. 1983, p. 1.
30. Leatherbury, L., et al.: Low dose bucindolol in children with congestive heart failure (CHF). AHA 1984.
31. Bengtsson, C.: The effect of metoprolol—a new selective adrenergic β_1-receptor blocking agent—in mild hypertension. Acta Med. Scand., 199:65, 1976.
32. Jaatela, A., and Pyorala, K.: A controlled study on the antihypertensive effect of a new β-adrenergic receptor blocking drug, metoprolol, in combination with chlorthalidone. Br. J. Clin. Pharmacol., 3:655, 1976.
33. Weiss, L., et al.: Effects of prolonged treatment with adrenergic β-receptor antagonists on blood pressure, cardiovascular design and reactivity in spontaneous hypertensive rats (SHR). Acta Physiol. Scand., 8:447, 1974.
34. Comerford, M.B., and Besterman, E.M.M.: An eighteen-month study of the clinical responses to metoprolol, a selective β-receptor blocking agent, in patients with angina pectoris. Postgrad. Med. J., 52:481, 1976.
35. Eklund, D., et al.: Effects of the cardioselective beta-adrenergic receptor blocking agent metoprolol in angina pectoris: subacute study with exercise tests. Br. Heart J., 38:155, 1976.
36. Hjalmarson, Å., et al.: Effect on mortality of metoprolol in acute myocardial infarction. Lancet, 2:823, 1981.

37. Wiest, W., et al.: Placental passage and distribution of metoprolol in the human fetus. Abstract presented at the Seventh International Symposium on Hypertension in Pregnancy, Milan, 1984.
38. Wichman, K., et al.: Metoprolol in the treatment of hypertension in pregnancy—effects on the newborn baby. Abstract presented at the Seventh International Symposium on Hypertension in Pregnancy, Milan, 1984.
39. Ryden, G., et al.: Metoprolol in the treatment of hypertension in pregnancy—effect on the mother and foetus. Abstract presented at the Seventh International Symposium on Hypertension in Pregnancy, Milan, 1984.
40. Johansson, K.A., et al.: Binding of two adrenergic beta-receptor antagonists, alprenolol and H93/26, to human serum proteins. Acta Pharm. Suec., 11:333, 1974.
41. Maron, B.J., et al.: Obstructive hypertrophic cardiomyopathy associated with minimal left ventricular hypertrophy. Am. J. Cardiol., 53:377, 1984.
42. Hicks, D.C., et al.: A comparison of intravenous pindolol and propranolol in normal man. J. Clin. Pharmacol., 12:212, 1972.
43. Carruthers, S.G.: Cardiac dose-response relationships of oral and intravenous pindolol. Br. J. Clin. Pharmacol., 13:193s, 1982.
44. Hill, R.C., and Turner, P.: Preliminary investigations of new beta-adrenoceptive receptor blocking drug, LB-46, in man. Br. J. Pharmacol., 36:368, 1969.
45. Aellig, W.H.: Beta-adrenoceptor blocking activity and duration of action of pindolol and propranolol in healthy volunteers. Br. J. Pharmacol., 3:251, 1976.
46. Dubois, D., et al.: Treatment of hypertension in pregnancy with β-adrenoceptor antagonists. Br. J. Clin. Pharmacol., 13:375s, 1982.
47. Johnson, G.L., et al.: Antihypertensive effects of labetalol. (Abstract.) Fed. Proc., 36:1059, 1977.
48. Brittain, R.T., and Levy, G.P.: A review of the animal pharmacology of labetalol, a combined α- and β-adrenoceptor blocking drug. Br. J. Clin. Pharmacol., 3 (Suppl. 3):681, 1976.
49. Frishman, W., and Halprin, S.: Clinical pharmacology of the new beta-adrenergic blocking drugs. Part 7. New horizons in beta-adrenoceptor blockade therapy: labetalol. Am. Heart J., 98:660, 1979.
50. Carey, B., and Whalley, E.T.: Labetalol, an alpha- and beta-adrenoceptor-agonist action on the rat isolated uterus. J. Pharm. Pharmacol., 31:791, 1979.
51. Michael, C.A.: The evaluation of labetalol in the treatment of hypertension complicating pregnancy. Br. J. Clin. Pharmacol., 49:127s, 1982.
52. Walker, J.J., et al.: The effect of maternal labetalol on the neonate. Abstract presented at the Seventh International Symposium on Hypertension in Pregnancy, Milan, 1984.
53. Macpherson, M., et al.: The effect of maternal labetalol on the new-born human infant. Abstract presented at the Seventh International Symposium on Hypertension in Pregnancy, Milan, 1984.
54. Scriabine, A., et al.: Some cardiovascular effects of timolol, a new beta-adrenergic blocking agent. Arch. Int. Pharmacodyn., 205:76, 1973.
55. Ulrych, M., et al.: Comparison of a new beta-adrenergic blocker (MK 950) and propranolol in man. Clin. Pharmacol. Ther., 13:232, 1972.
56. Achong, A.R., et al.: Comparison of cardiac effects of timolol and practolol. Clin. Pharmacol. Ther., 18:278, 1975.
57. Tocco, D.J., et al.: Physiological disposition and metabolism of timolol in man and laboratory animals. Drug. Metab. Dispos., 3:361, 1975.
58. Phillip, C.I. et al.: Propranolol as ocular hypotensive agent. Br. J. Ophthalmol., 51:222, 1967.
59. Boger, W.P., III, et al.: Clinical trial comparing timolol ophthalmic solution to pilocarpine in open-angle glaucoma. Am. J. Ophthalmol., 86:8, 1978.
60. Heel, R.C., et al.: Timolol: a review of its therapeutic efficacy in the topical treatment of glaucoma. Drugs, 17:38, 1979.

61. Frishman, W.: Appraisal and reappraisal of cardiac therapy: clinical pharmacology of the new beta-adrenergic blocking drugs. Part 1. Pharmacodynamic and pharmacokinetic properties. Am. Heart J., *97*:663, 1979.
62. Neuvonen, P.J., et al.: Prolonged QT interval and severe tachyarrhythmias, common beats. S. Afr. Med. J., *56*:295, 1979.

Section V
ANTIARRHYTHMIC AGENTS

Antiarrhythmic agents are drugs that terminate or prevent arrhythmias. To this general definition may be added that drugs that control the ventricular response to supraventricular arrhythmias are also antiarrhythmic drugs. The antiarrhythmic effect of these agents results from their electrophysiologic properties. The electrophysiologic effects on isolated myocardial fibers were correlated with the antiarrhythmic effect in intact animals and human subjects; the result is the modern classification of antiarrhythmic agents, which was suggested by Singh and Vaughan-Williams.

Antiarrhythmic agents are classified into four groups. To these should be added agents such as digitalis glycosides, which are not included in the classification, and drugs whose electrophysiologic properties and mechanism of action are not known, such as adenosine. The antiarrhythmic agents are classified mainly according to their mechanism of action, but this classification also has clinical use. The four classes are as follows:

Class I: Agents with membrane-stabilizing (local anesthetic) properties; these drugs primarily affect membrane depolarization.

Class II: Beta-adrenoreceptor blocking agents.

Class III: Agents that mainly affect repolarization, such as amiodarone.

Class IV: Calcium antagonists.

Some overlap exists in this classification. For example, sotalol is a beta-adrenoreceptor blocker that also has Class III antiarrhythmic properties. Several other beta-blocking drugs, such as propranolol, also have Class I antiarrhythmic properties (membrane-stabilizing effect), although the relevance of these properties to the clinical effect of these drugs is not known.

Although all agents in Classes I, II, and III have antiarrhythmic properties, not all calcium antagonists (Class IV) have such characteristics. For example, nifedipine, a calcium antagonist widely used for the treatment of angina pectoris and hypertension, has no significant electrophysiologic or antiarrhythmic properties.

The classification of antiarrhythmic drugs has some clinical use. The combination of two Class I agents is rarely beneficial, whereas the combination of Class I and Class II agents may produce an additive antiarrhythmic effect. Another important finding is that the response to a single Class I or Class II agent may predict the response to other agents of these classes. If a Class I agent is effective, but the patient cannot tolerate the side effects, it is reasonable to try another agent of this class.

Class I agents are useful for termination and prevention of atrial and ventricular arrhythmias. Class II agents have some effect on ectopic atrial and ventricular activity and a significant effect on re-entrant supraventricular arrhythmias involving the atrioventricular node. Calcium antagonists are effective mainly in re-entrant arrhythmias affecting the atrioventricular node. Class III agents are effective in all types of atrial and ventricular arrhythmias.

Class I Agents

Class I antiarrhythmic agents have membrane-stabilizing activity. They inhibit the fast membrane channels and the fast inward sodium current. Because this current is responsible for depolarization, the main effect of these agents is slowing of phase-0 depolarization. Class I agents thereby affect both cardiac excitability and conductivity. Class I agents also depress automaticity, as manifested by a decreased slope of phase-4 depolarization. These drugs have an inconsistent effect on action potential duration, and they prolong the effective refractory period. Class I agents may be further classified to Class Ia agents, which prolong both ventricular and atrial effective refractory periods, and Class Ib agents, which do not alter the atrial effective refractory period. The effect on the atrial effective refractory period makes Class Ia agents useful in patients with atrial fibrillation and flutter, whereas Class Ib agents are ineffective in patients with these arrhythmias.

Class II Agents

Class II antiarrhythmic agents are drugs with beta-adrenoreceptor blocking activity. They suppress arrhythmias that depend on adrenergic stimulation. Their main electrophysiologic effect is depression of automaticity, as seen by a reduction in the slope of phase-4 depolarization.

Class IV Agents

Class IV antiarrhythmic agents include some of the calcium antagonists. Their main effect is depression of phase-4 depolarization. They slow conduction and prolong refractoriness in the atrioventricular node. Therefore, these agents may slow the rapid ventricular response to atrial tachyarrhythmias and may terminate supraventricular re-entrant arrhythmias whose cycle incorporates the atrioventricular node. Verapamil and diltiazem are the most important agents in this group.

Digitalis Glycosides

Digitalis glycosides slow conduction in the atrioventricular node. Therefore, they are used for slowing the ventricular response to rapid atrial arrhythmias and for terminating supraventricular re-entrant arrhythmias involving the atrioventricular node. Digitalis glycosides are discussed in Chapter 1.

Chapter 20

Quinidine

Quinidine, the most widely used Class I antiarrhythmic agent, has been prescribed for suppression and prevention of ventricular and supraventricular arrhythmias for almost 70 years. It is given almost exclusively orally. In children, quinidine is used for termination and prevention of supraventricular tachycardia, atrial flutter and fibrillation, and premature ventricular beats and for prevention of malignant ventricular arrhythmias. This drug should not be used in patients with arrhythmias associated with digitalis toxicity or in patients with advanced conduction disturbances. Quinidine is not given intravenously because of serious adverse hemodynamic effects.

Structure

The molecule of quinidine is composed of a quinuclidine ring, containing a tertiary nitrogen, connected by an alcohol bridge to a quinoline ring. It is an optical isomer of quinine.

Pharmacologic Properties

Quinidine has membrane-stabilizing (local anesthetic) activity, which is responsible for its antiarrhythmic effect. It has also direct vagolytic and peripheral vasodilatory effects.[1] This drug has antimalarial and antipyretic effects similar to those of quinine.

Electrophysiologic Effects

The electrophysiologic effects of quinidine are the net result of its direct (local anesthetic) effect and its vagolytic effect. Quinidine decreases the maximal rate of rise and the amplitude of phase-0 action potential and decreases the rate of phase-4 action potential; that is, it decreases automaticity.[2,3] The duration of action potential is not changed, but the refractory periods of Purkinje and myocardial fibers are prolonged.[4] The effects of quinidine result in slowing of conduction and depression of automaticity in various cardiac tissues. Quinidine increases the spontaneous sinus rate because of its vagolytic effect. In patients with sick sinus syndrome, quinidine can cause marked bradycardia. Like other Class Ia antiarrhythmic agents, quinidine prolongs the atrial effective refractory period and slows intra-atrial conduction.[4]

Quinidine usually delays conduction in the atrioventricular node, mainly by prolonging the HV interval. Occasionally, however, a transient acceleration of atrioventricular nodal conduction may occur, as a result of the vagolytic effect of quinidine.[5] For this reason, quinidine administration should not be initiated alone in patients with atrial fibrillation, who may develop a rapid ventricular response from enhancement of atrioventricular nodal conduction. In patients with dual atrioventricular pathways, quinidine depresses retrograde conduction.[6] In patients with Wolff-Parkinson-White syndrome, quinidine usually prolongs the anterograde and retrograde refractory periods of the accessory atrioventricular pathways.[7] Quinidine prolongs the effective refractory period of ventricular myocardium and Purkinje system.[4,8] It also prolongs the HV interval in some patients. Therapeutic concentrations of quinidine increase the duration of the QRS interval by up to 25%. Prolongation of 50% or more requires prompt discontinuance of the drug. Quinidine prolongs the QTc interval.

Effects in Arrhythmias

Quinidine is effective in the termination and prevention of almost all ventricular and supraventricular arrhythmias.

Atrial Flutter

Atrial flutter is a rare cardiac arrhythmia in infancy and childhood. Congenital flutter usually responds to digoxin. In my experience, the additon of quinidine to digoxin converted atrial flutter to normal sinus rhythm in one infant; however, at least one case of the deleterious consequences of this combination in an infant with atrial flutter has been reported.

In adults, quinidine effectively converts atrial flutter to normal sinus rhythm. Treatment should not be initiated with quinidine alone, however, but in combination with digoxin, verapamil, or beta-blocking agents, to avoid acceleration of ventricular response due to the vagolytic effect of quinidine.

Atrial Fibrillation

Atrial fibrillation is rare in infancy and childhood. From the experience in adults, it may be concluded that quinidine effectively converts atrial fibrillation to normal sinus rhythm.[9] This conversion occurs within 1 to 6 days of treatment.

Prior administration of quinidine has no effect on the energy requirements or the success rate of D.C. electroversion in patients with atrial fibrillation.[10,11] Quinidine prevents recurrences of atrial fibrillation.[11,12]

Supraventricular Tachycardia

Quinidine prevents induction and spontaneous recurrences of paroxysmal supraventricular tachycardia. This effect is due to the suppression of atrial premature beats, which initiate the tachycardia, and to changes of conduction and refractoriness in various segments of the tachycardia cycle. Quinidine should not be used in patients with supraventricular tachycardia associated with digitalis toxicity.

My colleagues and I studied the effect of quinidine in the termination and prevention of supraventricular tachycardia in a large series of infants and children. Quinidine was ineffective in terminating the arrhythmia, but the combination of quinidine and digoxin effectively prevented recurrences.

Ventricular Arrhythmias

Quinidine suppresses premature ventricular beats and prevents ventricular fibrillation and ventricular tachycardia.[13-15] In most studies, quinidine has not been compared to placebo in well-controlled protocols. In some studies, quinidine has been compared to some investigational antiarrhythmic agents.[14, 16]

No well-controlled studies of the effect of quinidine on ventricular arrhythmias in infants and children have been reported. My colleagues and I studied 12 children with multiple complex premature ventricular beats; 6 of these patients had congenital heart disease. Quinidine, administered alone or with propranolol, completely abolished the complex forms in 8 of the patients and suppressed the overall number of premature beats by more than 90% in 7 of them. These results are about equal to those reported in adults, but the small number of children studied does not allow accurate interpretation. Short-term drug testing using electrophysiologic studies has been effective in predicting the long-term clinical results of quinidine therapy in adults.[17, 18] The antiarrhythmic effect of quinidine is comparable to that of procainamide and is greater than that of propranolol.

Hemodynamic Effects

Like other Class I antiarrhythmic agents, quinidine has a negative inotropic effect.[19] Not all investigators have been able to demonstrate this effect, however.[20] Quinidine also produces peripheral vasodilation. Sympathetic activation due to vasodilation can counteract the direct negative inotropic effect of the drug.[21] The combined negative inotropic and vasodilatory effects may cause hypotension and hemodynamic deterioration. Several investigators found no deleterious effect of quinidine on cardiac performance in healthy human subjects or in patients with congestive cardiomyopathy.[22, 23]

In patients who underwent cardiac transplantation, intravenously administered quinidine reduced stroke volume and cardiac output by about 20% and mean arterial pressure by about 11%.[5] These effects were attributed to venodilation.

Several cases of severe hypotension and even syncope after intravenous administration of quinidine have been reported. Therefore, the intravenous administration of quinidine should be avoided.

Clinical Pharmacology

Quinidine is given only orally. About 70% of the dose is absorbed from the gastrointestinal tract. The maximal plasma concentration is reached about an hour after oral administration.[24] In a study of children and young adults aged 4 to 22 years, the peak plasma concentration was achieved within 0.5 to 2.0 hours.[25] The rate of absorption was reduced in patients with congestive heart failure, probably because of intestinal wall congestion.[26] The bioavailability of orally administered quinidine is only about 70%, because of incomplete absorption and significant first-pass hepatic metabolism. The plasma protein binding of quinidine is about 60 to 80%.[27] Therapeutic plasma concentrations of quinidine range between 1.0 and 6.0 $\mu g/ml$.[18,28]

Quinidine is eliminated mainly by hepatic metabolism.[29] Three of the metabolites have some pharmacologic activity that contributes to the electrophysiologic effects of quinidine.[30] The metabolites and about 15% of the unchanged drug are excreted in the urine. The elimination half-life of quinidine in adults is 4.5 to 6.0 hours.[27] In children, a shorter elimination half-life has been reported.[25] The rate of elimination of quinidine is especially rapid in children under 12 years of age.

Total body clearance is 4.8 ± 0.8 ml/min/kg.[31] Lower values have been observed in patients with congestive heart failure. Quinidine and its metabolites may accumulate in patients with renal failure.

Drug Interactions

Several drug interactions with quinidine have been reported. The most important of them is the quinidine-digoxin interaction.

Interaction with Digoxin

Quinidine and digoxin are often given together. This combination is of greater relative importance in children than in adults because fewer Class I antiarrhythmic drugs are recommended for children than for adults, and quinidine is often used. When quinidine is given to patients who are already receiving digoxin, the plasma concentration of digoxin is increased by 20 to 300%.[32-35] The extent of the increase may depend on the dose of quinidine,[36] although this finding is controversial.[37] A quinidine plasma concentration of at least 2 µg/ml is necessary for a significant interaction. The elevation of the plasma digoxin concentration is evident within a day of quinidine administration. A new steady state is achieved in about a week. Almost all patients treated concomitantly with both agents develop this interaction.[34, 38]

The mechanism of this interaction may involve the displacement of digoxin from tissue binding sites, a decrease in renal and possibly also in non-renal clearance of digoxin, and an increase in absorption of digoxin from the gastrointestinal tract. Elevation of the plasma concentration of digoxin may increase the intensity of the effects of this drug. On the other hand, displacement from tissue binding sites may attenuate the effects of digoxin. At present, it is not clear whether the elevated plasma concentration of digoxin that results from interaction with quinidine is associated with increased inotropic and electrophysiologic effects. Digitalis toxicity is more common in patients treated concomitantly with quinidine, however.[33] Therefore, the dose of digoxin should be reduced if quinidine is added. The positive inotropic effect of digoxin is probably not altered by quinidine. This interaction also results in a slight elevation of quinidine plasma levels.[40]

Because of the interaction between quinidine and digoxin, one should not give quinidine to patients with arrhythmias associated with digoxin toxicity. The quinidine-digoxin interaction has only recently been investigated in infants and children. I have observed an elevation of plasma digoxin concentration in two children after the addition of quinidine to the therapeutic regimen.

Recently, Koren reported on 11 children who were treated with a combination of quinidine and digoxin.[41] All had normal renal function. The addition of quinidine to maintenance digoxin therapy caused an increase of about 100% in the mean digoxin serum concentration, from 1.3 ± 0.4 to 2.5 ± 1.1 ng/ml. The interaction was observed in 8 of the 11 children, aged 6 to 17 years. No interaction was observed in 3 infants aged 1 to 2 months. No correlation was found between quinidine serum concentrations and the percentage of increase in digoxin levels. In most of these children, the digoxin levels dropped after reduction of the digoxin dose. In a few children, however, reduction of dose was followed by a second increase in digoxin levels. One child had signs of digitalis toxicity. The interaction probably results from the displacement of digoxin from its receptors by quinidine. Infants have a higher density of digoxin receptors than older persons. Koren hypothesized that this higher density of receptor sites in the newborn makes displacement of digoxin by quinidine more difficult.[41]

If a patient is receiving both quinidine and digoxin, discontinuance of quinidine will reduce the digoxin plasma concentration.

Side Effects

Side effects of quinidine are common and require discontinuance of treatment in 10 to 30% of the patients. The classic syndrome of cinchonism includes headache, nausea, blurring of vision, ringing in the ears, and in extreme cases, vertigo tinnitus, confusion, delirium, diplopia, and disturbances of color perception. The syndrome may appear even after a single dose of quinidine.

The most serious adverse effects of quinidine are related to the cardiovascular system. They include syncope, myocardial depression, hypotension, asystole, and conduction disturbances. Like othe antiarrhythmic drugs, quinidine has an arrhythmogenic potential. Serious ventricular arrhythmias are associated with QT prolongation. An 0.5% incidence of sudden death has been associated with quinidine therapy.[42]

Quinidine may cause adverse gastrointestinal effects such as nausea, vomiting, diarrhea, and abdominal pain, hematologic hypersensitivity reactions such as thrombocytopenia, agranulocytosis, and hemolytic anemia, cutaneous reactions such as rash and edema, and drug fever.

Dosage and Administration

Quinidine should only be given orally. The doses in adults are 200 to 500 mg, 4 to 6 times daily. In children, doses of 15 to 60 mg/kg/day are used. One report suggested that children under 12 years of age should receive 15 mg/kg/day, in 4 to 6 divided doses, and children over 12 years of age should receive 10 mg/kg/day.[25] These doses are low. In some large series, including ours, doses of 30 to 40 mg/kg/day were given.

References

1. Motulsky, H.J., et al.: Quinidine binds to α_1- and α_2-adrenergic, and muscarinic cholinergic receptors. AHA 1983.
2. Klein, R.L., et al.: Quinidine and unidirectional cation fluxes in atria. Circ. Res., 8:246, 1960.
3. Hoffman, B.F.: The action of quinidine and procaine amide on single fibers of dog ventricle and specialized conduction systems. An. Acad. Bras. Cienc., 29:365, 1958.
4. Wallace, A.C., et al.: Electrophysiologic effects of quinidine. Circ. Res., 19:960, 1966.
5. Mason, J.W., et al.: Hemodynamic effects of intravenously administered quinidine on the transplanted human heart. Am. J. Cardiol., 40:99, 1977.
6. Wu, D., et al.: Effects of quinidine on atrioventricular nodal reentrant paroxysmal tachycardia. Circulation, 64:823, 1981.
7. Hein, J.J., et al.: Effect of procaine amide, quinidine and ajmaline in the Wolff-Parkinson-White syndrome. Circulation, 50:114, 1974.
8. Gettes, L.S., and Sandquest, V.: Effect of quinidine on the differences between Purkinje and ventricular fibers. Circulation, 40:88, 1969.
9. Lown, B., et al.: New method for terminating cardiac arrhythmias: use of synchronized capacitor discharge. JAMA, 182:548, 1962.
10. Szekely, P., et al.: Direct current shock and anti-dysrhythmic drug. Br. Heart J., 32:209, 1970.

11. Hillestad, L., et al.: Quinidine before direct current countershock: a controlled study. Br. Heart J., *34*:139, 1972.
12. Härtel, G., et al.: Value of quinidine in maintenance of sinus rhythm after electric conversion of atrial fibrillation. Br. Heart J., *32*:57, 1970.
13. Jelinek, M.V., et al.: Antiarrhythmic drug therapy for sporadic ventricular ectopic arrhythmias. Circulation, *49*:659, 1974.
14. Flecainide Quinidine Research Group: Flecainide versus nidine for treatment of chronic ventricular arrhythmias. Circulation, *67*:1117, 1983.
15. Gey, G.O., et al.: Quinidine plasma concentration and exertional arrhythmias. Am. Heart J., *90*:19, 1975.
16. Sami, M., et al.: Antiarrhythmic efficacy of encainide and quinidine: validation of a model for drug assessment. Am. J. Cardiol., *48*:147, 1981.
17. Horowitz, L.N., et al.: Recurrent sustained ventricular tachycardia. III. Role of the electrophysiologic study in selection of antiarrhythmic regimens. Circulation, *58*:986, 1978.
18. DiMarco, J.P., et al.: Quinidine for ventricular arrhythmias: value of electrophysiologic testing. Am. J. Cardiol., *51*:90, 1983.
19. Engler, R.L., et al.: Depressant effects of quinidine gluconate on left ventricular function in conscious dogs with and without volume overload. Circulation, *60*:828, 1979.
20. Markiewicz, W., et al.: Normal myocardial contractile state in the presence of quinidine. Circulation, *53*:101, 1976.
21. Darby, T.D., et al.: Evaluation of sympathetic reflex effects on the inotropic action of nitroglycerin, quinidine, papaverine, aminophylline and isoproterenol. J. Pharmacol. Exp. Ther., *157*:1, 1967.
22. Holford, N.H.G., et al.: The effect of quinidine and its metabolites on the electrocardiogram and systolic time intervals: concentration-effect relationship. Br. J. Clin. Pharmacol., *11*:187, 1981.
23. Crawford, M.H., et al.: Effects of oral quinidine on left ventricular performance in normal subjects and patients with congestive cardiomyopathy. Am. J. Cardiol., *44*:714, 1979.
24. Conn, H.L.: Quinidine as an antiarrhythmic agent. *In* Advances in Cardiopulmonary Disease. Edited by A.L. Banyai and B.L. Gordon. Chicago, Year Book, 1964, p. 286.
25. Szefler, S.J., et al.: Rapid elimination of quinidine in pediatric patients. Pediatrics, *70*:370, 1982.
26. Ueda, C.T., and Dzindzio, B.S.: Bioavailability of quinidine in congestive heart failure. Br. J. Clin. Pharmacol., *11*:571, 1981.
27. Carliner, N.H., et al.: Quinidine therapy in hospitalized patients with ventricular arrhythmias. Am. Heart J., *98*:708, 1979.
28. Carliner, N.H., et al.: Relation of ventricular premature beat suppression to serum quinidine concentration determined by a new and specific assay. Am. Heart J., *100*:483, 1980.
29. Guentert, T.W., et al.: Determination of quinidine and its major metabolites by high-performance liquid chromatography. J. Chromatogr., *162*:59, 1979.
30. Drayer, D.E., et al.: Steady-state serum levels of quinidine and active metabolites in cardiac patients with varying degrees of renal function. Clin. Pharmacol. Ther., *24*:31, 1978.
31. Denes, P., et al.: Clinical, electrocardiographic and follow-up observations in patients having ventricular fibrillation during Holter monitoring. Am. J. Cardiol., *48*:9, 1981.
32. Doering, W., and König, E.: Anstieg der Digoxinkonzentration im Serum unter Chinidinmedikation. Med. Klin., *73*:1085, 1978.
33. Ejvinsson, G.: Effect of quinidine on plasma concentrations of digoxin. Br. Med. J., *1*:279, 1978.
34. Leahey, E.B., Jr., et al.: Interaction between quinidine and digoxin. JAMA, *240*:533, 1978.
35. Bussey, H.I.: The influence of quinidine and other agents on digitalis glycosides. Am. Heart J., *104*:289, 1982.

36. Risler, T., et al.: Quinidine-digoxin interaction. (Letter.) N. Engl. J. Med., *302*:175, 1980.
37. Friedman, H.S., and Chen, T.S.: Use of steady-state serum digoxin levels for predicting serum digoxin concentrations after quinidine administration. (Abstract no. 696.) Circulation, *62 (Suppl. III)*:183, 1980.
38. Doering, W.: Quinidine-digoxin interaction: pharmacokinetics, underlying mechanism and clinical implications. N. Engl. J. Med., *301*:400, 1979.
39. Cody, R.J., Jr., et al.: Increased digoxin toxicity during quinidine administration. (Abstract no. 697.) Circulation, *62 (Suppl. III)*:183, 1980.
40. Mungall, D.R., et al.: Effects of quinidine on serum digoxin concentration: a prospective study. Ann. Intern. Med., *93*:689, 1980.
41. Koren, G.: Interaction between digoxin and commonly coadministered drugs in children. Personal communication.
42. Lown, B., and Wolf, M.: Approaches to sudden death from coronary heart disease. Circulation, *44*:130, 1971.

Chapter 21

Procainamide

Procainamide is a Class I antiarrhythmic drug resembling quinidine in its structure, electrophysiologic properties, and antiarrhythmic effect. It has been available for clinical use for 25 years and has a high rate of efficacy, as well as a considerable incidence of serious side effects. Procainamide is used for to suppress ventricular arrhythmias not responsive to lidocaine. It has the advantage of efficacy by both intravenous and oral routes. To a lesser extent, the drug is also used in patients with supraventricular arrhythmias.

Several factors limit the therapeutic use of procainamide, such as its low therapeutic-to-toxic ratio, its short elimination half-life, which requires short dosing intervals, and its common side effects, the most important of which is a drug-induced syndrome resembling systemic lupus erythematosus.

About 40% of the dose of procainamide is metabolized in the liver. The most important metabolite is N-acetylprocainamide (NAPA), which has antiarrhythmic properties resembling those of the parent drug and fewer side effects. NAPA is under investigation for clinical use and is discussed at the end of this chapter.

The experience with procainamide in children is limited to several patients with ventricular arrhythmias. Infants and small children require high doses of the drug for control of arrhythmias. This phenomenon may result from altered pharmacokinetics of the drug at young ages or from decreased sensitivity of immature cardiac tissues to procainamide. Procainamide may be used in children for control of ventricular arrhythmias resistant to lidocaine and quinidine or for oral treatment of ventricular arrhythmias responsive to intravenous lidocaine. Procainamide is a Class Ia antiarrhythmic agent.

Structure

Procainamide is para-aminobenzoic acid bound by an amide bridge to diethylaminoethanol. In procaine, a local anesthetic agent with some antiarrhythmic properties, the para-aminobenzoic acid is bound to the diethylaminoethanol by an ester rather than by an amide bridge. Because this ester bridge is rapidly hydrolyzed, systemic administration of procaine is not effective.

Pharmacologic Properties

Procainamide has membrane-stabilizing (local anesthetic) properties, which are responsible for the direct effect of procainamide on cardiac tissues, as described later in this chapter. The drug also affects the heart indirectly, by its vagolytic effect. The precise site of exertion of this vagolytic effect is not known.

Electrophysiologic Effects

Effect on the Action Potential

The effect of procainamide on the action potential in isolated Purkinje fibers resembles that of quinidine. It reduces the rate of rise and the amplitude of phase-0 depolarization with little alteration in the resting membrane potential.[1-3]

Effect on the Sinus Node

In most patients studied, procainamide has had no significant effect on the sinus rate. Occasionally, a slight slowing of the sinus rate has been observed.[4] One study showed that procainamide increased heart rate and decreased the sinoatrial conduction time.[5] These data are derived from studies in adults because no large series of children have been studied. Interesting and different findings were obtained in a study of the effect of procainamide on the immature canine heart. In a group of 8 nonsedated puppies, aged 12 to 28 days, which had undergone long-term instrumentation, procainamide decreased the spontaneous sinus rate and the sinus node recovery time and increased the sinoatrial conduction time.[6] Procainamide has both direct and indirect (vagolytic) effects on the sinus node. Slowing of the rate of the immature heart appears to result from predominance of the direct effect. The apparent shortening of the sinus node recovery time is probably produced by enhancement of sinoatrial entrance block by procainamide. Slowing of the spontaneous sinus rate may be expected in infants treated with procainamide.

Effect on the Atria

Procainamide has been reported not to change or to increase atrial effective refractory periods and not to alter atrial conduction time.[4,7] In the immature canine heart, procainamide caused a significant lengthening of atrial refractory periods.[6]

Effect on the Atrioventricular Node

Procainamide has little effect on anterograde conduction and refractoriness in the atrioventricular node. At therapeutic concentrations, the drug may prolong the AH and PR intervals, or it may not alter these intervals at all. In a group of patients with ventricular arrhythmias, procainamide prolonged the PR interval by about 8% in 59% of the patients; the prolongation was greater in the patients with shorter pretreatment PR intervals than in the other patients.[8] In another series of 13 patients with ventricular arrhythmias, the AH interval was not altered by the drug.[4]

In a study of the effect of procainamide on the immature canine heart, the drug did not alter the PR interval or the effective and functional refractory periods of the atrioventricular node.[6] In several children treated with procainamide, no change in the PR interval was seen, although high doses of the drug were administered.

Although procainamide does not alter anterograde refractoriness of the atrioventricular node, it depresses retrograde atrioventricular nodal refractoriness and conduction in patients with re-entrant tachycardia due to dual atrioventricular nodal pathways.[9,10] The drug may even produce a complete retrograde block.

Effect on Accessory Atrioventricular Pathway

Procainamide can prolong the anterograde effective refractory period of accessory atrioventricular pathways and may even produce a complete anterograde block. This effect is more pronounced in patients with a long pretreatment effective refractory period of the accessory pathway than on other patients.[11-13] Procainamide usually also increases the retrograde effective refractory period.

Effect on the Ventricles

Procainamide slows conduction in the His-Purkinje system and thus prolongs the HV interval. Conduction is slowed in both anterograde and retrograde directions.[4,14,15] Procainamide may either increase or not alter the duration of the QRS interval. For example, in a series of 32 patients with ventricular arrhythmias, procainamide prolonged the QRS interval in 11 patients, from 0.080 ± 0.017 to 0.093 ± 0.016 sec, and did not alter it in 21 patients.[8] In a study of the immature canine heart, procainamide did not much alter the duration of the QRS interval.[6] In children, the duration of this interval was not altered.[16]

Procainamide usually increases or does not alter the effective refractory period of the ventricular myocardium. For example, Kastor and associates reported that, in adult human patients, procainamide increased the ventricular effective refractory period from 237 ± 7 to 279 ± 16 msec.[17] In the immature canine heart, the drug prolonged the ventricular effective refractory period from 148 ± 6 to 157 ± 6 msec.[6] Therapeutic concentrations of procainamide prolong the QTc interval by up to 25%. A greater prolongation is associated with a high incidence of arrhythmias especially polymorphous ventricular tachycardia. In a study of the immature canine heart, procainamide prolonged the QTc interval from 295 ± 4 to 305 ± 9 msec.[6] In the few studied children treated with procainamide, no significant prolongation of this interval was observed.[16, 18, 19]

Effect on Arrhythmias

Experimental animal studies and studies in human adults have shown that procainamide is effective in terminating and preventing various ventricular and supraventricular arrhythmias. In several studies in adults, procainamide suppressed premature ventricular beats in about 90% of the patients and ventricular tachycardia in about 60%.[20-22] In some small series, procainamide completely suppressed ventricular tachycardia.[23]

Procainamide has only a limited effect in preventing the induction of ventricular arrhythmias during electrophysiologic studies. For example, Waxman and co-workers reported that procainamide, administered intravenously or orally, prevented the induction of ventricular tachycardia in only 33% of 126 patients.[24] Because the response to procainamide predicted the response to other conventional Class I antiarrhythmic agents, however, it was suggested that if procainamide does not prevent the induction of ventricular tachycardia in a certain patient, no further studies with other conventional Class I antiarrhythmic agents should be performed in this patient, and Class III or investigational agents should be tried. Procainamide also suppresses ventricular arrhythmias associated with acute myocardial infarction. Procaine can suppress and prevent supraventricular arrhythmias in patients with Wolff-Parkinson-White syndrome.[14]

Only a few cases of treatment of arrhythmias with procainamide in infancy and childhood have been reported, and a common finding was the need for high doses of the drug.

As early as 1960, Mortimer and Rakita reported successful control of ventricular tachycardia in children with large doses of procainamide.[19] In 1971 Gelband and colleagues reported on an 18-month-old infant with ventricular tachycardia.[16] He had no structural heart disease, and the origin of the arrhythmia was unknown. The arrhythmia, which was resistant to quinidine, was controlled only by procainamide, 3600 mg/day. The plasma procainamide concentration achieved with this dose was 9 µg/ml, a concentration within the therapeutic range in adults. Several other investigators have reported the use of procainamide in infants and children with various arrhythmias.

In summary, procainamide may be tried in infants and children with ventricular or supraventricular arrhythmias resistant to lidocaine and quinidine or in those wth ventricular arrhythmias responsive to short-term intravenous lidocaine and requiring continued oral treatment. The long-term risk of treatment with procainamide should be weighed against the potential benefit. One should not treat children with procainamide for long periods. The antiarrhythmic effect of procainamide is comparable to that of quinidine, but quinidine is better tolerated.[14] Procainamide is more effective and is better tolerated than phenytoin.[25]

Hemodynamic Effects

Like other Class I antiarrhythmic agents, procainamide has a negative inotropic effect.[26, 27] This effect may be of no clinical significance in the normal heart, but it may cause hemodynamic deterioration in patients with impaired myocardial function. Procainamide also relaxes vascular smooth muscle by an adrenergic-mediated mechanism and produces peripheral vasodilation.[28] The negative inotropic effect and the peripheral vasodilatory effect may result in a marked decrease in systemic arterial pressure.[29] In patients wth peripheral vasoconstriction, the peripheral vasodilatory effect of procainamide makes it superior to antiarrhythmic agents with a vasoconstricting effect.

Clinical Pharmacology

Most studies of the clinical pharmacology of procainamide have been conducted in adults. The pharmacologic profile of the drug in children may be different from that in adults, as shown by a few studies in children and in immature animals. Procainamide may be administered intravenously, intramuscularly, or orally. Intramuscular administration is rare, although one may thereby achieve maximal plasma concentrations in under 30 min.[30, 31] After oral administration, procainamide is rapidly and completely absorbed from the gastrointestinal tract; the maximal plasma concentration is reached in under 75 min. The drug undergoes only minimal or no first-pass hepatic metabolism.[32, 33] The range of therapeutic plasma levels is usually 4 to 10 µg/ml, although some patients require plasma concentrations as high as 20 µg/ml.[8, 34, 35] A correlation between plasma levels and the drug's therapeutic and toxic effects has been found.

Procainamide is distributed in all body tissues, except the brain. About 60% of a dose of the drug is excreted unchanged in the urine and the remainder undergoes hepatic metabolism. The most important metabolite is NAPA, which has antiarrhythmic properties. The elimination half-life is about 3 hours.[1]

The pharmacokinetics and pharmacodynamics of procainamide have not specifically been studied in infants and children. Animal experiements have shown, however, that the pharmacokinetic profile of procainamide in the immature animal may be different from that in adults. For example, Singh and associates studied the pharmacokinetics of procainamide in 5 puppies, 5 to 8 weeks of age, and compared it to that in 5 adult dogs.[36] The drug was given intravenously as loading infusions followed by maintenance infusions. The distribution half-life was 12.5 ± 14 min in puppies and 4.6 ± 2.4 min in adults, and the elimination half-life was 166 ± 46 min in puppies and 117 ± 36 min in adults. These differences were not statistically significant. The volume of distribution was 5.0 ± 2.7 L/kg in puppies and 2.1 ± 0.55 L/kg in adults. Plasma clearance was 1.192 ± 324 mg/kg/hour in puppies and 747 ± 121 mg/kg/hour in adults. These values were statistically significant. Thus, the plasma clearance and volume of distribution of procainamide are greater in the immature dog than those in the adult. This finding suggests that higher or more frequent doses are required in immature animals, and probably also in human infants, to achieve therapeutic plasma concentrations. Clinical studies are still required.

In several case reports, high doses of procainamide were required to achieve therapeutic effects in infants and children.[16,18,19] The findings in dogs partially explain this need. Other factors that may contribute to the need for higher doses are decreased sensitivity of cardiac tissues to procainamde and delayed absorption of the drug from the gastrointestinal tract.[19]

In neonates, the opposite condition may occur, namely, accumulation of procainamide because of delayed elimination resulting from immaturity of the liver and slow hepatic metabolism of the drug.[37] For example, in a neonate born to a mother treated with procainamide, the half-life of elimination of the drug given to the mother from the neonate's plasma was 13.5 hours.[38] In this neonate, the plasma concentrations of procainamide and NAPA were higher than in umbilical cord and maternal blood. Renal clearances of procainamide and NAPA 2 days after birth were 400 and 300 ml/min, respectively, in the mother. In the neonate, these values were 0.7 and 1.65 ml/min, respectively, 8 hours after birth. The half-life of NAPA was 19.5 hours.[38]

In a child who inadvertently ingested a high dose of procainamide, 28 mg/kg, elimination of the drug was delayed. This delay did not result from immaturity of the liver, but from procainamide-induced hypotension with reductions in hepatic blood flow and in the rate of hepatic metabolism.

Singh and co-workers studied the pharmacokinetics of procainamide in 5 children after a single intravenous dose of 5.5 ± 0.9 mg/kg.[39] The following values were found: distribution half-life, 10.3 ± 3.4 minutes; elimination half-life, 1.7 ± 0.1 hours; plasma clearance, 19.4 ± 2.0

ml/min/kg; and steady-state volume of distribution, 2.2 ± 0.3 L/kg. NAPA was found in the plasma shortly after the intravenous administration of procainamide, and its peak plasma concentration was attained 1 to 2 hours after administration. The plasma levels of the metabolite were usually lower than those of the parent drug. These findings, and especially the short elimination half-life, confirm the results of animal studies and suggest that continuous intravenous infusion may be required to maintain therapeutic plasma levels.[39]

Side Effects

Procainamide frequently produces side effects, the most serious of which are cardiovascular effects and a syndrome resembling systemic lupus erythematosus. Some of the side effects are dose-dependent. Side effects have been observed in 87% of patients treated with procainamide.[40]

Cardiovascular Effects

Like other Class I antiarrhythmic drugs, procainamide may produce or may aggravate congestive heart failure or hypotension. This effect is discussed in the section of this chapter on hemodynamic effects of procainamide. At least one child has developed hypotension after a high dose of procainamide. Like other Class I antiarrhythmic agents, procainamide also has an arrhythmogenic potential. This effect is evident especially at low doses.[15, 41] Although procainamide may cause or may aggravate intraventricular conduction disturbances, this effect has not been reported in children.

Lupus Erythematosus

Drug-induced systemic lupus erythematosus is the most disturbing side effect of prolonged treatment with procainamide. It is found in about 50% of patients treated for long periods, but its incidence has varied among reported series.[40, 42, 43] The patient's lungs are consistently involved, but the elevation of body temperature and the cutaneous and renal lesions are more limited than those observed in idiopathic systemic lupus erythematosus. Although antinuclear factor commonly develops in these patients, antibodies to native DNA are rarely observed.[44-46] This syndrome is probably produced by procainamide itself and not by its metabolite NAPA; slow acetylators develop a lupus-like syndrome after shorter periods of treatment than fast acetylators.[47, 48] This syndrome is resolved when procainamide is replaced with NAPA.[49]

Agranulocytosis

Procainamide, given at high doses for long periods, rarely causes agranulocytosis. Fifteen such cases have been reported.[50]

Other Effects

Procainamide may cause anorexia, nausea, vomiting, diarrhea, dizziness, hallucinations, mental depression, and psychosis.[51]

Dosage and Administration

Intravenous Administration

A loading dose of 15 mg/kg is given over an hour and is followed by a maintenance dose of 2.5 to 3.0 mg/kg.

Oral Administration

In adults, 250 to 600 mg are given every 6 hours. Some patients require doses as high as 12.0 g/daily. Infants and children require high doses.

N-acetylprocainamide (NAPA)

N-acetylprocainamide (NAPA), the most important metabolite of procainamide, has electrophysiologic and antiarrhythmic properties resembling those of the parent drug. NAPA may be responsible for some of the effects of procainamide. In contrast, NAPA is devoid of some of procainamide's adverse effects. Treatment with NAPA is associated with a much lower incidence of drug-induced systemic lupus erythematosus than treatment with procainamide. The hemodynamic effects of NAPA differ from those of procainamide; NAPA is less prone to produce hemodynamic deterioration. Because NAPA has a longer half-life than procainamide, it can be given three times daily, instead of the six times daily necessary with procainamide. The compliance of patients is thereby improved.

Because of these properties, NAPA has been evaluted for use as an independent antiarrhythmic agent. A favorable response was found in the short-term treatment of ventricular arrhythmias. NAPA completely abolished complex ventricular arrhythmias and almost completely suppressed premature ventricular beats in five patients.[52] In another study, NAPA suppressed exercise-induced ventricular arrhythmias by about half.[37] An important problem is recurrent arrhythmias in patients with an initially favorable response to the drug.

References

1. Singer, D.H., Strauss, H.C., and Hoffman, B.F.: Biphasic effects of procainamide on cardiac conduction. Bull. N.Y. Acad. Med., 43:1194, 1968.
2. Bigger, J.T., Jr., and Heissenbuttel, R.H.: The use of procaine amide and lidocaine in the treatment of cardiac arrhythmias. Prog. Cardiovasc. Dis., 11:515, 1969.
3. Hoffman, B.G.: The action of quinidine and procaine amide on single fibers of dog ventricle and specialized conduction systems. An. Acad. Bras. Cienc., 29:365, 1958.
4. Shenasa, M., et al.: Procainamide and retrograde atrioventricular nodal conduction in man. Circulation, 65:355, 1982.

5. Wyse, D.G., et al.: Influence of plasma drug level and the presence of conduction disease on the electrophysiologic effects of procainamide. Am. J. Cardiol., *43*:619, 1979.
6. Shih, J.Y., et al.: The electrophysiologic effects of procainamide in the immature heart. Pediatr. Pharmacol., *2*:65, 1982.
7. Sellers, T.D. et al.: Effects of procainamide and quinidine sulfate in the Wolff-Parkinson-White syndrome. Circulation, *55*:15, 1977.
8. Lima, J.J., et al.: Safety and efficacy of procainamide infusions. Am. J. Cardiol., *43*:98, 1979.
9. Gomes, J.A., et al.: Simultaneous anterograde fast-slow atrioventricular nodal pathway conduction after procainamide. Am. J. Cardiol., *46*:677, 1980.
10. Wu, B., et al.: Effect of procainamide on atrioventricular nodal re-entrant paroxysmal tachycardia. Circulation, *57*:1171, 1978.
11. Mandel, W.J., et al.: Tachycardia in Wolff-Parkinson-White syndrome: alterations by ouabain and procainamide. Clin. Res., *21*:435, 1973.
12. Wellens, H.J.J., et al.: Use of procainamide in patients with the Wolff-Parkinson-White syndrome to disclose a short refractory period of the accessory pathway. Am. J. Cardiol., *50*:1087, 1982.
13. Mandel, W.J. et al.: The Wolff-Parkinson-White syndrome: pharmacological effects of procaine amide. Am. Heart J., *90*:744, 1975.
14. Wellens, J.J.H., and Durrer, D.: Effect of procaine amide, quinidine, and ajmaline in the Wolff-Parkinson-White syndrome. Circulation, *50*:114, 1974.
15. Reddy, C.P., and Lynch, M.: Abolition and modification of reentry within the His-Purkinje system by procainamide in man. Circulation, *58*:1010, 1978.
16. Gelband, H., Steeg, C.N., and Bigger, J.T., Jr.: Use of massive doses of procainamide in the treatment of ventricular tachycardia in infancy. Pediatrics, *48*:110, 1971.
17. Kastor, J.A., et al.: Human ventricular refractoriness. Circulation, *56*:462, 1977.
18. Dimich, I., et al.: Treatment of recurrent paroxysmal tachycardia. Am. Heart J., *79*:811, 1970.
19. Mortimer, E.A., Jr., and Rakita, L.: Ventricular tachycardia in childhood controlled with large doses of procainamide. N. Engl. J. Med., *262*:615, 1960.
20. Giardina, E.V., Helssenbuttel, R.H., and Bigger, T.J.: Intermittent intravenous procainamide to treat ventricular arrhythmias. Ann. Intern. Med., *78*:183, 1973.
21. Koch-Weser, J., et al.: Antiarrhythmic prophylaxis with procainamide in acute myocardial infarction. N. Engl. J. Med., *281*:1253, 1969.
22. Kayden, H.J., Brodle, B.B., and Skele, J.M.: Procainamide: a review. Circulation, *15*:118, 1957.
23. Myerburg, R.J. et al.: Antiarrhythmic drug therapy in survivors of prehospital cardiac arrest: comparison of effects on chronic ventricular arrhythmias and recurrent cardiac arrest. Circulation, *59*:855, 1979.
24. Waxman, H.D., et al.: The response to procainamide during electrophysiologic study for sustained ventricular tachyarrhythmias predicts the response to other medications. Circulation, *67*:30, 1983.
25. Karlsson, E.: Procainamide and phenytoin: comparative study of their antiarrhythmic effects at apparent therapeutic plasma levels. Br. Heart J., *37*:731, 1975.
26. Harrison, D.C., Sprouse, J.H., and Morrow, A.G.: The antiarrhythmic properties of lidocaine and procaine amide. Circulation, *28*:486, 1963.
27. Giardina, E.V., Heissenbuttel, R.H., and Bigger, J.T., Jr.: Intermittent intravenous procaine amide to treat ventricular arrhythmias. Ann. Intern. Med., *78*:183, 1973.
28. Koch-Weser, J.: Clinical application of the pharmacokinetics of procaine amide. Cardiovasc. Clin., *6(2)*:63, 1974.
29. Woske, H., et al.: The effect of procainamide on excitability refractoriness and conduction in the mammalian heart. J. Pharmacol. Exp. Ther., *107*:134, 1953.
30. Koch-Weser, J.: Pharmacokinetics of procainamide in man. Ann. N.Y. Acad. Sci., *179*:370, 1971.
31. Mark, L.C., et al.: The physiological disposition and cardiac effects of procaine amide. J. Pharmacol. Exp. Ther., *102*:5, 1951.

32. Karlsson, E., and Molin, L.: Polymorphic acetylation of procainamide in healthy subjects. Acta Med. Scand., *197*:299, 1975.
33. Karlsson, E., and Sonnhag, C.: Comparative evaluation of procainamide and its main metabolite, N-acetylprocainamide, in the acute treatment of ventricular arrhythmias. Br. J. Clin. Pharmacol., *4*:632, 1977.
34. Myerburg, R.J. et al.: Relationship between plasma levels of procainamide, suppression of premature ventricular complexes and prevention of recurrent ventricular tachycardia. Circulation, *64*:280, 1981.
35. Bellet, S., Zeeman, S.E., and Hirsh, S.A.: The intramuscular use of Pronestyl. Am. J. Med., *31*:145, 1952.
36. Singh, S., et al.: The pharmacokinetics of procainamide in the immature canine. Pediatr. Cardiol., *4*:315, 1983.
37. Sonnhag, C., and Karlsson, E.: Comparative antiarrhythmic efficacy of intravenous N-acetylprocainamide and procainamide. Eur. J. Clin. Pharmacol., *15*:311, 1979.
38. Lima, J.J., et al.: Fetal uptake and neonatal disposition of procainamide and its acetylated metabolite: a case report. Pediatrics, *61*:491, 1978.
39. Singh, S., et al.: Procainamide elimination kinetics in pediatric patients. Clin. Pharmacol. Ther., *32*:607, 1982.
40. Kosowsky, B.D., et al.: Long-term use of procaine amide following acute myocardial infarction. Circulation, *47*:1204, 1973.
41. Greenspan, A.M., et al.: Large dose procainamide therapy for ventricular tachyarrhythmia. Am. J. Cardiol., *46*:453, 1980.
42. Bellet, S.: Essentials of cardiac arrhythmias: diagnosis and management. Philadelphia, W.B. Saunders, 1972, p. 358.
43. Henningsen, N.C., et al.: Effects of long-term treatment with procaine amide: a prospective study with special regard to ANF and SLE in fast and slow acetylators. Acta. Med. Scand. *198*:475, 1975.
44. Fakhro, A.M., Ritchie, R.F., and Lown, B.: Lupus-like syndrome induced by procainamide, Am. J. Cardiol., *20*:367, 1967.
45. Winfield, J.B., Koffler, D., and Kundel, H.G.: Development of antibodies to ribonucleoprotein following short-term therapy with procainamde. Arthritis Rheum., *18*:531, 1975.
46. Atkinson, A. J., Jr., et al.: Dose-ranging trial of N-acetylprocainamide in patients with premature ventricular contractions. Clin. Pharmacol. Ther., *21*:575, 1977.
47. Reidenberg, M.M., et al.: Polymorphic acetylation of procainamide in man. Clin. Pharmacol. Ther., *17*:722, 1975.
48. Drayer, D.E., et al.: Cumulation of N-acetylprocainamide, an active metabolite of procainamide, in patients with impaired renal function. Clin. Pharmacol. Ther., *22*:63, 1979.
49. Kluger, J., et al.: Clinical phamacology of N-acetylprocainamide (NAPA) the major metabolite of procainamide in man. Clin. Res., *26*:244A, 1978.
50. Lertora, J.J., et al.: Long-term antiarrhythmic therapy with N-acetylprocainamide. Clin. Pharmacol. Ther., *25*:273, 1979.
51. Nagesh, K.G., et al.: Procainamide induced agranulocytosis. J. Kans. Med. Soc., *81*:8, 1980.
52. Boccardo, D., Pitchon, R., and Wiener, I.: Adverse reactions and efficacy of high-dose procainamide therapy in resistant tachyarrhythmias. Am. Heart J., *102*:797, 1981.
53. Crawford, M.H., et al.: Hemodynamic effects of N-acetylprocainamide in heart disease. Clin. Pharmacol. Ther., *31*:459, 1982.

Chapter 22

Disopyramide

Disopyramide is a Class I antiarrhythmic agent with electrophysiologic properties and an antiarrhythmic profile resembling those of quinidine and procainamide. It also has potent anticholinergic characteristics, which are responsible for some of its side effects. Disopyramide is effective in suppression and prevention of both ventricular and supraventricular arrhythmias.

In adults, disopyramide is widely used, usually as a second-line antiarrhythmic agent. The experience in children is limited; only a few cases have been reported in the literature. A few adolescents and young adults under 19 years of age have been included in electrophysiologic studies of patients with Wolff-Parkinson-White syndrome.

Structure

Disopyramide is 4-disopropylamino-2-(2-pyridyl)-butyramide.

Pharmacologic Properties

The most important properties of disopyramide are a membrane-stabilizing effect, resembling that of procainamide and quinidine, and an anticholinergic effect. Disopyramide, a Class Ia antiarrhythmic agent,[1-3] may have a calcium-antagonistic effect.[4]

Electrophysiologic Effects

The electrophysiologic effects of disopyramide in intact animals and human subjects are the net result of the direct membrane-stabilizing effect, the anticholinergic effect, and sympathetic-mediated responses to the actions of the drug on the peripheral vasculature.

Disopyramide decreases the rate of rise and the amplitude of phase-0 depolarization, prolongs the duration of the action potential, depresses membrane responsiveness, and slows conduction.[5,6] The drug also decreases automaticity, as evident by a decrease in slope of phase-4 depolarization.

The effect of disopyramide on the sinus node is inconsistent. One study showed that intravenously administered disopyramide slowed heart rate 5 minutes after injection because of a direct depressant effect and accelerated it after 15 minutes because of the drug's anticholinergic effect.[7] Other studies did not show any significant effect of intravenously or orally administered disopyramide on spontaneous sinus rate.[8–10] The effect of disopyramide on sinus node recovery time is usually insignificant,[11] although a slight prolongation may be observed.[12] The effect on sinoatrial conduction time is inconsistent. In patients with sick sinus syndrome, disopyramide may prolong the length of the sinus cycle, sinus node recovery time, and sinoatrial conduction time.[9–13] This feature should be remembered when disopyramide is considered for treatment of arrhythmias in children after cardiac operations involving the interatrial septum.

Disopyramide prolongs or does not alter the atrial refractory periods.[11, 14] It may prolong the duration of the P wave.

Disopyramide either prolongs or does not alter atrioventricular nodal conduction time.[11, 13] For example, in a group of 12 patients with Wolff-Parkinson-White syndrome, 5 of them under 18 years of age, the drug prolonged the AH interval from 64 ± 11 to 71 ± 23 msec.[15] In another group, the AH interval increased in 9 patients, decreased in 5, and was unaltered in 1 patient. The effect on atrioventricular nodal refractoriness is inconsistent.

Disopyramide prolongs retrograde and, to a lesser extent, anterograde conduction time and effective refractory period of accessory atrioventricular pathways. This phenomenon has been demonstrated in adults as well as in adolescents and children.[15]

Disopyramide may prolong or may not alter the intraventricular conduction time, as evident by prolongations of the HV and QRS intervals. The drug lengthens the ventricular effective refractory period and the QTc interval. It may prolong the refractoriness of the His-Purkinje system.[16]

Effects in Arrhythmias

Disopyramide is used mainly for suppression and prevention of ventricular arrhythmias. Several large-scale studies have shown that the efficacy of disopyramide for this indication is moderate to high. For example, Nichols and Willis reported that orally administered disopyramide reduced the number of premature ventricular beats by more than 90% in 52% of 55 patients with multiple premature ventricular beats.[17] Other investigators have reported lower success rates of 30 to 50%.[18–20] Disopyramide has also been effective in preventing the induction of ventricular tachycardia in patients with recurrent ventricular tachycardia and fibrillation. In one study, patients in whom tachycardia could be induced after disopyramide, the cycle length was prolonged.[21] Electrophysiologic studies predicted the clinical response to disopyramide in about 80% of these patients. In the study by Manz and co-workers, disopyramide prevented the induction of sustained ventricular tachycardia in only 1 of 25 patients.[22]

The experience in treating ventricular arrhythmias in children with disopyramide is limited, and only a few cases have been reported. In my experience, with a few children with ventricular arrhythmias resistant to other Class I antiarrhythmic agents, disopyramide was effective, especially in combination with beta-adrenoreceptor blocking agents.

Several studies have shown that disopyramide can terminate paroxysmal supraventricular tachycardia.[23,24] In a study of patients with Wolff-Parkinson-White syndrome, this effect was mainly due to prolongation of retrograde conduction time and refractory period in the accessory pathway.[15] An important effect of disopyramide in patients with Wolff-Parkinson-White syndrome and atrial fibrillation is prevention of rapid ventricular response.[15] Disopyramide also prevents the induction and spontaneous recurrences of various supraventricular arrhythmias. This property has also been demonstrated in children and adolescents.[15,25] Disopyramide also controls arrhythmias resulting from dual atrioventricular nodal pathways.[26]

Disopyramide may convert atrial fibrillation and flutter to normal sinus rhythm. In a series of 53 patients with these arrhythmias, the conversion rate was 42%.[27]

Comparison with Other Antiarrhythmic Agents

Disopyramide causes more infranodal conduction disturbances and has more adverse hemodynamic effects than lidocaine. Lidocaine is the drug of first choice of immediate termination of ventricular arrhythmias. Several cases of ventricular arrhythmias resistant to lidocaine but responsive to disopyramide have been reported, however.[28,29] Procainamide is reported to be more effective than disopyramide.[30] Disopyramide may control ventricular arrhythmias resistant to quinidine.[31] In a comparative study, the effect of both drugs was comparable.[32]

Hemodynamic Effects

Disopyramide has a negative inotropic effect. It may depress left ventricular function even in patients without pre-existing dysfunction,[7,33] although this subject is controversial.[34] In patients with heart disease and myocardial damage, disopyramide has decreased ejection fraction and cardiac output.[33,34] Disopyramide may increase peripheral vascular resistance.

Effects in Hypertrophic Cardiomyopathy

Pollick reported that disopyramide reduced the resting and provokable pressure gradients and increased exercise duration in patients with hypertrophic cardiomyopathy.[35] These phenomena may result from the negative inotropic effect of disopyramide and possibly also from a direct effect on diastolic properties of the heart.

Clinical Pharmacology

Disopyramide may be given intravenously or orally. It is rapidly and almost completely absorbed from the gastrointestinal tract. The onset of action occurs within 1 to 3 hours of oral administration and 1 min after intravenous administration. The systemic bioavailability of disopyramide is about 80%.[36] About 15% of the dose undergoes first-pass hepatic metabolism. The volume of distribution of disopyramide is reported to be 0.78 ± 0.26 L/kg in healthy human subjects.[37] The therapeutic plasma concentration ranges between 2 and 7 μg/ml.[38,39] The protein binding of disopyramide is about 80%.[40] The drug is bound mainly to alpha-1-acid glycoprotein,[41] but it is also bound to albumin.

Disopyramide is eliminated by renal excretion and hepatic metabolism. The elimination half-life ranges between 6 and 10 hours.[36] The total body clearance of disopyramide is 1.30 ± 0.70 ml/min/kg. The elimination rate may be reduced in patients with impaired renal function.

The monodealkylated metabolite of disopyramide may be responsible for the anticholinergic properties of this drug.

Side Effects

Disopyramide may cause hemodynamic deterioration, especially when the drug is administered intravenously to patients with impairment of myocardial function.[20,24] Electromechanical dissociation has been described in patients with congestive heart failure and impairment of renal function. Like other Class Ia antiarrhythmic agents, disopyramide has an arrhythmogenic potential. It may also produce or may aggravate conductive disturbances. The anticholinergic properties of disopyramide may cause urinary retention, visual disturbances, and gastrointestinal disorders.

Contraindications

Contraindications to disopyramide administration are severe congestive heart failure, shock, glaucoma, and urinary retention.

Dosage and Administration

Pediatric dosage recommendations are not available. In adults, an infusion rate of 0.4 mg/kg/hour and oral doses of 100 to 150 mg 3 to 4 times daily are used. An initial loading dose may be given.

References

1. Giacomini, K.M., et al.: Comparative anticholinergic potencies of R and S disopyramide in longitudinal muscle strips from guinea pig ileum. Life Sci., 27:1191, 1980.
2. Mokler, C.M. and Van Arman, C.G.: Pharmacology of a new antiarrhythmic agent: gamma-disopropylamino-2-phenyl-(2-pyridyl)-butyramide (SC-7031). J. Pharmacol. Exp. Ther., 136:114, 1962.
3. Baines, M.W., et al.: Some pharmacological effects of disopyramide and a metabolite. J. Int. Med. Res., 4(Suppl. 1), 1976.
4. Mayler, W.G.: The pharmacology of disopyramide. J. Int. Med. Res., 4 (Suppl. 1): 8, 1976.
5. Kus, T., and Sasvniuk, B.L.: Electrophysiological actions of disopyramide phosphate on canine ventricular muscle and Purkinje fibers. Circ. Res., 37:844, 1975.
6. Danilo, P., et al: Effects of disopyramide phosphate (Norpace) on electrophysiologic properties of isolated canine cardiac Purkinje fibers. Am. J. Cardiol., 35:130, 1975.
7. Pollick, C., et al.: The cardiac effects of d- and l-disopyramide in normal subjects: a noninvasive study. Circulation, 66:447, 1982.
8. Jansesn, C., et al.: Haemodynamic effects of intravenous disopyramide in heart failure. Eur. J. Clin. Pharmacol., 8:167, 1975.
9. Marrot, P.K., et al.: A study of the acute electrophysiological and cardiovascular action of disopyramide in man. Eur. J. Cardiol., 4:303, 1976.
10. Heel, R.C., et al.: Disopyramide: a review of its pharmacological properties and therapeutic use in treating cardiac arrhythmias. Drugs, 25:331, 1978.
11. Desai, J.M., et al.: Electrophysiological effects of disopyramide in patients with bundle branch block. Circulation, 59:215, 1979.
12. Katoh, T., et al.: The cellular electrophysiologic mechanism of the dual actions of disopyramide on rabbit sinus node function. Circulation, 66:1216, 1982.
13. LaBarre, A., et al.: Electrophysiologic effects of disopyramide phosphate on sinus node function in patients with sinus node dysfunction. Circulation, 59:226, 1979.
14. Wilkinson, P.R., et al.: Electrophysiologic effects of disopyramide in patients with atrioventricular nodal dysfunction. Circulation, 66:1211, 1982.
15. Kerr, C.R., et al.: Electrophysiologic effects of disopyramide phosphate in patients with Wolff-Parkinson-White syndrome. Circulation, 65:869, 1982.
16. Befeler, B., et al.: Electrophysiological effects of the antiarrhythmic agent disopyramide phosphate. Am. J. Cardiol., 35:282, 1975.
17. Nichols, A.B., and Willis, P.W.: Efficacy of oral disopyramide phosphate for long-term treatment of ventricular arrhythmias. (Abstract.) Am. J. Cardiol., 37:159, 1976.
18. Denes, P., et al.: Chronic long-term electrophysiologic study of paroxysmal ventricular tachycardia. Chest, 77:478, 1980.
19. Swiryn, S., et al.: Prediction of response to class I antiarrhythmic drugs during chronic electrophysiologic study of ventricular tachycardia. (Abstract.) Circulation, 62(Suppl. III):III-85, 1980.
20. Benditt, D.C., et al.: Recurrent ventricular tachycardia in man: evaluation of disopyramide therapy by intracardiac electrical stimulation. Eur. J. Cardiol., 9:255, 1979.
21. Lerman, B.B., et al.: Disopyramide: evaluation of electrophysiologic effects and clinical efficacy in patients with sustained ventricular tachycardia or ventricular fibrillation. Am. J. Cardiol., 51:759, 1983.
22. Manz, M., et al.: Treatment of recurrent sustained ventricular tachycardia with disopyramide: control by programmed ventricular stimulation. Br. Heart J., 49:222, 1983.
23. Spurrell, R.A.J., et al.: Effects of disopyramide on electrophysiological properties of atrioventricular pathway in Wolff-Parkinson-White syndrome. Br. Heart J., 37:861, 1975.
24. Deano, D., et al.: The antiarrhythmic efficacy of intravenous therapy with disopyramide phosphate. Chest, 72:597, 1977.
25. Kou, H.C., et al.: Effects of oral disopyramide phosphate on induction and sustenance of atrioventricular reentrant tachycardia incorporating retrograde accessory pathway conduction. Circulation, 66:454, 1982.

26. Sethi, K.K., et al.: Selective blockage of retrograde fast pathway by intravenous disopyramide in paroxysmal supraventricular tachycardia mediated by dual atrioventricular nodal pathways. Br. Heart. J., 49:532, 1983.
27. Luoma, P.V., et al.: Efficacy of intravenous disopyramide in the termination of supraventricular arrhythmias. J. Clin. Pharmacol., 18:293, 1978.
28. Green, S.C.H.: Disopyramide—an effective treatment for lignocaine-resistant arrhythmias Scott. Med., J., 24:21, 1979.
29. Deano, D.A., et al.: Comparative efficacy of intravenous disopyramide and lidocaine in ventricular dysrhythmias. (Abstract.) Am. J. Cardiol., 41:416, 1978.
30. Hiejima, K., et al.: Electrophysiologic evaluation of antiarrhythmic drugs on supraventricular tachyarrhythmias. Jpn. Circ. J., 47:98, 1983.
31. Swiryn, S., et al.: Prediction of response to class I antiarrhythmic drugs during electrophysiologic study of ventricular tachycardia. Am. Heart J., 104:43, 1982.
32. Oshrain, C., et al.: A double-blind comparison of disopyramide and quinidine sulphate as antiarrhythmic agents. Report of the Scientific Exhibit, Fortieth Scientific Sessions, American Heart Associations, Miami, 1976.
33. Gottdiener, J.S., et al.: Effects of disopyramide on left ventricular function assessment by radionuclide cineangiography. (Abstract.) Circulation, 62(Suppl. III):III-47, 1980.
34. Sutton, R.: Hemodynamics of intravenous disopyramide. J. Int. Med. Res., 4(Suppl. 1):46, 1976.
35. Pollick, C.: Muscular subaortic stenosis; hemodynamic and clinical improvement after disopyramide. N. Engl. J. Med., 307:997, 1982.
36. Bryson, S.M., et al.: Disopyramide serum and pharmacological effect kinetics applied to the assessment of bioavailability. Br. J. Clin. Pharmacol., 6:409, 1978.
37. Landmark, K., et al.: Pharmacokinetics of disopyramide in patients with imminent to moderate cardiac failure. Eur. J. Clin. Pharmacolol, 19:187, 1981.
38. Niarchos A.P.: Disopyramide: serum level and arrhythmia conversion. Am. Heart J., 92:57, 1976.
39. Koch-Weser, J.: Drug therapy: disopyramide. N. Engl. J. Med., 300:957, 1979.
40. Aitio, M.L.: Plasma concentrations and protein binding of disopyramide and mono-n-delayldisopyramide during chronic oral disopyramide therapy. Br. J. Clin. Pharmacol., 11:369, 1981.
41. Lima, J.J., and Salzer, L.B.: Contamination of albumin by alpha$_1$-acid glycoprotein. Biochem. Pharmacol., 30:2633, 1981.

Chapter 23
Lidocaine

Lidocaine, a Class Ib antiarrhythmic agent, is the drug of first choice for rapid suppression of ventricular arrhythmias. It has been used for this indication for the past 35 years. Lidocaine is especially suitable for emergency treatment because of its rapid onset of action. Moreover, the effect of lidocaine disappears soon after discontinuance of the intravenous infusion. A major limitation is that lidocaine is not effective orally. Lidocaine is ineffective in patients with supraventricular arrhythmias.

In children, lidocaine is used primarily to suppress ventricular arrhythmias after cardiac operations or myocardial injury. Because lidocaine does not interact with digitalis glycosides and does not impair atrioventricular nodal conduction, it is especially suitable for suppression of ventricular arrhythmias associated with digitalis toxicity in infants and children.

Structure

The molecule of lidocaine consists of a hydrophilic group, diethylglycine, which contains a tertiary nitrogen, connected by an amide link to an aromatic ring, 2,6-xylidide.

Pharmacologic Properties

The most important pharmacologic property of lidocaine is its membrane-stabilizing effect, which is responsible for the Class I antiarrhythmic and local anesthetic activities of this drug.[1] Lidocaine may have also a vagolytic effect.[2]

Electrophysiologic Effects

Lidocaine reduces the maximal rate of rise of phase-0 depolarization in partially damaged Purkinje fibers, but not in normal fibers.[3,4] It also reduces the rate of rise of phase-4 depolarization and the duration of the action potential. Lidocaine prolongs the effective refractory period of ischemic myocardium and shortens the effective refractory period of normal fibers. It decreases the inhomogeneity of refractory periods between Purkinje fibers and the myocardium. The drug does not alter conduction in normal atrioventricular node and Purkinje fibers.[4,5] Lidocaine increases the threshold for ventricular fibrillation.[6]

In patients with a normal sinus node, lidocaine accelerates the spontaneous sinus rate.[7] This effect may result from sympathetic activation secondary to peripheral vasodilation or from the vagolytic action of lidocaine. In patients with sick sinus syndrome, lidocaine shortens the cycle length of the sinus node and the sinus node recovery time and prolongs the sinoatrial conduction time.[7]

Lidocaine has an inconsistent effect on accessory atrioventricular pathways. It usually does not alter, but may accelerate, the ventricular response to atrial fibrillation in these patients.[8]

Lidocaine does not usually alter the duration of the QRS interval. It may shorten or may not alter the QTc interval.

Effect on Ventricular Arrhythmias

In adults, lidocaine is mainly used for immediate suppression of ventricular fibrillation, ventricular tachycardia, and premature ventricular beats, especially in patients with acute myocardial infarction. In children, lidocaine is used for immediate suppression of ventricular arrhythmias that appear early after cardiac surgical procedures or myocardial damage or that are associated with digitalis toxicity. The rate of suppression of arrhythmias in adults may reach 90%. In my experience with children, the success rate of lidocaine is high, but results are less favorable than in adults. The small number of children studied limits the interpretation of these results.

Although lidocaine is safer than Class Ia antiarrhythmic agents in patients with conduction disturbances, in patients with conduction disturbances and escape rhythms, lidocaine may depress these rhythms. In patients with acute myocardial infarction, ventricular arrhythmias, and advanced conduction disturbances, lidocaine may be given only after insertion of an endocardial pacemaker.

Phenytoin has traditionally been considered the drug of first choice for treatment of ventricular arrhythmias associated with digitalis toxicity. Lidocaine is at least as effective as phenytoin for this indication, however, and it has a more favorable pharmacokinetic profile than phenytoin. Like phenytoin, lidocaine does not interact with digitalis glycosides and does not enhance, and may even improve, the atrioventricular nodal conduction disturbances associated with digitalis toxicity. Therefore, lidocaine may be preferred in patients with serious ventricular arrhythmias associated with digitalis toxicity.

Clinical Pharmacology

Lidocaine is administered intravenously, and rarely also intramuscularly, for treatment of arrhythmias, and subcutaneously or topically for local anesthesia. This lipid-soluble drug undergoes rapid distribution. Therefore, its onset of action is rapid, from 1 to 5 min after intravenous administration.[9] Lidocaine is not given orally because it undergoes extensive first-pass hepatic metabolism and because the oral administration of lidocaine is associated with a high incidence of adverse gastrointestinal effects.

About 70% of the amount of lidocaine in the plasma is protein-bound, mainly to alpha-1-acid glycoprotein.[10] Therapeutic plasma levels range between 2 and 5 µg/ml.

The elimination of lidocaine is biphasic. The first phase represents distribution, with a half-life of 10 min; the second phase is actual elimination, with a half-life of 1 to 3 hours. Lidocaine is eliminated mainly by hepatic metabolism and urinary excretion of metabolites.[11,12]

Mihaly and co-workers reported that the elimination half-life of lidocaine is 3.5 hours.[13] Data on the elimination half-life in infants and children are not available. Lidocaine crosses the placenta. Fetuses and neonates can metabolize the drug.[14] Lidocaine has two pharmacologically active metabolites.

Side Effects

Effects related to the central nervous system, such as sedation, confusion, and nausea, are the most common side effects of lidocaine. In children, prolonged seizures have been associated with the oral use of viscous lidocaine, prescribed for sore throat or upper respiratory tract infections.[15]

Adverse cardiovascular effects, including depression of myocardial contractility, hypotension, conduction disturbances, and arrhythmias, may also occur.

Dosage and Administration

An initial intravenous loading dose of 1 mg/kg, given as a bolus injection, followed by a constant infusion of 20 to 50 µg/kg/min, is used in adults and in older children.

References

1. Gintant, G.A., et al.: The influence of molecular form of local anesthetic-type antiarrhythmic agents on reduction of the maximum upstroke velocity of canine cardiac Purkinje fibers. Circ. Res., 52:735, 1983.
2. Liberman, N.A., et al.: The effects of lidocaine on the electrical and mechanical activity of the heart. Am. J. Cardiol., 22:375, 1968.
3. Bigger, J.T., Jr., and Mandel, W.J.: Effects of lidocaine on the electrophysiological properties of ventricular muscle and Purkinje fibers. J. Clin. Invest., 49:63, 1970.
4. Davis, L.D., and Temte, J.V.: Electrophysiological actions of lidocaine on acanine ventricular muscle and Purkinje fibers. Circ. Res., 24:639, 1969.
5. Aravindakshan, V., et al.: Effect of lidocaine on escape rate in patients with complete atrioventricular block. Am. J. Cardiol., 40:177, 1977.

6. Spear, J.F., et al.: The effect of lidocaine on the ventricular fibrillation threshold during acute coronary ligation. Circulation, 43-44 (II):86, 1971.
7. Dhingra, R.C., et al.: Electrophysiologic effects of lidocaine on sinus node and atrium in patients with and without sinoatrial dysfunction. Circulation, 57:448, 1978.
8. Akhtar, M., et al.: Effect of lidocaine on atrioventricular response via the accessory pathway in patients with Wolff-Parkinson-White syndrome. Circulation, 63:435, 1981.
9. Sung, C.Y., and Truant, A.P.: The physiological disposition of lidocaine and its comparison in some respects with procaine. J. Pharmacol. Exp. Ther., 112:432, 1975.
10. LeLorier, J., et al.: Pharmacokinetics of lidocaine after prolonged intravenous infusions in uncomplicated myocardial infarction. Ann. Intern. Med., 87:700, 1977.
11. Hullunger, G.: On the metabolism of lidocaine. II. The biotransformation of lidocaine. Acta Pharmacol. Toxicol., 17:365, 1960.
12. Collinsworth, K.A., et al.: Clinical pharmacology of lidocaine as an antiarrhythmic drug. Circulation, 50:1217, 1974.
13. Mihaly, G.W., et al.: The pharmacokinetics and metabolism of the anilide local anesthetics in neonates. 1. Lignocaine. Eur. J. Clin. Pharmacol., 13:143, 1978.
14. Kuhnert, B.A., et al.: Maternal, fetal, and neonatal metabolism of lidocaine. Clin. Pharmacol. Ther., 26:213, 1979.
15. Rothstein, P., et al.: Prolonged seizures associated with the use of viscous lidocaine. J. Pediatr., 101:461, 1982.

Chapter 24
Phenytoin

Phenytoin (diphenylhydantoin) is an anticonvulsant and antiarrhythmic agent. Its electrophysiologic and antiarrhythmic properties resemble those of lidocaine, but it is superior to lidocaine because it is also effective orally. Phenytoin is used to suppress ventricular arrhythmias resulting from various causes and supraventricular and ventricular arrhythmias resulting from digitalis toxicity. Phenytoin is important in the treatment of arrhythmias associated with digitalis toxicity because it does not aggravate, and even improves, the atrioventricular nodal conduction disturbances induced by digitalis and because no adverse pharmacokinetic interaction occurs between phenytoin and digoxin. Quinidine, on the other hand, elevates the plasma levels of digoxin and can enhance conduction disturbances; it is therefore unsuitable for treatment of arrhythmias associated with digoxin toxicity.

In infants and children, phenytoin is used for treatment of arrhythmias associated with digitalis toxicity, as well as for treatment of ventricular arrhythmias occurring after surgical procedures for congenital heart disease.

Structure
Phenytoin structurally resembles the barbiturates.

Pharmacologic Properties
Phenytoin is a Class I antiarrhythmic agent with local anesthetic properties. These properties result from inhibition of the fast membranous channels and the fast sodium inward current.[1-3] At high concentrations, phenytoin may also inhibit the fast outward potassium current and the slow inward calcium current.[1] The resultant electrophysiologic effects are discussed in the following section of this chapter.

Phenytoin has a specific antiepileptic effect, without causing depression. The drug also decreases the efferent sympathetic activity of the central nervous system.[4] This effect contributes to phenytoin's antiarrhythmic properties.

Electrophysiologic Effects
The electrophysiologic effects of phenytoin resemble those of lidocaine and, at high concentrations, those of other Class I antiarrhythmic

agents. In isolated His-Purkinje fibers, phenytoin increases the duration of the action potential and the effective refractory periods.[5] In damaged fibers, in which the maximal rate of rise of phase-0 depolarization is partially depressed, phenytoin can increase the maximal rate of rise of phase-0 depolarization. This effect is especially common in the presence of hypokalemia and is considered to be partially responsible for the high efficacy of phenytoin in arrhythmias induced by digitalis toxicity because these arrhythmias are generated in fibers in which the rate of phase-0 depolarization is partially depressed and are frequently associated with hypokalemia.

In normal fibers and in the presence of normokalemia or hyperkalemia, phenytoin has no effect or even a depressant effect on the maximal rate of phase-0 depolarization. This effect slows conduction velocity and membrane responsiveness.[5,6]

Phenytoin slows the rate of spontaneous phase-4 depolarization in Purkinje and atrial fibers and, to a lesser extent, in the sinoatrial node.[7]

Phenytoin does not usually alter the resting membrane potential, but in the presence of hypokalemia, it may increase the resting potential. The effect of phenytoin also depends on the rate of stimulation. In atrial fibers, at a stimulation rate below normal sinus rhythm, phenytoin may increase the rate of rise of phase-0 depolarization. When the stimulation rate is equal to or higher than normal sinus rhythm, phenytoin may depress the rate of rise of phase-0 depolarization. These findings partially explain the mechanism of the antiarrhythmic effect of phenytoin. By enhancing conduction in partially damaged fibers, the drug decreases the likelihood of unidirectional block, an important factor in re-entrant arrhythmias. Phenytoin also increases the threshold for ventricular and atrial fibrillation.[8]

Effect on the Sinoatrial Node

Usually, phenytoin has no effect on the spontaneous rate of the sinoatrial node. In patients with sick sinus syndrome, however, high concentrations of phenytoin may cause bradycardia.[9] The solvent of commercially available phenytoin may depress the sinoatrial nodal function.

Effect on the Atria

Phenytoin may slow intra-atrial conduction; the drug has no consistent effect on the atrial effective refractory period.[8,10,11]

Effect on the Atrioventricular Node

Phenytoin either enhances or does not alter atrioventricular nodal conduction.[7,11-14] In a study of dogs with digitalis toxicity and atrioventricular conduction disturbances, phenytoin improved atrioventricular nodal conduction.[15] This effect is probably mediated by the autonomic nervous system.[7] Rarely, phenytoin toxicity impairs atrioventricular nodal conduction.

Effect on Accessory Atrioventricular Pathway

Phenytoin does not alter the electrophysiologic properties of accessory atrioventricular pathways.

Effect on the Ventricles

Phenytoin has no significant effect on the intraventricular conduction of normal beats,[12, 15] but it has enhanced the intraventricular conduction of premature beats.[16] Phenytoin shortens the ventricular effective refractory period and the QTc interval.[11] The QRS interval is not altered by the drug.

Effects in Arrhythmias

Phenytoin is a second- or third-line antiarrhythmic agent, except for arrhythmias associated with digitalis toxicity, in which the drug plays a more primary role. It is especially effective in suppression and prevention of ventricular arrhythmias, but it also controls supraventricular arrhythmias associated with digitalis toxicity and electrolytic disturbances. In children, phenytoin is used for suppression of arrhythmias after cardiac surgical procedures.

Effects in Ventricular Arrhythmias

Phenytoin is effective in suppression and prevention of various ventricular arrhythmias, including those resistant to other Class I antiarrhythmic agents such as quinidine and procainamide.[17, 18] It suppressed ventricular arrhythmias in a study of patients with acute myocardial infarction and reduced the incidence of sudden death after acute myocardial infarction,[19] although this subject is controversial. Bigger and associates reviewed the experience in the treatment of premature ventricular beats in adults.[20] Phenytoin was the most effective and the safest drug when plasma levels were adequate.

Phenytoin is especially effective and safe in suppression of ventricular arrhythmias associated with digitalis toxicity.[21, 22] For example, Rosen and co-workers reported that up to 92% of patients of various ages with these arrhythmias responded to phenytoin.[22] The drug has also been found effective in children with these arrhythmias. Because ventricular arrhythmias associated with digitalis toxicity are rare in children, no well-controlled studies have been performed. Phenytoin is safer than quinidine and procainamide in such children because it does not impair atrioventricular nodal conduction. Moreover, unlike quinidine, phenytoin does not interact with digoxin to elevate the plasma digoxin concentration.

Lidocaine is at least as effective as phenytoin in suppression of ventricular arrhythmias associated with digitalis toxicity. This subject is further discussed in Chapter 1.

Garson and colleagues studied the effect of phenytoin on ventricular arrhythmias in the late postoperative period in children and young adults.[23] This study included 6 patients, aged 7 to 27 years (mean 16.5 years) who had had cardiac operations a mean of 10.7 years before the arrhythmias were recognized. The patients received phenytoin orally, at doses sufficient to maintain a plasma concentration of 15 to 20 μg/ml. Before treatment, 2 patients had ventricular tachycardia, 2 had pairs of premature ventricular beats, and 2 had multiple premature ventricular beats. During treatment, 5 of the patients had complete suppression of ventricular arrhythmias. The remaining patient required combined treatment with phenytoin and disopyramide. Only 1 of the 5 responding patients had premature ventricular beats during or after exercise in the treatment period, although all of them had such arrhythmias before treatment.

In another study, the effect of phenytoin was elevated in 19 patients with ventricular arrhythmias that developed late after corrective operations for congenital heart diseases.[24] Four patients had ventricular tachycardia, 3 had couplets, 6 had frequent multiform premature ventricular beats, 4 had infrequent multiform premature ventricular beats, and 2 had frequent uniform premature ventricular beats. Sixteen of the patients had tetralogy of Fallot. In 9 of the patients, the arrhythmias were resistant to several Class I antiarrhythmic agents, including quinidine, disopyramide, and procainamide, or to propranolol. Phenytoin completely suppressed the ventricular arrhythmias in 15 of the patients and partially suppressed them in the remaining 4 patients, who had only a few uniform premature ventricular beats during treatment.

Thus, phenytoin appears to be effective in suppressing ventricular arrhythmias in the late postoperative period in patients undergoing corrective operations for congenital heart diseases. Phenytoin may even be the drug of choice for this group of patients.

An important problem with phenytoin is inadequate dosing. Many arrhythmias are diagnosed as resistant to phenytoin when adequate doses of the drug have not been given.

Effects in Supraventricular Arrhythmias

Because phenytoin has only a limited effect on atrial myocardium, and because it does not slow atrioventricular nodal conduction, the drug is ineffective in patients with most supraventricular arrhythmias. It is effective in controlling supraventricular arrhythmias associated with digitalis toxicity, however.[25-27]

Phenytoin has terminated digitalis-induced supraventricular tachycardia, with normal or impaired atrioventricular nodal conduction, and has converted it to normal sinus rhythm. Occasionally, phenytoin has also converted digitalis-induced atrial fibrillation or flutter to normal sinus rhythm; however, this drug, which can enhance atrioventricular nodal conduction, may accelerate the ventricular response to atrial fibrillation or flutter. Phenytoin is ineffective in patients with atrioventricular junctional tachycardia.[25]

Hemodynamic Effects

Phenytoin may depress myocardial contractility, especially in patients with impaired myocardial function. Phenytoin can also produce peripheral vasodilation.[28-30] Because of both these effects, the drug may cause hypotension and may aggravate congestive heart failure.

Clinical Pharmacology

Phenytoin is given either intravenously or orally. Absorption from the gastrointestinal tract after oral administration is slow, incomplete, and varies among patients. The drug is concentrated in the kidney, liver, brain, salivary gland, and muscles. The myocardial concentration is about equal to the plasma concentration.[31,32] In adults and children, the protein binding of phenytoin in the plasma is 90%. It is lower in neonates and in patients with renal dysfunction.

Bigger and associates reported that the antiarrhythmic effect of phenytoin is exerted at plasma concentrations of up to 20 μg/ml in adults.[14] Garson and co-workers, studying children and young adults, reported that the mean effective phenytoin concentration was 15.7 μg/ml, but it varied from 8.5 to 20.0 μg/ml.[23] Webb Kavey and colleagues reported that, in a larger group of patients in whom phenytoin was given for this indication, the mean serum level of the drug (which has been effective in these patients) was 16.8 μg/ml, and the range was from 12 to 25 μg/ml;[24] these levels were reported to be effective.

Phenytoin is eliminated almost exclusively by hepatic metabolism, by the mixed-function oxidase system. The predominant metabolite is paradihydroxyphenyl phenytoin. It is excreted in the bile and, after undergoing enterohepatic metabolism and conjugation with glucuronic acid or sulfate, it is excreted in the urine. The metabolites of phenytoin are pharmacologically inactive.[33,34] The metabolic pathways may be saturated by high doses.[35] A few patients have genetically determined rapid metabolism of phenytoin or impaired drug metabolism.[36,37] The elimination half-life of phenytoin is about 24 hours, with marked variability among patients.

Side Effects

Some disagreement exists concerning the incidence of side effects associated with phenytoin therapy in adults. In children, however, phenytoin is definitely associated with a low incidence of adverse effects.

Effects on the Central Nervous System

Cerebellar and vestibular effects, lethargy, blurring of vision, and nystagmus are the most common side effects of phenytoin therapy in adults.[33]

Peripheral Neuropathy

This adverse effect, which appears in up to 20% of elderly patients treated with phenytoin,[38] is rare in children.

Gingival Hyperplasia

This effect occurs mainly in the labial gingivae of the anterior maxillary and mandibular teeth. The hyperplastic gingivae are pale, and the surface may be nodular or smooth. Microscopic examination shows epithelial hyperplasia, mild hyperkeratosis, and inflammatory infiltration in the subepithelial connective tissue.[39] These changes may result from impairment of collagen metabolism. Until a few years ago, gingival hyperplasia was thought to be a specific effect of phenytoin; however, a form of gingival hyperplasia with similar histologic changes may be caused also by nifedipine. Gingival hyperplasia is considered to be the most frequent adverse effect of phenytoin in children. In several series of young patients treated with phenytoin, this effect was not reported, but in these series, the drug was given for short periods. The development and extent of gingival hyperplasia may be limited by a reduction in dose and by maintenance of proper oral hygiene.

Skin Rash

This effect is rare, but it may appear, even in young patients, after short periods of treatment. For example, in a series of 19 young patients with postoperative ventricular arrhythmias treated for short periods with phenytoin, skin rash appeared in 1 patient. It was the only side effect observed in this series.

Osteomalacia

By impairing vitamin D metabolism, phenytoin may produce osteomalacia and hypocalcemia and may increase serum alkaline phosphatase activity.

Cardiovascular Side Effects

Phenytoin may accelerate the ventricular response to atrial fibrillation and flutter. The drug rarely causes hypotension and hemodynamic deterioration from myocardial depression and peripheral vasodilation.

Dosage and Administration

Intravenous Administration

Phenytoin is given intravenously, preferably as bolus injections, but not as a continuous infusion, to avoid phlebitis, which may be produced by the solvent of the drug. The bolus should be injected over 2 to 3 min. No well-defined criteria exist for dosage in children. A loading dose can be given, if required, by repeated injections every 5 min. A slow infusion of 2 to 10 mg/kg/day has been recommended for patients with digitalis toxicity. The total dose should not exceed 400 mg/day.

Oral Administration

In adults, a loading dose of 10 to 15 mg/kg is given on the first day, divided into 3 to 4 doses, followed by 7.5 to 10 mg/kg on the second day, with a maintenance dose of 2 to 6 mg/kg/day, divided into 3 to 4 doses.

In children and young adults, a regimen consisting of a loading dose of 3.75 mg/kg every 6 hours for 4 consecutive doses, followed by 1.9 mg/kg for 4 doses, has been suggested.[23] Another suggested regimen for children and young adults is 3 to 3.5 mg/kg twice daily.[24]

References

1. Helfant, R.H., et al.: Effect of diphenylhydantoin sodium (Dilantin) on myocardial A-V potassium difference. Am. J. Physiol., *214*:880, 1968.
2. Goldstein, R.E., et al.: Correlation of antiarrhythmic effects of diphenylhydantoin with digoxin-induced changes on myocardial contractility, sodium-potassium adenosine triphosphate activity and potassium efflux. Circ. Res., *33*:175, 1973.
3. Spain, R.C., and Chidsey, C.A.: Myocardial Na/K adenosine triphosphate activity during reversal of ouabain toxicity with diphenylhydantoin. J. Pharmacol. Exp. Ther., *179*:594, 1971.
4. Gillis, R.A.: Cardiac sympathetic nerve activity: changes induced by ouabain and propranolol. Science, *166*:508, 1969.
5. Bigger, J.T., Jr., et al.: Electrophysiological effects of diphenylhydantoin on canine Purkinje fibers. Circ. Res., *22*:221, 1968.
6. El-Sherif, N., and Lazzara, R.: Re-entrant ventricular arrhythmias in the late myocardial infarction period. V. Mechanism of action of diphenylhydantoin. Circulation, *57*:465, 1978.

7. Rozati, R.A., et al.: Influence of diphenylhydantoin on electrophysiological properties of the canine heart. Circ. Res., *21*:757, 1967.
8. Bigger, J.T., Jr., et al.: Effect of diphenylhydantoin on excitability and automaticity in the canine heart. Carc. Res., *26*:1, 1970.
9. Unger, A.H., and Sklaroff, H.J.: Fatalities following intravenous use of sodium diphenylhydantoin for cardiac arrhythmias: report of two cases. JAMA, *200*:159, 1967.
10. Wit, A.L., et al.: Electrophysiology and pharmacology of cardiac arrhythmias. VIII. Cardiac effects of diphenylhydantoin. Am. Heart J., *90*:397, 1975.
11. Caracta, A.R., et al.: Electrophysiological properties of diphenylhydantoin. Circulation, *47*:1234, 1973.
12. Damato, A.N., et al.: The effect of diphenylhydantoin on atrioventricular and intraventricular conduction in man. Am. Heart J., *79*:51, 1970.
13. Helfant, R.H., et al.: Use of diphenylhydantoin sodium to dissociate the effects of procainamide on automaticity and conduction in the normal and arrhythmic heart. Am. J. Cardiol., *20*:820, 1967.
14. Bigger, J.T., Jr., et al.: Relationship between the plasma level of diphenylhydantoin sodium and its cardiac antiarrhythmic effects. Circulation, *38*:363, 1968.
15. Helfant, R.H., et al.: The electrophysiological properties of diphenylhydantoin sodium as compared to procaine amide in the normal and digitalis intoxicated heart. Circulation, *36*:108, 1967.
16. Bissett, J.K., et al.: Improved intraventricular conduction of premature beats after diphenylhydantoin. Am. J. Cardiol., *33*:493, 1974.
17. Leonard, W.A.: The use of diphenylhydantoin (Dilantin) sodium in the treatment of ventricular tachycardia. Arch. Intern. Med., *101*:714, 1958.
18. Eddy, J.D., and Singh SP: Treatment of cardiac arrhythmias with phenytoin. Br. Heart J., *4*:270, 1969.
19. Vajda, F.J.E., et al.: The possible effect on long-term high plasma levels of phenytoin on mortality after acute myocardial infarction. Eur. J. Clin. Pharmacol., *5*:138, 1973.
20. Bigger, J.T., et al.: Ventricular arrhythmias in ischemic heart disease: mechanism, prevalence, significance and management. Prog. Cardiovasc. Dis., *19*:255, 1977.
21. Conn, R.D.: Newer drugs in the treatment of cardiac arrhythmia. Med. Clin. North Am., *51*:1223, 1967.
22. Rosen, M., et al.: Diphenylhydantoin in cardiac arrhythmias. Am. J. Cardiol., *20*:674, 1967.
23. Garson, A., et al.: Control of late postoperative ventricular arrhythmias with phenytoin in young patients. Am. J. Cardiol., *46*:290, 1980.
24. Webb Kavey, R.E., et al.: Phenytoin therapy for ventricular arrhythmias occurring late after surgery for congenital heart disease. Am. Heart J., *104*:794, 1982.
25. Bigger, J.T., Jr., and Strauss, H.C.: Digitalis toxicity: drug interactions promoting toxicity and the management of toxicity. Semin. Drug Treat., *2*:147, 1972.
26. Mercer, E.N., and Osborn, J.A.: The current status of diphenylhydantoin in heart disease. Ann. Intern. Med., *67*:1084, 1967.
27. Helfant, R.H., et al.: The clinical use of diphenylhydantoin (Dilantin) in the treatment and prevention of cardiac arrhythmias. Am. Heart J., *77*:315, 1969.
28. Mixter, C.G., et al.: Cardiac and peripheral vascular effects of diphenylhydantoin sodium. Am. J. Cardiol., *17*:332, 1966.
29. Leiberson, A.D., et al.: Effects of diphenylhydantoin on left ventricular function in patients with heart disease. Circulation, *36*:692, 1969.
30. Puri, P.S.: The effect of diphenylhydantoin sodium (Dilantin) on myocardial contractility and hemodynamics. Am. Heart J., *82*:62, 1971.
31. Dill, W.A., et al.: Studies on 5,5'-diphenylhydantoin (Dilantin) in animals and man. J. Pharmacol. Exp. Ther., *118*:363, 1956.
32. Svensmark, O., et al.: 5,5'-diphenylhydantoin (Dilantin) blood levels after oral or intravenous dosage in man. Acta Pharmacol. Toxicol., *16*:331, 1960.
33. Kutt, H: Biochemical and genetic factors regulating Dilantin metabolism in man. Ann. N.Y. Acad. Sci., *179*:704, 1971.
34. Noach, E.L. et al.: Studies on the absorption, distribution, fate and excretion of 4-C^{14}-labeled diphenylhydantoin. J. Pharmacol. Exp. Ther., *122*:301, 1958.

35. Atkinson, A.J., and Shaw, J.M.: Pharmacokinetic study of a patient with diphenylhydantoin toxicity. Clin. Pharmacol. Ther., *14*:521, 1973.
36. Kutt, H., et al.: Some causes of ineffectiveness of diphenylhydantoin. Arch. Neurol., *14*:489, 1966.
37. Josephson, M.E., et al.: The electrophysiological effects of intramuscular quinidine on the atrioventricular conducting system in man. Am. Heart J., *87*:55, 1974.
38. Symposium on phenytoin, New York, 1972.
39. Shafer, W.G., et al.: A Textbook of Pathology. 3rd Ed. Philadelphia, W.B. Saunders, 1974, p. 733.

Chapter 25

Mexiletine

Mexiletine is a new Class I antiarrhythmic agent with features resembling those of lidocaine. Because it is effective both intravenously and orally, an effective course of short-term intravenous treatment with mexiletine may be followed by oral treatment with the same drug. Mexiletine is effective in controlling supraventricular and ventricular arrhythmias and has been useful in some conditions resistant to other antiarrhythmic agents. In clinical practice, mexiletine is usually administered orally, to treat ventricular arrhythmias that have responded to intravenous lidocaine.

Administration of mexiletine is associated with a high incidence of adverse effects on the cardiovascular, gastrointestinal, and central nervous systems and the skin. These adverse effects have restricted the use of the drug. This incidence of side effects is one reason that the experience with mexiletine in children is so limited.

At present, mexiletine is recommended for pediatric use only in children with malignant arrhythmias resistant to conventional antiarrhythmic agents. Although only a few cases of mexiletine use in children have been reported, the pediatric cardiologist should be familiar with the potential effectiveness of this drug.

Structure

Mexiletine is 1-(2',6'-dimethylphenoxy)-2-aminopropane. This structure resembles that of lidocaine.

Pharmacologic Properties

Mexiletine is a Class I antiarrhythmic drug with a local-anesthetic effect equal to that of lidocaine. It is possible that mexiletine has also a calcium-antagonist effect,[1] but such an action, even if present, would be unlikely to play role in the mechanism of the drug's antiarrhythmic effect. Mexiletine also has vagolytic activity, which contributes to its electrophysiologic effects.

Electrophysiologic Effects

Like other Class I antiarrhythmic agents, the main effect of mexiletine is reduction of the rate of phase-0 depolarization in His-Purkinje and myocardial fibers. The duration of the action potential is decreased, increased, or unchanged. The resting potential is usually unchanged.[1, 1] Like lidocaine, but unlike quinidine and procainamide, mexiletine depresses phase-0 depolarization to a greater extent at low membrane potentials than at high potentials.[5] Therefore, mexiletine acts primarily in damaged tissues. Although mexiletine can shorten both the duration of the action potential and the effective refractory period of Purkinje fibers, the ratio of effective refractory period to action potential duration is always prolonged.[4]

Mexiletine has also increased the uniformity of the action potential's duration in the various segments of the conduction system,[6] although this finding is controversial.[4] At high concentrations, mexiletine may prolong the effective refractory period of Purkinje fibers.[7] Mexiletine may decrease or may not alter the slope of phase-4 action potential.[8, 3] The effect on phase 4 may depend on the concentration of the drug.

Effect on the Sinus Node

In human patients, the effect of mexiletine on the sinoatrial node is variable, but in most patients with normal sinus function, the drug does not alter the spontaneous sinus cycle length.[10–13] In some cases, however, mexiletine may slow the sinus rate to the point of sinus arrest.[14, 15] Mexiletine-induced bradycardia may be resistant to atropine,[2] but such is not usually the case in human subjects. In only one study did mexiletine increase the spontaneous sinus rate.[16] Shakibi and Moezzi evaluated the effect of intravenous administration of mexiletine, 3 mg/kg followed by 1 mg/kg/hour, on the sinus rate in 10 children with heart diseases.[17] The drug increased the spontaneous sinus rate in this group of children, in contrast to the findings of most studies in adults. All other electrophysiologic effects in these patients were similar to those observed in adults. The different effect on the sinoatrial node was attributed to a stronger vagolytic effect of mexiletine in children.[17]

Effect on the Atria

Mexiletine does not usually alter the refractory period and the duration of conduction in the atria.[16] In a group of 10 children, the atrial functional refractory period increased in 3, decreased in 2, and was not altered in 5 of the children.[17] The atrial effective refractory periods increased in 3, decreased in 3, and were not altered in 4 of the 10 children. The overall effect in this group was not significant.

Effect on the Atrioventricular Node

The atrioventricular nodal conduction time, as measured by the AH and PR intervals, and refractory periods may be shortened, not altered, or prolonged by mexiletine.[11, 12, 16, 18] The limited effect on the atrioventricular node explains the limited effect of mexiletine on re-entrant arrhythmias incorporating this node. In children, the changes in the AH interval were not generally significant, although mild and inconsistent changes were observed in a few children.[17]

Effect of Accessory Atrioventricular Pathways

Mexiletine may prolong, may not alter, or may shorten the effective refractory period for anterograde conduction in patients with pre-excitation.[10, 11, 13, 16] The use of this drug is uncommon in such patients. No data are available in children with Wolff-Parkinson-White syndrome.

Effect on the Ventricles

The most important electrophysiologic effects of mexiletine are exerted on the His-Purkinje system and on the ventricular myocardium. The HV interval is usually unaltered or undergoes a slight increase.[11, 12, 13, 18] In 10 children, mexiletine had no significant effect on the HV interval. The duration of this interval increased in 4, decreased in 2, and showed no change in 4 of the 10 children studied.[17] In several patients with conduction disturbances, mexiletine increased the grade of block distal to the atrioventricular node.[10, 11, 16]

The duration of the QRS interval is not usually altered by mexiletine. The effect of the drug on the refractory periods of the His-Purkinje system and the ventricular myocardium is minimal in the normal heart. In a diseased conduction system, mexiletine prolongs the refractory periods of the His-Purkinje system, as does quinidine.[13] Mexiletine has no significant effect on the QTc interval.[19] In a study of children, mexiletine had no important effect on the ventricular effective refractory periods.[17]

Effects in Arrhythmias

Mexiletine has controlled several types of cardiac arrhythmias, but it is most effective and usually used in patients with ventricular arrhythmias. The drug is not generally given as a first-line agent, but rather is administered orally following successful intravenous treatment with lidocaine, or in patients with arrhythmias resistant to other Class I agents. The experience in children is limited, and to the best of any knowledge, only 2 reports of its use in infants and small children have been published. Several reported series have included children and adolescents over 15 years of age, however.

Effects in Ventricular Arrhythmias

Mexiletine has effectively suppressed experimentally induced ventricular arrhythmias.[2, 20, 21] In some animal experiments, mexiletine was more effective than several conventional Class I antiarrhythmic agents.

In human patients, the effect of mexiletine on termination of ventricular tachycardia induced by electrical stimulation has been disappointing,[15, 22-24] although the drug is more effective in preventing recurrent episodes of ventricular tachycardia.[16] Favorable results have also been obtained in studies of the suppression of premature ventricular beats.[22, 25] For example, in a group of 58 patients with premature ventricular beats, intravenous administration of mexiletine completely suppressed the arrhythmia in 88%.[26] In another large series of patients with complex ventricular arrhythmias that were, in many cases, resistant to several antiarrhythmic drugs, mexiletine suppressed the arrhythmia in 65% of the patients during short-term drug testing and in 65.4% of the patients during continued therapy.[27] In children over the age of 15 years, mexiletine has been used to treat ventricular arrhythmias unassociated with structural heart disease as well as ventricular associated with mitral valve prolapse, various congenital cardiac lesions, and cardiac surgical procedures.

Lidocaine is used in adults as well as in children to suppress ventricular arrhythmias. Oral treatment following intravenous lidocaine therapy in children has traditionally been limited mainly to phenytoin. Like lidocaine and phenytoin, mexiletine has little negative inotropic effect in patients with impaired myocardial function, in contrast to other Class I antiarrhythmic agents.

Moak and co-workers studied the effect of mexiletine in 25 pediatric and young-adult patients, ranging in age from 5.5 months to 34 years.[28] Eighteen patients had recently undergone operations for congenital heart disease, 3 had cardiomyopathy, and 4 had normal hearts. All had ventricular arrhythmias; 11 patients had ventricular tachycardia, 7 had couplets, 3 had multiform premature ventricular beats, and 3 had uniform premature ventricular beats. Mexiletine was given at oral doses of 1.4 to 5.1 mg/kg, 3 times daily, for up to 24 hours of treatment (mean 6 months). Eighteen of the 25 patients had a significant reduction in level of ventricular arrhythmias. The suppression of ventricular arrhythmias was more dramatic in the postoperative patients with congenital heart diseases (89%) than in the other patients (29%). In 11 of 16 patients followed for more than 3 months, long-term control of the arrhythmias was achieved. In 2 of 16 patients, mexiletine was discontinued because of late drug failure.[28]

In summary, one may give mexiletine to children and adolescents with complex ventricular arrhythmias in whom conventional antiarrhythmic agents have failed. Short-term drug testing can predict the long-term response to the agent in the majority of the patients,[27] although electrophysiologic studies are of limited use in evaluating the long-term clinical response. The effect of mexiletine is comparable to that of lidocaine. In one study, all patients who responded to lidocaine responded to mexiletine, and some patients resistant to lidocaine responded to mexiletine.[29] The only reported case of treatment of arrhythmia in an infant with mexiletine is that of a 10-day-old female infant with tachycardia at a rate of 250 beats/min.[30] Electrophysiologic studies identified this arrhythmia as an ectopic upper His-bundle tachycardia, resistant to electrical conversion and to lidocaine and disopyramide administration.

Effects in Supraventricular Arrhythmias

Mexiletine may be effective in terminating and preventing supraventricular tachyarrhythmias in patients with or without pre-excitation syndromes. For example, in a series of 6 patients with Wolff-Parkinson-White syndrome and inducible supraventricular tachycardia, mexiletine prevented the reinduction of the arrhythmias in 3 patients and made it nonsustained in 2 other patients.[31] The experience in the pediatric age group is limited. Joseph and Kelly reported that mexiletine prevented the induction of arrhythmias in a 17-year-old patient with Wolff-Parkinson-White syndrome, but not in another 17-year-old patient with LGL syndrome.[32] Holt and colleagues reported on a 20-month-old boy with paroxysmal supraventricular tachycardia that developed during a febrile illness and that was resistant to digoxin, lidocaine, and disopyramide.[30] The arrhythmia was controlled by the combination of oral mexiletine, 15 mg/kg, and disopyramide, 20mg/kg.

In patients with Wolff-Parkinson-White syndrome and atrial fibrillation, mexiletine may produce deleterious effects, including acceleration of ventricular rate and syncope.[32]

Hemodynamic Effects

Mexiletine has a negative inotropic effect,[33] and at high concentrations, it may cause hemodynamic deterioration. In patients with coronary artery disease or valval heart diseases, the drug has had a direct depressant effect on myocardial contractility, has decreased the stroke work index and the cardiac index, and has increased the pulmonary capillary wedge pressure.[34, 35] The negative inotropic effect of mexiletine is comparable to that of lidocaine,[34] whereas it is less than that of disopyramide, propafenone,[36] and propranolol.[34] It is not clear whether mexiletine has a direct effect on peripheral vascular resistance.

In several studies, hypotension occurred in about 10% of the patients treated with intravenous mexiletine and in up to 2% of those treated with oral mexiletine.[15,37] Aggravation of the symptoms and signs of congestive heart failure during mexiletine therapy were reported in a few patients.[15] All these studies were performed in adults. In a group of 10 children with various congenital heart diseases, intravenous administration of mexiletine did not have any adverse hemodynamic effects.[17]

Clinical Pharmacology

Mexiletine may be given intravenously or orally. Rapid infusion of appropriate doses can achieve therapeutic plasma levels within several minutes.[38] After oral administration, the drug is rapidly and almost completely absorbed from the gastrointestinal tract.[39] The antiarrhythmic effect may be evident within 15 min, and the maximal plasma concentration is evident within 1.5 to 4 hours of oral administration.[33,40] The systemic bioavailability of orally administered mexiletine is about 90%.[39,41] The drug has a large volume of distribution of about 5.5 L/kg.[41] The therapeutic plasma levels of mexiletine range between 0.5 and 2.0 $\mu g/ml$.[37,42] A strong correlation between plasma level and antiarrhythmic effect of mexiletine has been observed.

Mexiletine is eliminated by hepatic metabolism. The elimination half-life is about 12 hours. Usually, under 10% of the administered dose is found unchanged in the urine.[39] An increase in urinary pH causes a decrease in renal clearance of mexiletine,[43,44] and marked changes in the pH of the urine should be prevented in patients treated with this agent. The metabolites of mexiletine, which probably are pharmacologically inactive, may accumulate in patients with hepatic or renal dysfunction.[45] The drug may be administered to patients with renal diseases.

Side Effects

From 20 to 66% of adults treated with intravenous or oral mexiletine have side effects.[15,46] No specific report on side effects of this drug in children has been published. In a study of intravenous mexiletine therapy in 10 children with various congenital heart diseases, no adverse effect was observed.[17] The side effects consist of cardiovascular disorders such as bradycardia, hypotension, congestive heart failure, and conduction disturbances, gastrointestinal disorders such as nausea and vomiting, effects on the central nervous system such as dizziness, tremor, nystagmus, confusion, and visual disturbances and an erythematous rash.[46,47]

Mexiletine is usually well tolerated in young age groups. Minor side effects were observed in 9 of 25 children and young adults (mean age 16 years) during oral treatment with mexiletine.[28] Five of these patients had headache, 2 had rash, 3 had tremor, and 7 had nausea. All these side effects diminished with a reduction in dosage. No cardiovascular side effects were observed in this group.

Drug Interactions

To the best of my knowledge, no specific drug interactions with mexiletine have been reported. Mexiletine may potentiate the effects of other Class I antiarrhythmic drugs and the cardiodepressant effect of beta-adrenoreceptor blocking agents. Antacids may diminish the bioavailability of mexiletine,[48] whereas cimetidine may increase the plasma level of mexiletine by about 40%.[49]

Dosage and Administration

Until recently, no dosage recommendation had been made for children. The doses used in adults are given as follows.

Intravenous Administration

An initial loading dose of 2 to 3 mg/kg is recommended for adults, followed by maintenance doses of 250 to 500 mg 2 to 3 times daily. The bolus should be injected slowly, over at least 3 min, preferably over 10 min.

No recommendations for use in small children and infants are available.

Oral Administration

The usual adult oral dose is 600 to 1200 mg daily, given in 2 to 4 divided doses. One should usually give a loading dose of 400 mg, followed by 200 to 400 mg at 2 hours and the first maintenance dose at 8 hours. No strict pediatric dosage regimen has been suggested. In a 1-year-old girl with ventricular arrhythmia, a daily maintenance dose of up to 25 mg/kg was used.[30] The monitoring of plasma levels may be beneficial in determining dosage regimens in small children. Recently, oral doses of 1.4 to 5.1 mg/kg 3 times daily have been found to be effective in infants and children. At present, this is the only recommended dosage regimen for pediatric patients.

References

1. Haap, K., and Antoni, H.: Mexiletine—tierexperimentelle Befunde uber die antiarrhythmichen und elektrophysiologischen Effekte am Herzen. Klin. Wochenschr., 56:169, 1978.
2. Singh, B.N., and Vaughan Williams, E.M.: Investigation of the mode of action of a new antidysrhythmic drug, Kö-1173. Br. J. Pharmacol., 44:1, 1972.

3. Weld, F.M., et al.: Effects of mexiletine (Kö 1173) on electrophysiological properties of sheep cardiac Purkinje fibers. (Abstract.) Am. J. Cardiol., *39*:292, 1977.
4. Yamaguchi, I., et al.: Electrophysiological effects of mexiletine on isolated cardiac tissue. *In* Management of Ventricular Tachycardia—Role of Mexiletine. Edited by E. Sandoe et al. Amsterdam, Excerpta Medica, 1978, p. 197.
5. Hohnloser, S. et al. Effects of mexiletine on steady-state characteristics and recovery kinetics of V_{max} and conduction velocity in guinea pig myocardium. J. Cardiovasc. Pharmacol., *4*:232, 1982.
6. Vaughan Williams, E.M.: Mexiletine in isolated tissue models. Postgrad. Med. J., *53* (Suppl. 1):30, 1977.
7. Yamada, K., et al.: Electrophysiological action of mexiletine on dog Purkinje and papillary muscle fibers studied in both in vitro and in situ experiments. *In* Management of Ventricular Tachycardia—Role of Mexiletine. Edited by E. Sandoe et al. Amsterdam, Excerpta Medica, 1978, p. 210.
8. Iwamura, N., et al.: Electrophysiological actions of a new antiarrhythmic agent on isolated preparations of the canine Purkinje fiber and ventricular muscle. Cardiologia (Basel), *61*:329, 1976.
9. Weld, F.M., et al.: Electrophysiological effects of mexiletine (Kö 1173) on bovine cardiac Purkinje fibers. In preparation.
10. Roos, J.C., et al.: Electrophysiological effects of mexiletine in man. Br. Heart J., *38*:1262, 1976.
11. Lang, K.F., et al.: Untersuchungen über die Einwirkung von mexiletine (Kö 1173) auf die AV-überleitungszeit und die Sinusimpulsautomatie bei Herzgesunden und Patienten mit Erkrankung des Reizleitungssystems. Z. Kardiol., *64*:389, 1975.
12. Probst, P., and Joskowics, G.: Die Wirkung von Mexiletine auf die AV-überleitung. Herz Kreislauf, *8*:81, 1976.
13. Roos, J.C., and Dunning, A.J.: Electrophysiological effects of mexiletine, a new antiarrhythmic drug, in man. (Abstract.) Circulation, 52 *(Suppl. II)*:233, 1975.
14. Waleffe, A., and Kulbertus, H.E.: The efficacy of intravenous mexiletine on ventricular ectopic activity. Acta Cardiol. (Brux.), *32*:269, 1977.
15. Campbell, N.P.S., et al.: Mexiletine in the management of ventricular dysrhythmias. Eur. J. Cardiol., *6*:245, 1977.
16. Seipel, L., and Breithardt, G.: Electrophysiological effects of mexiletine in man: influence on stimulus-induced ventricular arrhythmias. *In* Management of Ventricular Tachycardia—Role of Mexiletine. Edited by E. Sandoe et al. Amsterdam, Excerpta Medica, 1978, p. 219.
17. Shakibi, J.G., and Moezzi, B.: Electrophysiologic effects of mexiletine in children. Jpn. Heart J., *23*:733, 1982.
18. McComish, M., et al.: Clinical electrophysiological effects of mexiletine and its mechanism of antidysrhythmic action. (Abstract.) Br. Heart J., *38*:311, 1976.
19. Waspe, L.E., et al.: Mexiletine for control of drug-resistant ventricular tachycardia: clinical and electrophysiologic results in 44 patients. Am. J. Cardiol., *51*:1175, 1983.
20. Allen, J.D., et al.: The effect of Ko 1173, a new anticonvulsant agent, on experimental cardiac arrhythmias. Br. J. Pharmacol., *45*:561, 1972.
21. Allen, J.D., et al.: Comparison of the effects of lignocaine and mexiletine on experimental ventricular arrhythmias. Postgrad. Med. J., 53 *(Suppl. 1)*:35, 1977.
22. Westveer, D.C., et al.: The ineffectiveness of mexiletine for malignant ventricular arrhythmias. ACC 1983.
23. Palileo, E., et al.: Failure of mexiletine in drug-refractory paroxysmal, sustained ventricular tachycardia, ACC 1982.
24. Manz, M., et al.: Treatment of recurrent sustained ventricular tachycardia with mexiletine and disopyramide. Br. Heart J., *49*:222, 1983.
25. Talbot, R.G., et al.: Treatment of ventricular arrhythmias with mexiletine (Ko 1173). Lancet, *2*:399, 1973.
26. Esser, H., and Kikis, D.: Mexiletine in the suppression of ventricular ectopic activity: short and long term treatment. *In* Management of Ventricular Tachycardia—Role of Mexiletine. Edited by E. Sandoe et al. Amsterdam, Excerpta Medica, 1978, p. 585.

27. Podrid, P.J. and Lown, B.: Mexiletine for ventricular arrhythmias. Am. J. Cardiol., 47:895, 1981.
28. Moak, J.P., et al.: Mexiletine: an alternative to dilantin for pediatric ventricular arrhythmias. AHA 1984.
29. Duff, H.J., et al.: Mexiletine for resistant ventricular tachycardia: comparison with lidocaine and enhancement of efficacy by combination with quinidine. (Abstract.) Clin. Res., 28:878A, 1980.
30. Holt, D.W., et al.: Paediatric use of mexiletine and disopyramide. Br. Med. J., 2:1476, 1979.
31. Discussion. *In* Management of Ventricular Tachycardia—Role of Mexiletine. Edited by E. Sandoe et al. Amsterdam, Excerpta Medica, 1978, p. 604.
32. Joseph, S.P., and Kelly, H.B.: Mexiletine: studies with intracardiac electrography in the pre-excitation syndromes. *In* Management of Ventricular Tachycardia—Role of Mexiletine. Edited by E. Sandoe et al. Amsterdam, Excerpta Medica, 1978, p. 260.
33. Danneberg, P.B., and Shelley, J.H.: The pharmacology of mexiletine. Postgrad. Med. J., 53(Suppl. I):25, 1977.
34. Shaw, T.R.D.: The effect of mexiletine on left ventricular ejection: a comparison with lignocaine and propranolol. Postgrad. Med. J., 53 (Suppl. I):69, 1977.
35. Saunamaki, K.I.: Haemodynamic effects of a new antiarrhythmic agent, mexiletine (Ko 1173) in ischaemic heart disease. Cardiovasc. Res., 9:788, 1975.
36. Böcker, K., et al.: The influence of disopyramide, mexiletine, and propafenone of intravenous and oral application on left ventricular function assessed by M-mode echocardiography. Z. Kardiol., 71:839, 1982.
37. Campbell, R.W.F., et al.: Comparison of procainamide and mexiletine in prevention of ventricular arrhythmias after acute myocardial infarction. Lancet, 1, 1975.
38. Jewitt, D.: Clinical electrophysiological effects of mexiletine. *In* Management of Ventricular Tachycardia—Role of Mexiletine. Edited by E. Sandoe et al. Amsterdam, Excerpta Medica, 1978, p. 237.
39. Prescott, L.F., et al.: Absorption, distribution and elimination of mexiletine. Postgrad. Med. J., 53(Suppl I):50, 1977.
40. Herzog, P., et al.: Absorption of mexiletine after treatment with gastric antacid. Br. J. Clin. Pharmacol., 14:746, 1982.
41. Haoelbarth, V., et al.: Kinetics and bioavailability of mexiletine in healthy subjects. Clin. Pharmacol. Ther., 29(6):729, 1981.
42. Merx, W., et al.: Mexiletine in acute myocardial infarction. *In* Management of Ventricular Tachycardia—Role of Mexiletine. Edited by E. Sandoe, et al. Amsterdam, Excerpta Medica, 1978, p. 472.
43. Kiddie, M.A., et al.: The influence of urinary pH on the elimination of mexiletine. Br. J. Clin. Pharmacol., 1:229, 1974.
44. Kiddie, M.A., et al.: Preliminary studies on the pharmacology of an antidysrhythmic—Ko 1173 in man. Br. J. Pharmacy, 47:674, 1973.
45. Shelley, J.H.: Harmony and discord: a review of interactions with mexiletine. *In* Management of Ventricular Tachycardia—Role of Mexiletine. Edited by E. Sandoe et al. Amsterdam, Excerpta Medica, 1978, p. 341.
46. Graeme Sloman, J., et al.: Tolerance and side effects of oral mexiletine. *In* Management of Ventricular Tachycardia—Role of Mexiletine. Edited by E. Sandoe et al. Amsterdam, Excerpta Medica, 1978, p. 329.
47. Talbot, R.G., et al: Long-term treatment of ventricular arrhythmias with oral mexiletine. Am. Heart J., 91:58, 1976.
48. Affrime, M.B., et al.: Drug interaction study of oral mexiletine and digoxin. ACCP 1982.
49. Nitsche, J., and Luderitz, B.: Interaction of mexiletine and cimetidine—delayed elimination of an antiarrhythmic agent. Unpublished data.

Chapter 26

Flecainide

Flecainide, a recently developed Class II antiarrhythmic agent, slows phase-0 action potential without affecting repolarization and may be classified as a Class Ic antiarrhythmic drug. It slightly slows the sinus rate and prolongs the sinus node recovery time and the PR interval.[1-4] The drug usually prolongs the refractory periods of the atrioventricular node. It slows intraventricular conduction and prolongs the HV and QRS intervals by 10 to 30%.[3,5,6] The duration of the QTc interval may also be prolonged. Flecainide slows conduction in accessory atrioventricular pathways.[7]

Flecainide is effective in terminating and preventing supraventricular and ventricular arrhythmias. For example, the drug terminated supraventricular tachycardia in 12 of 14 patients with accessory pathways.[7] The rate of suppression of ventricular arrhythmias has been 90%.[8] The drug's antiarrhythmic effect has been sustained throughout long periods of treatment.[6] Flecainide is at least as potent as conventional Class I antiarrhythmic drugs. For example, a recent comparative study showed that flecainide suppressed chronic multiple premature ventricular beats in 85% of the patients, whereas quinidine was effective in only 57% of these patients.

Flecainide has a negative inotropic effect. It has also a significant arrhythmogenic effect that may limit its use. The drug may produce or may aggravate conduction disturbances and may cause visual disorders.

The only experience with flecainide in pediatric patients is that of the pediatric cardiology group at St. George Hospital in London. Ward and co-workers studied the effect of intravenous and oral flecainide in 5 children, aged 4.5 to 11.7 years, with refractory junctional tachycardia.[9] Electrophysiologic studies identified atrioventricular re-entry junctional tachycardia in 4 of the children and fast-slow ("unusual") junctional tachycardia in 1 child. Flecainide, 2 mg/kg injected intravenously over 5 to 10 min during junctional tachycardia, prolonged the cycle length of the arrhythmia from 298 ± 38 to 393 ± 76 msec and then terminated it, within 3 to 6 min of the onset of the drug infusion. In all patients, the arrhythmia was terminated by a retrograde block. Reinduction of junctional tachycardia was possible in only 1 patient 15 min after administration of flecainide.

Oral flecainide, 100 to 200 mg daily, was given to all 5 children in this group. Repeated studies in 4 patients showed nonsustained junctional tachycardia in 2 patients, slow-junctional tachycardia in 1 patient, and no arrhythmia in the remaining patient. Serum flecainide levels at the time of the repeat study were 215 to 680 μg/L (412 ± 168). Oral flecainide therapy was continued in all patients. One patient has had 3 episodes of the arrhythmia in 26 months, at periods of low serum levels of the drug, and 2 patients have had a single episode at 6 and 10 months, respectively. One patient remained in incessant junctional tachycardia. These workers concluded that flecainide is useful in short- and long-term therapy of junctional tachycardia in children.[9]

References

1. Hodess, A.B., et al.: Electrophysiological effects of a new antiarrhythmic agent, flecainide, on the intact canine heart. J. Cardiovasc. Pharmacol., *1*:427, 1979.
2. Seipel, L., et al.: Electrophysiological effects of flecainide (R-818) in man. (Abstract.) Circulation, *62(Suppl. III)*:III-153, 1980.
3. Legrand, V., et al.: Hemodynamic effects of a new antiarrhythmic agent, flecainide (R-818), in coronary heart disease. Am. J. Cardiol., *51*:422, 1983.
4. Anderson, J.L., et al.: Oral flecainide acetate for the treatment of ventricular arrhythmias. N. Engl. J. Med., *305*:473, 1981.
5. Vik-Mo, H., et al.: Electrophysiologic effects of flecainide acetate in patients with sinus nodal dysfunction. Am. J. Cardiol., *50*:1090, 1982.
6. Duff, H.J., et al.: Suppression of resistant ventricular arrhythmias by twice daily dosing with flecainide. Am. J. Cardiol., *48*:1133, 1981.
7. Hellestrand, K.J., et al.: Cardiac electrophysiologic effects of flecainide acetate for paroxysmal reentrant junctional tachycardias. Am. J. Cardiol., *51*:770, 1983.
8. Hodges, M., et al.: Suppression of ventricular ectopic depolarizations by flecainide acetate, a new antiarrhythmic agent. Circulation, *65*:879, 1982.
9. Ward, D., et al.: The use of flecainide acetate for control of junctional tachycardias in children. AHA 1984.

Chapter 27

Propafenone

Propafenone, a recently developed and important antiarrhythmic agent, is effective in patients with various ventricular and supraventricular arrhythmias. Results in children have been favorable, and the drug is considered to be especially promising in the control and prevention of arrhythmias associated with pre-excitation syndromes.[1,2] Propafenone may be particularly important in patients with junctional ectopic tachycardia, a resistant arrhythmia in children.

Although propafenone is a Class I antiarrhythmic agent, it also has beta-blocking properties that make it a Class II agent as well. Among Class I antiarrhythmic agents, propafenone is further defined as Class Ib by some investigators and Ic by others. At high concentrations, propafenone also has calcium-antagonist properties.

Structure

Propafenone is 2'-(2-hydroxy-3-propyl amino-propoxy)-3-phenyl-proplophenone hydrochloride.

Pharmacologic Properties

Like other Class I antiarrhythmic agents, the main effect of propafenone is a membrane-stabilizing (local anesthetic) activity, inhibition of the fast inward current. Propafenone may interact with negatively charged groups of the selectivity filter of the fast inward channels, possibly resulting in competitive inhibition between propafenone and sodium.[3] This theory has not been confirmed.

At therapeutic plasma concentrations, propafenone also blocks beta-adrenoreceptors. This nonselective effect is more potent for beta-2 adrenoreceptors, as evident by inhibition of beta-adrenoreceptors in the trachea and isolated coronary arteries to a greater extent than in the myocardium.[4-7] At high plasma concentrations, propafenone also has calcium-antagonist properties. This effect is much less potent than that of the clinically used calcium antagonists. The concentrations required for effective blockade of the slow (calcium) channels are 20 times higher than those required for blockade of the fast channels.[6]

Electrophysiologic Effects

Propafenone mainly has the electrophysiologic effects of Class I antiarrhythmic agents, related to membrane-stabilizing activity.

Effect on the Action Potential

Like other Class I antiarrhythmic agents, propafenone reduces the rate of rise of phase-0 depolarization of the action potential. At high concentrations, the drug completely suppresses excitability. The effect of propafenone on phase-0 depolarization is more pronounced in Purkinje fibers than in myocardial fibers.[3,8] This effect depends on the rate of stimulation.

Propafenone also has some Class IV antiarrhythmic properties that result in reduction of the plateau of the action potential to less positive potentials.[9] The drug shortens the duration of the action potential. In this respect, it resembles lidocaine and differs from quinidine and procainamide. At high concentrations, propafenone also alters the resting membrane potential.[9] In contrast to conventional local anesthetic agents, the inhibitory effect of propafenone on the fast inward current (the membrane-stabilizing effect) develops slowly. About 30 min are required to attain the maximal effect.[3]

Effect on the Sinoatrial Node

In the intact animal and in human subjects, propafenone has an inconsistent effect on the spontaneous sinus node rate. It may decrease this rate by a direct depressant effect and beta-adrenergic blockade, it may not alter it at all, or it may increase it because of sympathetic stimulation activated by a propafenone-induced decrease in blood pressure.[4,10,11] In a series of 23 children with arrhythmias, propafenone produced a mean increase of 9.1% in the minus cycle length during spontaneous sinus rhythm.[12]

The reduction of heart rate by propafenone is different from that produced by beta-blocking agents because this effect is greater during the day than during the night, but the ratio of mean heart rate between day and night is not altered.[10] The effect of propafenone on the sinus node recovery time is also inconsistent. In series of patients with supraventricular arrhythmias, propafenone increased the sinus node recovery time,[11,13] whereas in a series of patients with ventricular arrhythmias, propafenone did not alter this parameter. Weber and coworkers reported that propafenone increased the frequency-corrected sinus node recovery time by 1.0% in children with arrhythmias.[12]

Effect on the Atria

In a study of adult patients with arrhythmias, propafenone increased the intra-atrial conduction time by up to about 50% and increased functional and effective refractory periods by about 10%.[14] On the electrocardiogram, these effects are evident by prolongation of the P wave, or the F wave in cases of flutter.

Effect on the Atrioventricular Node

Propafenone slows conduction in the atrioventricular node in the majority of patients. In studies of healthy volunteers and of adult patients with arrhythmias, propafenone prolonged the AH interval by up to 25%.[10, 11, 14, 15] The Wenckebach point, or the rate of atrial pacing at which Wenckebach-type atrioventricular block appears, either becomes evident at slower rates or is not altered by propafenone.[11, 15]

In a study of children with arrhythmias, propafenone delayed conduction in the atrioventricular node. The functional refractory period of the atrioventricular node was increased by 11.8%, and the effective refractory period was increased by 14.1%, by a mean intravenous dose of 39.7 mg/m^2 body surface area.[12] In a study of adults with arrhythmias, the anterograde functional refractory period of the atrioventricular node was unchanged.[15]

Effect on Accessory Atrioventricular Pathways

Propafenone has a significant effect on accessory atrioventricular pathways in the majority of patients with pre-excitation syndromes. It slows conduction and prolongs the effective refractory period of accessory pathways in both anterograde and retrograde directions.[11, 15] The significant inhibitory effect of propafenone on anterograde conduction in accessory pathways became evident by the disappearance of the pre-excitation pattern on electrocardiograms in eight of ten patients with Wolff-Parkinson-White syndrome who were treated with propafenone.[16]

Effect on the Ventricles

Propafenone depresses conduction and prolongs the effective refractory periods in the intraventricular conduction system and ventricular myocardium. The HV interval is either prolonged or not altered. In 2 series of patients with arrhythmias, the HV interval was prolonged by about 10 and 30%, respectively.[11, 15] In another group of patients, propafenone did not alter the HV interval.[17] Therapeutic doses of propafenone often prolong the QRS interval by up to 20%,[10, 18] but more pronounced prolongations have been observed.[16] The QTc interval may be prolonged, mainly because of prolongation of the QRS complex. The ventricular myocardial effective refractory period is either prolonged or not altered.[11, 14, 16, 17]

In summary, propafenone delays conduction and prolongs refractoriness in several segments of the normal and abnormal conduction system and atrial and ventricular myocardium. These effects underlie the mechanism of the antiarrhythmic effect of propafenone.

Effects in Arrhythmias

Propafenone has been effective against a variety of supraventricular and ventricular arrhythmias in animal experiments and in human patients, adults as well as children.

Effects in Experimentally Induced Arrhythmias

Propafenone has controlled a variety of arrhythmias experimentally induced in animals by several stimuli, including myocardial ischemia.[19, 20]

Effects in Supraventricular Tachyarrhythmias

Propafenone effectively suppresses, whether by termination or by prevention, a variety of supraventricular tachyarrhythmias in adults and in children. In adults, the drug has been especially effective in supraventricular re-entrant tachycardia. For example, in a group of 13 adult patients with atrioventricular nodal re-entrant tachycardia, the intravenous administration of propafenone immediately terminated the arrhythmia in 11 of the patients. In 10 of these 11 patients, this effect was achieved by a block in the retrograde limb of the tachycardia circle. Reinitiation of the arrhythmia was impossible in 8 of the patients after propafenone administration.[11] In another group of 23 adult patients with supraventricular tachycardia, intravenous administration of propafenone terminated the arrhythmia in all cases.[16] In a study of 16 adult patients with various forms of supraventricular tachyarrhythmias, oral propafenone prevented recurrences of the arrhythmia in 11 of the patients for at least several months.[21]

At least comparable results have been obtained in children. Weber and colleagues evaluated the effect of propafenone in 66 children and young adults up to 23 years of age who had various forms of supraventricular tachyarrhythmias.[12] During oral treatment lasting from 36 days to almost 4 years, 44 patients (66.6%) were free of arrhythmias and complaints, and 11 patients (16.6%) experienced significant improvement. In 4 patients, the response was unsatisfactory, and in the remaining 7 patients, no favorable effect was observed. The favorable results were obtained in patients with all forms of supraventricular tachycardia. Thirty-three children had paroxysmal supraventricular tachycardia and an accessory atrioventricular pathway. During treatment with orally administered propafenone, 22 of these patients were free of arrhythmias, 7 patients experienced significant improvement, and the remaining 4 patients had either an unsatisfactory response or no response. Three of 4 children with atrioventricular nodal re-entrant tachycardia were free of arrhythmias during treatment with propafenone. The arrhythmia could be terminated in these patients by a block in the accessory pathway.

Propafenone is also effective in preventing atrial flutter in patients with accessory atrioventricular pathways. In 4 of 6 young patients with this arrhythmia reported by Weber and associates, propafenone achieved favorable results.[12] In 3 of 4 children, propafenone converted atrial flutter to sinus rhythm. In a more recent report, Weber and co-workers studied 96 infants and children, aged 1 day to 15.5 years (mean 5.3 years) who required treatment for paroxysmal supraventricular tachycardia (59 patients), ventricular extrasystoles (18 patients), atrial flutter (14 patients), sustained ventricular tachycardia (16 patients), nodal tachycardia (11 patients), and ventricular fibrillation or flutter (4 patients).[22] In 39 of these 96 patients, the arrhythmias could not be controlled with another antiarrhythmic agent, such as digoxin, verapamil, ajmaline, propranolol, pindolol, lidocaine, phenytoin, or flecainide.

Oral propafenone, 300 mg/m^2/day, was given to all patients. In addition, 53 of them received the drug intravenously as well, at doses of 36.2 to 63.8 mg/m^2, prior to oral therapy. Propafenone abolished or reduced the arrhythmia in 81 of 96 children (84.4%). Propafenone was ineffective in 5 patients with supraventricular tachycardia; in 4 other patients, propafenone was discontinued because of the development of atrioventricular conduction disturbances.

Although this study was not controlled, the results are impressive. Propafenone appears to be an important antiarrhythmic agent for pediatric patients. Recently, several investigators have reported that propafenone effectively suppresses and prevents various supraventricular and ventricular arrhythmias in newborns, infants, and children. The drug has even proved to be superior to several conventional antiarrhythmic agents.

The success of propafenone is especially significant in patients with junctional ectopic tachycardia. This arrhythmia can be fatal when it occurs immediately after intracardiac surgical correction of congenital lesions. This arrhythmia is not affected by cardioversion and responds poorly to cardiac pacing and antiarrhythmic agents.

Garson and colleagues studied 4 infants with junctional ectopic tachycardia (rate of 210 to 300 beats/min) that occurred within 24 hours of cardiac operations. The patients ranged in age from 11 days to 9 months.[23] Propafenone was given in a loading dose of 0.2 mg/kg intravenously every 10 min up to 2.0 mg/kg. Once the ventricular rate decreased below 150 beats/min, a constant infusion of 0.004 to 0.007 mg/kg/min was given. In all 4 patients, a loading dose of 1.6 to 1.8 mg/kg caused an immediate decrease in ventricular rate to 120 to 140 beats/min, with alternating sinus and junctional rhythm. In all 4 infants, the arrhythmia reverted to sinus rhythm. Continued propafenone infusion for up to 48 hours was given to 3 of these children. The remaining patient, an 11-day-old infant, died of low cardiac output. In summary, propafenone is effective in infants and children with junctional ectopic tachycardia.

Salice and associates evaluated the potential usefulness of short-term oral drug testing for selection of antiarrhythmic drugs in children.[24] In 5 children, aged 8 months to 13 years, with chronic supraventricular arrhythmias and no detectable heart disease, short-term testing of propafenone, propranolol, verapamil, quinidine, and disopyramide was performed. Propafenone suppressed over 90% of the arrhythmias in 4 of the 5 children. It was the single most effective drug in this group of children.[24] Despite these favorable results, the use of propafenone in supraventricular arrhythmias is associated with some problems. For example, propafenone has been ineffective in patients with vagal atrial fibrillation and flutter; it may even aggravate these arrhythmias.[18] This phenomenon may be attributed to the beta-blocking activity of the drug.[10] Another problem, reported by Waleffe and Kulbertus, is that propafenone may not prevent recurrences of supraventricular tachycardias associated with an accessory atrioventricular pathway, although it prevents atrioventricular nodal re-entrant arrhythmias.[15]

In summary, propafenone is among the few antiarrhythmic agents effective in the termination and prevention of supraventricular tachyarrhythmias in infancy and childhood.

Effects in Ventricular Arrhythmias

Propafenone has been useful in controlling a variety of ventricular arrhythmias in adults and in children, with or without an organic heart disease, at rest and during exercise. Electrophysiologic studies performed in adults have shown a limited efficacy of the drug. For example, propafenone given in a loading dose of 2 mg/kg intravenously, followed by 1 mg/min, prevented the induction of sustained ventricular tachycardia in only 1 of 13 patients with this arrhythmia. These poor results should not, however, discourage the clinician from trying propafenone in children with ventricular arrhythmias because (1) the causes of ventricular arrhythmias in adults and children may be different and (2) as in amiodarone, the results of electrophysiologic studies of propafenone with programmed electrical stimulation do not predict the clinical response to the drug.[25] Moreover, a preliminary report on the inducibility of ventricular arrhythmias after intravenous administration of propafenone in children and young adults has had favorable results.[12]

The clinical response to short- or long-term propafenone treatment of adults with ventricular arrhythmias has been favorable. For example, in a group of 40 Chinese patients with ventricular or junctional premature beats, propafenone suppressed the arrhythmia in 39 of the patients 2 hours after administration of the drug.[16] In another study performed by Podrid and Lown, control of premature ventricular beats was satisfactory in 8 of 13 patients after a single oral dose of propafenone, 450 mg, and in 9 of 13 patients after 3 days of treatment with 450 to 900 mg daily.[26] Results in children have also been encouraging, although the number of patients treated is too small to draw general conclusions. Weber and co-workers reported that propafenone effectively controlled premature ventricular beats in 4 of 5 children and had an unsatisfactory effect in 1 patient.[12] Eight of 9 children with ventricular tachycardia were free of the arrhythmia during treatment with propafenone, while the remaining child showed significant improvement. Children with postmyocarditic arrhythmias responded poorly to propafenone.

Comparison with Other Antiarrhythmic Drugs

No controlled comparative studies of propafenone and other antiarrhythmic drugs have been performed in infants and children. Some comparative data are available from studies in adults, however.

Flecainide

Flecainide, 400 mg daily, was more effective than propafenone, 900 mg daily, in a study of adults with ventricular arrhythmias due to coronary artery disease.[27]

Mexiletine

In a series of 12 patients with ventricular arrhythmias due to coronary artery disease, propafenone, 900 mg daily, was more effective than mexiletine, 600 mg daily.[27] The superiority of propafenone was also confirmed in another study.[28]

Lidocaine

In children, lidocaine is the drug of choice for immediate suppression of ventricular arrhythmias associated with myocarditis, myocardial infarction, and cardiac catheterization. In adults with acute myocardial infarction, propafenone is at least as effective as lidocaine. For example, in one series, both drugs suppressed ventricular arrhythmias in patients with acute myocardial infarction by about 80%.[29] In another series, propafenone suppressed multiform ventricular tachycardia in 8 of 10 patients, whereas lidocaine suppressed this arrhythmia in only 1 of 13 patients.[30] In a study of children with myocarditis-induced arrhythmias, however, propafenone was ineffective,[12] whereas in my experience, lidocaine is effective in patients with this condition. Moreover, lidocaine is safer than propafenone in patients with atrioventricular and intraventricular conduction disturbances.

Disopyramide

The antiarrhythmic and negative inotropic effects of propafenone and disopyramide are about equal.[11,13] In some patients, propafenone requires shorter dosage intervals than disopyramide.[11] In a controlled study in adults with ventricular arrhythmias, the effect of propafenone was more potent and longer lasting than that of disopyramide.[32]

Procainamide

The response to procainamide predicted the response to propafenone in 8 of 10 patients.[35] Therefore, propafenone may be useful in treating arrhythmias responsive to procainamide in children who cannot tolerate procainamide for long periods because of side effects.

Quinidine

No formal, well-controlled comparative studies of quinidine and propafenone have been performed. The antiarrhythmic effect of propafenone was comparable to that of a combination of quinidine and beta-blockers in one study.[10] In certain patients, propafenone has been more effective than quinidine.[10] In a study of healthy volunteers, the negative inotropic effect of both drugs was about equal.[31]

Clinical Pharmacology

Propafenone may be given intravenously or orally. It is rapidly absorbed from the gastrointestinal tract after oral administration, in a concentration-dependent manner. Its extensive first-pass hepatic metabolism results in a bioavailability of about 50%. Plasma levels reach a maximum within 2 to 3 hours. The effect is evident within an hour of oral administration.[10,33-36]

One report noted that, during continued oral administration of propafenone in children, the serum level rose until the fourth day. It then ranged between 112 and 2706 ng/ml (mean 447 ng/ml). Relapses of arrhythmias occurred in children and young adults whose serum levels were below 150 ng/ml. No correlation was found between serum levels and side effects, even at the high concentration range.[12] In some adults, a linear correlation between the log of plasma level and the antiarrhythmic effect has been seen.[37]

In adults, the antiarrhythmic effect is evident at concentrations of 0.2 to 5.3 μg/ml.[33, 36, 38] Many therapeutic failures, especially in children, have resulted from inadequate compliance.[12]

The plasma protein binding of propafenone is about 90%.[33, 34, 39] Propafenone is extensively metabolized in the liver, mainly by oxidation and conjugation. The metabolites are excreted in the feces and in the urine.[39] The elimination half-life of propafenone is usually less than 4 hours.[39] Propafenone displays polymorphic metabolism, which correlates with the genetically determined debrisoquin oxidative phenotype.[40]

Side Effects

Propafenone is usually well tolerated, and serious side effects are rare. Most side effects of propafenone resemble those of other Class I antiarrhythmic agents. In one series of children and young adults, almost half the patients complained of side effects during treatment; most of these side effects were mild.

In a series of 96 infants and children reported by Weber and associates, no major side effects were observed during treatment with intravenously and orally administered propafenone.[22]

Cardiovascular Effects

Cardiovascular side effects occur in many adults treated with propafenone. In a review of 1723 patients, 38 had depression of the sinus node and 46 had atrioventricular conduction disturbances; overall cardiovascular side effects were found in 223 of these patients.[11] In other series, sinus bradycardia was the most common cardiovascular side effect; it occurred in about 20% of patients. Intraventricular conduction disturbances have been noted in 5 to 10% of patients.[10, 18]

In children, slowing of heart rate has often been observed, but to the best of my knowledge, significant intraventricular conduction disturbances in children have not been reported to be induced by propafenone.[12] Orthostatic symptoms, mainly fatigue, were observed in 7.6% of young patients in a study.[12] Dizziness was observed in 4% of these patients.

Gastrointestinal Effects

Gastrointestinal side effects have been reported in about 20% of adults treated with propafenone. In children, nausea is the most common reported side effect, with an incidence of 25%. Vomiting or anorexia has been observed in about 8% of patients. Other adverse gastrointestinal effects are a bitter taste in the mouth and constipation.[11, 41] The gastrointestinal side effects may gradually subside during continued administration of the drug.[10]

Disturbances of Sexual Function

Animal experiments have shown that prolonged intravenous treatment with propafenone may inhibit spermatogenesis. This effect is reversed several weeks after discontinuance of the drug. A single case of a man who developed impotence has been reported.[42, 43]

Other Effects

Blurring of vision and cholestatic jaundice rarely develop.[11]

Abnormal Laboratory Findings

A positive antinuclear antibody test result was seen in 2 of 16 patients treated with propafenone.[21] In a study of 66 infants, children, and young adults, 1 infant developed an elevation of gamma globulin, and 2 other patients developed elevated serum glutamic-oxaloacetic transaminase levels.

Drug Interactions

Class I Antiarrhythmic Agents

Propafenone may potentiate the effect of other Class I antiarrhythmic agents.

Amiodarone

Amiodarone may potentiate the bradycardia produced by propafenone.[44] This subject is further discussed in Chapter 29. When an arrhythmia can be controlled only by this combination, and when excessive bradycardia is produced, an artificial pacemaker should be inserted.

Propranolol

One report noted that propafenone plasma levels increased after administration of propranolol in 1 of 4 patients.[44]

Anticoagulant Agents

Propafenone may potentiate the anticoagulant effect of warfarin.[45]

Dosage and Administration

Intravenous Administration

In children, the active intravenous dose of propafenone ranges between 11.5 and 63.8 mg/m^2 body surface area (mean 39.7 mg/m^2). An infusion of 1 mg/kg, injected over 5 min, has been used in electrophysiologic studies.

Garson and colleagues suggested a loading dose of 0.2 mg/kg, repeated every 10 min up to 2.0 mg/kg, followed by a maintenance infusion of 0.004 to 0.007 mg/kg/min in infants and children.[23]

Oral Administration

The active oral dose is between 200 and 600 mg/m^2 body surface area per day, in 3 to 4 divided doses.

References

1. Rudolph, W., et al.: Effects of propafenon on the accessory pathway (AP) in patients with WPW syndrome. (Abstract.) Am. J. Cardiol., 43:430, 1979.
2. Waleffe, A., et al.: Electrophysiological effects of propafenone studied with programmed electrical stimulation of the heart in patients with recurrent paroxysmal supraventricular tachycardia. Eur. Heart J., 2:345, 1980.
3. Kohlhardt, M.: Der Einflub von Propafenon auf der transmembranaren Na$^+$ und Ca^{++}- Strom der Warmblutler Myokardfasermembran. In Fortschritte in der Pharmakotherapie von Herzrhythmusstorungen. Edited by H. Hochrein, H.-J. Hapke, and O.A. Beck. Stuttgart, Fischer, 1977, p. 91.
4. Kukovetz, W.R., et al.: Wirkung von Propafenon auf Phosphodiesterase, Koronararterien und Herz. In Fortschritte in der Pharmakotherapie von Herzrhythmusstorungen. Edited by H. Hochrein, H.-J. Hapke, and O.A. Beck. Stuttgart, Fischer, 1977, p. 9.
5. Paietta, E., Poch, G., and Kukovetz, W.R.: Analyse der B-Blockerwirkung von Propafenon (SA 79). In Fortschritte in der Pharmakotherapie von Herzrhythmusstorungen. Edited by H. Hochrein, H.-J. Hapke, and O.A. Beck. Stuttgart, Fischer, 1977, p. 20.
6. Ledda, F., et al: Electrophysiological and antiarrhythmic properties of propafenone in isolated cardiac preparations. J. Cardiovasc. Pharmacol., 3:1162, 1981.
7. Philipsborn, G. von: Uberblick uber pharmakologische Arbeiten mit Propafenon. Internal report VPFBP 8109. Ludwigshafen, Knoll, 1981.
8. Bergmann, M., and Bolte, H.D.: Elektrophysiologische Untersuchungen mit Propafenon and myokardialen Einzelfasen. In Fortschritte in der Pharmakotherapie von Herzrhythmusstorungen. Edited by H. Hochrein, H.-J. Hapke, and O.A. Beck. Stuttgart Fischer, 1977, p. 29.
9. Kohlhardt, M.: Der Einflub von Propafenon auf den transmembranaren Na$^+$- und Ca^{++}- Strom der Warmbluter-Myokardfasermembran. In Fortschritte in der Pharmakotherapie von Herzrhythmusstorungen. Edited by H. Hochrein, H.-J. Hapke, and O.A. Beck. Stuttgart, Fischer, 1977, p. 35.
10. Coumel, P., and Leclercq, J.-F.: Efficacy of oral propafenone in supraventricular and ventricular arrhythmias: experience with 47 cases. In Cardiac Arrhythmias: Diagnosis, Prognosis, Therapy. Edited by M. Schlepper and B. Olsson. Berlin, Springer, 1983, p. 21.
11. Neuss, H., and Schlepper, M.: Clinical pharmacology of propafenone. In Cardiac Arrhythmias: Diagnosis, Prognosis, Therapy. Edited by M. Schlepper and B. Olsson. Berlin, Springer, 1983, p. 113.

12. Weber, H., Elgster, G., and Wesselhooft, H.: Experience with propafenone in the treatment of arrhythmias in pediatric patients. *In* Cardiac Arrhythmias: Diagnosis, Prognosis, Therapy. Edited by M. Schlepper and B. Olsson. Berlin, Springer, 1983, p. 185.
13. Breithardt, G., et al.: Pharmakologische Beeinflussung der "sinus-atrialen Leitungszeit" und der Sinusknotenautomatie beim Menschen. Z. Kardiol., 64:895, 1975.
14. Conolly, S.J., et al.: Clinical efficacy and electrophysiology of oral propafenone for ventricular tachycardia. Am. J. Cardiol., 52:1208, 1983.
15. Waleffe, A., and Kulbertus, H.: Electrophysiologic effects and antiarrhythmic efficacy of rhytmonorm evaluated with programmed electrical stimulation of the heart in patients with recurrent reentrant supraventricular tachycardia. *In* Cardiac Arrhythmias: Diagnosis, Prognosis, Therapy. Edited by M. Schlepper and B. Olsson. Berlin, Springer, 1983, p. 113.
16. Fu-sheng, K., et al.: Observations on the antiarrhythmic effects of rytmonorm. *In* Cardiac Arrhythmias: Diagnosis, Prognosis, Therapy. Edited by M. Schlepper and B. Olsson. Berlin, Springer, 1983, p. 151.
17. Shen, E., et al.: Electrophysiologic and antiarrhythmic properties of propafenone in patients with recurrent ventricular tachycardia. American Heart Association, 1982.
18. Salerno, D., et al.: Efficacy of propafenone for treatment of ventricular ectopic depolarizations. American Heart Association, 1982.
19. Peter, T., et al.: On the mechanism of action of propafenone, a new antiarrhythmic agent, during acute myocardial infarction in the dog. (Abstract.) Clin. Res. 30:213A, 1982.
20. Zeiler, R.H., et al.: Electrophysiologic effects of propafenone on canine ischemic cardiac cells. (Abstract.) Am. J. Cardiol., 47:483, 1981.
21. Shen, E., et al.: Efficacy and safety of oral propafenone in chronic treatment of recurrent supraventricular tachycardia. American Heart Association, 1983.
22. Weber, H., et al.: Anti-arrhythmic drug therapy propafenone in the newborn, infants and children. Abstract submitted to the First International Symposium on Cardiovascular Pharmacotherapy, Geneva, 1985.
23. Garson, A., et al.: Control of postoperative junctional ectopic tachycardia with propafenone. J. Am. Coll. Cardiology, In press.
24. Salice, P., et al.: Acute oral drug testing in children with chronic arrhythmias. Abstract submitted to the first International Symposium on Cardiovascular Pharmacotherapy, Geneva, 1985.
25. Chilson, D.A., et al.: Propafenone: discriminant analysis of electrophysiologic results in patients with ventricular tachycardia predicts clinical outcome. American Heart Association, 1983.
26. Podrid, P.J., and Lown, B.: Propafenone—an effective antiarrhythmic agent for ventricular tachycardia. American Heart Association, 1982.
27. Klempt, H.-W., and Nayebagha, A.: Propafenone, flecainide and mexiletine in the treatment of stable ventricular premature beats. *In* Cardiac Arrhythmias: Diagnosis, Prognosis, Therapy. Edited by M. Schlepper and B. Olsson. Berlin, Springer, 1983, p. 171.
28. Bethge, K.-P., and Lichtlen, P.R.: Die beurteilung der antiarrhythmischen Therapie durch Langzeit-Elektrokardiographie. *In* Ventrikulaere Herzrhythmusstörungen. Edited by B. Luederitzo. Berlin, Springer, 1981, p. 170.
29. Rehnqvist, N.: Comparison of the efficacy of propafenone and lidocaine in patients with acute myocardial infarction and ventricular extrasystoles: result of a 24-h holter monitoring. *In* Cardiac Arrhythmias: Diagnosis, Prognosis, Therapy. Edited by M. Schlepper and B. Olsson. Berlin, Springer, 1983, p. 149.
30. Zilcher, H., Glogar, D., and Kaindl, F.: Torsades de pointes: occurrence in myocardial ischemia as a separate entity. Multiform ventricular tachycardia or not? Eur. Heart J., 1:63, 1980.
31. Breithardt, G., et al.: Die Wirkung verschiedener antiarrhythmika auf die systolischen Zeitintervalle bei Normalpersonen. Z. Kardiol., 67:680, 1978.
32. Clementy, J., Dalloccio, M., and Bricaud, H.: Comparative study of the therapeutic effect of propafenone and disopyramide in the oral treatment of chronic ventricular

premature beats. In Cardiac Arrhythmias: Diagnosis, Prognosis, Therapy. Edited by M. Schlepper and B. Olsson. Berlin, Springer, 1983, p. 159.
33. Blanke, H., et al.: Plasmaspiegel-wirkungs-beziehung und Organverteilung von Propafenon. Dtsch. Med. Wochenschr., *104*:587, 1979.
34. Brode, E., and Buhler, V. Zur Pharmakokinetik von Propafenon. Internal report. Ludwigshafen, Knoll, 1981.
35. Meyer-Estorf, G., et al.: Antiarrhythmische Wirksamkeit von Propafenon in Abhängigkeit von Serumkonzentration und Erregungsleitungshemmung. Z. Kardiol., *67*:352, 1978.
36. Meyer-Estorf, G., et al.: Serumkonzentration und AV-überleitungszeit unter mehrtägiger oraler Behandlung mit Propafenon. Z. Kardiol., *69*:417, 1980.
37. Connolly, S.J., et al.: Clinical pharmacology of propafenone. American Heart Association, 1982.
38. Keller, K., et al.: Correlation between serum concentration and pharmacological effect on atrioventricular conduction time of the antiarrhythmic drug propafenone. Eur. J. Clin. Pharmacol., *13*:17, 1978.
39. Hollmann, M., et al.: Pharmacokinetic and metabolic studies on propafenone in volunteers. In Cardiac Arrhythmias: Diagnosis, Prognosis, Therapy. Edited by M. Schlepper and B. Olsson. Berlin, Springer, 1983, p. 125.
40. Siddoway, L.A., et al.: Polymorphic oxidative metabolism of propafenone in man. American Heart Association, 1983.
41. deSoyza, N., et al.: The safety and efficacy of propafenone in suppressing ventricular ectopy. In Cardiac Arrhythmias: Diagnosis, Prognosis, Therapy. Edited by M. Schlepper and B. Olsson. Berlin, Springer, p. 217.
42. Kleinsorge, H., and Pfenningsdorf, G.: Potenz- und Spermiogenesestörungen durch Propafenon. Dtsch. Med. Wochenschr., *105*:395, 1980.
43. Korst, H.A., Brandes, J.-W., and Littmann, K.-P.: Potenz- und Spermiogenesestörungen durch Propafenon. Dtsch. Med. Wochenschr., *105*:1187, 1980.
44. Steinbach, K., et al.: Interaction between propafenone and other drugs. In Cardiac Arrhythmias: Diagnosis, Prognosis, Therapy. Edited M. Schlepper and B. Olsson. Berlin, Springer, 1983, p. 141.
45. Korst, H.A., Brandes, J.W., and Littmann, K.P.: Propafenon potenziert Wirkung von oralen Anti-koagulanzien. Med. Klin., *51*:349, 1981.

Chapter 28

Ethmozin

Ethmozin, a phenothiazine derivative studied in the Soviet Union, has antiarrhythmic properties resembling those of lidocaine, as well as a suppressant effect on abnormal automaticity. Several studies in the United States and Europe have confirmed the efficacy of ethmozin in patients with ventricular arrhythmias. Recently, the case of a child with atrial ectopic focus tachycardia, successfully treated with ethmozin, has been reported. This drug may play a role in the future treatment of this serious and resistant arrhythmia in infants and children.

Structure

Ethmozin is 10-(3-morpholinopropionyl)-phenothiazine-2-carbonic acid ethylester.

Pharmacologic Properties

The antiarrhythmic effect of ethmozin may result from its membrane-stabilizing activity or from phenothiazine's effect on the nervous system.[1-4]

Electrophysiologic Effects

Ethmozin decreases the maximal rate of rise of phase-0 depolarization, depresses phase-4 depolarization in ischemic fibers, and shortens repolarization. The drug also shortens the duration of the action potential and refractoriness, and it slows conduction in Purkinje fibers. In human subjects, ethmozin prolongs the AH and HV intervals, although only during long-term treatment; it may prolong the QRS interval, and it uncommonly alters the QTc interval and the atrial and ventricular refractory periods.[1-6]

Effects in Arrhythmias

Ethmozin is especially effective in suppressing ventricular arrhythmias. The largest study, published by Podrid and Lown, included 62 patients with malignant ventricular arrhythmias.[3] Of these patients, 56% responded to ethmozin therapy, with complete abolition of ventricular tachycardia, over 90% suppression of couplets, and over 50% suppression of premature ventricular beats. Ethmozin has also been reported to be more effective and more easily tolerated than disopyramide.[5]

Garson and co-workers reported a case of effective suppression by ethmozin of automatic atrial ectopic focus tachycardia in a child.[7] This arrhythmia is one of the few potentially lethal supraventricular arrhythmias in children. The rapid heart rate, persisting over long periods, may lead to the development of cardiomyopathy. This arrhythmia often resists conventional antiarrhythmic agents. A 9-month-old infant had atrial ectopic focus tachycardia at rates of 160 to 300 beats/min. The arrhythmia was resistant to combinations of digoxin, quinidine, verapamil, and propranolol. By the age of 3 years, the child had developed cardiomyopathy. He underwent surgical ablation of an ectopic focus in the right atrial appendage, but the arrhythmia persisted. Amiodarone was then tried, but was ineffective. Ethmozin, 11 mg/kg/day, given in 4 daily doses, almost abolished the arrhythmia. At a daily dose of 15 mg/kg/day this patient was completely free of the arrhythmia. Thus, ethmozin appears to play a role in the suppression of atrial ectopic focus tachycardia in infants and children.

Clinical Pharmacology

Ethmozin is well absorbed from the gastrointestinal tract after oral administration. The onset of the drug's antiarrhythmic effect may be delayed by 24 hours.[8,9] The mean maximal plasma concentration in adults is 0.66 ± 0.8 µg/ml. In the child studied by Garson and associates, this concentration was 0.234 µg/ml.[7] The drug's elimination half-life in adults is 2 to 6 hours; in the foregoing child, it was 1.2 hours. Intrinsic clearance of ethmozin in this child was high, 2.3 L/min.[7]

Side Effects

Ethmozin is usually well tolerated. Only about 10% of patients treated on a long-term basis develop side effects, which are usually mild. These adverse effects include headache, dizziness, nausea, and epigastric distress.[3] Ethmozin has a small arrhythmogenic potential.

Dosage and Administration

Ethmozin is given orally. The usual dose is 5 to 14 mg/kg/day, in 3 to 4 divided doses. The child reported by Garson and colleagues required 15 mg/kg/day, divided into 4 doses.[7]

References

1. Rosenshtraukh, L.V. et al.: Study of the effects of ethmozin on the force of contractions, transmembranal action potential and sodium flow of the muscles, of the

frog precordium. In Proceedings of the First U.S.-U.S.S.R. Symposium on Sudden Death, Yalta, October 3 to 5, 1977. Washington, D.C., United States Department of Health, Education and National Institutes of Health, DHEW Publication No. (NIH) 78-1470, 1978, p. 291.
2. Podrid P.J., et al.: Ethmozin, a new antiarrhythmic drug for suppressing ventricular premature complexes. Circulation, 61:450, 1980.
3. Podrid, P.J. & Lown, B.: Ethmozin therapy for malignant ventricular arrhythmia. American College of Cardiology, 1982.
4. Danilo, P., et al.: Effects of phenothiazine analog, EN131, on ventricular arrhythmias in the dog. Eur. J. Pharmacol., 45:127, 1977.
5. Pratt, C.M., et al.: Comparative effect of disopyramide and ethmozin in suppressing complex ventricular arrhythmias by use of a double-blind, placebo-controlled, longitudinal crossover design. Circulation, 69:288, 1984.
6. Mann, D.E., et al.: Electrophysiologic effects of ethmozin in patients with ventricular tachycardia. Am. Heart J., 17:674, 1984.
7. Garson, A., et al.: Ethmozine: a promising drug for "automatic" atrial ectopic focus tachycardia. Abstract submitted to the First International Symposium on Cardiovascular Pharmacotherapy, Geneva, 1985.
8. Zaslovskaya, R.M., et al.: Ethmozin therapy of patients with rhythm disturbances in heart activity. Sov. Med., 5:50, 1969.
9. Gomzyakova, T.G.: Results of clinical study of the antiarrhythmic drug carbazine (ethmozin). Vrach. Delo, 4:62, 1970.

Chapter 29

Amiodarone

Amiodarone is the most widely used Class III antiarrhythmic agent. It is a benzofuran derivative originally developed to treat angina pectoris. Over the past 15 years, the antiarrhythmic properties of this drug have been recognized, and it is now mainly used for treating supraventricular arrhythmias, as well as for controlling ventricular arrhythmias.

The mechanism of the antiarrhythmic effect of amiodarone is related to prolongation of refractory periods in all cardiac tissues, slowing of conduction, suppression of automaticity in some fibers, or an effect mediated by the autonomic nervous system. An important advantage of amiodarone, especially in pediatric practice, is the drug's long elimination half-life of about 2 months. Because of this long half-life, amiodarone may be given once daily. Important disadvantages of amiodarone are its slow onset of action and a high incidence of adverse effects.

In infants and children, amiodarone is used primarily to treat supraventricular arrhythmias, especially those associated with Wolff-Parkinson-White syndrome, the Mustard and Blalock-Hanlen procedures, congestive cardiomyopathy, and endocardial fibroelastosis.

Structure

Amiodarone is an amphophilic molecule composed of a nonpolar ring with a hydrophilic polar side chain. It contains about 40% iodine.

Pharmacologic Properties

Amiodarone lacks the membrane-stabilizing activity of Class I antiarrhythmic drugs and possesses the electrophysiologic properties of Class III antiarrhythmic drugs. These properties are discussed later in this chapter, in the section on electrophysiologic effects. Amiodarone reduces the outward potassium current and the rapid inward sodium current without being a membrane-stabilizing agent. In addition, the effect of amiodarone may be mediated by several other mechanisms. The drug may have features of a Class IV antiarrhythmic agent because of its calcium-antagonist properties,[1] although this subject is controversial.

Amiodarone also has a vasodilatory effect both because of a direct effect on blood vessels and because of alpha-adrenergic blocking activity. Moreover, amiodarone is a weak nonselective beta-adrenoreceptor blocking agent that can also block myocardial metabolic pathways, such as mitochondrial activity, which depend on thyroid hormones.[2] All these effects may be involved in the antiarrhythmic and antianginal effects of the drug. The predominant pharmacologic property of amiodarone is not known.

Electrophysiologic Effects

The most important electrophysiologic effects of amiodarone are prolongation of refractory periods of various cardiac tissues and depression of the sinoatrial and atrioventricular nodes. The drug has minimal effect on conduction in the His-Purkinje system or in the myocardium.

Microelectrode studies and studies of monophasic action potential have shown that amiodarone prolongs the duration of the action potential of His-Purkinje fibers and of ventricular and atrial myocardium, mainly by delaying repolarization. In atrial myocardium, amiodarone also shows the rate of rise of phase-0 depolarization.[3] The amplitude of the action potential and the resting potential are not altered by amiodarone. The increased duration of the action potential prolongs refractoriness and the QTc interval.[4] Amiodarone also depresses the function of the sinoatrial and atrioventricular nodes, as evident by prolongation of the sinus node cycle length and recovery time and the AH interval. The effective refractory periods of the sinoatrial and atrioventricular nodes are also prolonged.[4-7] In children, the most significant and consistent effect of amiodarone on the sinus node is slowing of its spontaneous rate, a change also observed in adults.[8]

Occasionally, amiodarone causes symptomatic sinus bradycardia that is resistant to atropine. This effect on the sinus node is not uniform. For example, Touboul and co-workers reported that amiodarone, 5 mg/kg intravenously, slowed the sinus rate in 12 of 24 patients and increased the sinus node recovery time (a mean increase of 110 msec) in 17 of these patients.[9] Rapid injection of amiodarone may cause a transient increase in heart rate because of the effect of the diluent of the drug.[10] Coumel and Fidelle reported that the sinus rate was steadily reduced in 135 children treated with amiodarone, but in only 10 patients was it less than 60 beats/min at rest.[11] Seven of these 10 children had a pre-existing atrial rhythm disturbance.

The drug also affects the atrioventricular node, as seen by prolongation of the AH and PR interval. Coumel and Fidelle observed PR prolongation from 40 to 80 msec in 41 children and the appearance of Wenckebach periods in 3 children.[11] Hesslein and colleagues reported worsening of an already compromised sinus node or atrioventricular node in 4 of 15 children, 3 of whom required implantation of a pacemaker.[12] Amiodarone also has some depressant effect on conduction in the His-Purkinje system, manifested by prolongation of the HV interval. This effect is more pronounced with oral than with intravenous drug administration.[4, 8, 9] Occasionally, the QRS interval is prolonged by amiodarone.[13] In 2 children with incomplete right bundle branch block, the duration of the QRS interval increased by 20 and 40 msec.[11] Amiodarone prolongs the effective refractory periods of accessory atrioventricular pathways in both anterograde and retrograde directions.[10] This effect is responsible for the high efficacy of amiodarone in suppressing arrhythmias associated with the Wolff-Parkinson-White syndrome.

Amiodarone may cause T-wave changes. I studied a patient in whom amiodarone caused T-wave inversion resembling that seen in subendocardial myocardial infarction. The patient's electrocardiogram returned to normal when the drug was discontinued. Oreto and associates reported a similar case.[14] Minimal changes in the configuration of the T wave have been observed in children treated with amiodarone. Occasionally, a large U wave appears during treatment. In a report of a large series of infants and children treated with amiodarone, it was suggested that before one decides that treatment has failed, one must have electrophysiologic evidence of the effect of amiodarone on repolarization, mainly QTc prolongation and a U wave.[11]

Although a few adolescents have been included in studies of the electrophysiologic effects of amiodarone, these effects have not specifically been studied in the pediatric age group, especially not in the immature human heart. Results of an animal experiment showed that intravenous administration of amiodarone produces electrophysiologic changes in the neonate that are qualitatively similar to those in adults.[15] Seven neonatal puppies aged 5 to 14 days and 6 adult dogs were studied. Amiodarone depressed sinus node cycle length, sinus node recovery time, and atrioventricular nodal conduction in both groups and prolonged atrial and ventricular refractory periods in a dose-dependent fashion. The immature dogs were more sensitive to amiodarone in prolongation of atrial refractory periods and in depression of sinus node recovery time, but they were more resistant to amiodarone-induced depression of atrioventricular nodal conduction. Thus, higher doses of amiodarone may be required in the neonate to produce a degree of depression of atrioventricular nodal conduction similar to that in adults. At these higher doses the sinus node may be more severely depressed, however.[15]

Amiodarone may be safely used in patients with intraventricular conduction disturbances complicating organic heart disease. Therefore, the drug may be given to children with bundle branch block and arrhythmias following cardiac operations. In a group of 52 children with right bundle branch block, 15 of whom also had a left anterior hemiblock, amiodarone did not cause any advanced distal atrioventricular conduction disturbance.[11]

Effects in Arrhythmias

Amiodarone is effective in terminating and, especially, in preventing various supraventricular and ventricular arrhythmias. The drug is also beneficial in infants and children with arrhythmias. For example, Coumel and Fidelle treated 135 children (mean age 10.2 years) with oral amiodarone for a mean duration of 4.1 months.[11] The children had idiopathic and postoperative arrhythmias. Complete control of arrhythmias was achieved in 60% of the patients, and partial control was obtained in 33%. This effect was evidence regardless of the location of the arrhythmia, its mechanism, resistance or sensitivity to other drugs, and the presence of cardiomyopathy or clinical signs of heart failure.

Effects in Experimentally Induced Arrhythmias in Animals

Amiodarone has suppressed arrhythmias induced in animals by coronary ligation and by administration of strophanthin, aconitine, and acetylcholine.[17, 18]

Effects in Supraventricular Tachycardia

Amiodarone is effective in termination and conversion of supraventricular tachycardia in adults. In a series of patients who had undergone cardiac operations, intravenous amiodarone converted supraventricular tachycardia to sinus rhythm in 13 of 17 patients.[19] Oral amiodarone prevented recurrences of supraventricular tachycardia in 15 of 21 patients, 13 of whom had Wolff-Parkinson-White syndrome and 8 of whom had concealed accessory pathway.[20] This effect of amiodarone was closely related to the extent of increase in the effective refractory periods of the accessory atrioventricular pathway and the atrioventricular node.[21] This effect was especially pronounced in patients with Wolff-Parkinson-White syndrome. The success rate in patients with this syndrome has ranged between 50 and 100%.[22-24]

Amiodarone is useful in the treatment of supraventricular tachycardia in infants and children. Hesslein and co-workers reported favorable results in 7 children with supraventricular arrhythmias.[12] In my experience, orally administered amiodarone prevented recurrences of paroxysmal supraventricular tachycardia in 3 of 4 children with Wolff-Parkinson-White syndrome and in a child without this syndrome. Shahar and colleagues, of the Sheba Medical Center, reported the experience of 2 medical centers in the treatment of 10 children, aged 3 months to 15 years, who had recurrent episodes of supraventricular tachycardia associated with Wolff-Parkinson-White syndrome.[25] Two of these children had tricuspid atresia, 1 had Ebstein's anomaly, 1 had a single ventricle, 1 had a ventricular septal defect, and the remaining children had no structural heart disease. In 9 of the children, amiodarone was administered following the failure of oral digoxin, quinidine, verapamil, and propranolol therapy. Each patient received an oral loading dose of 10 to 15 mg/kg, followed by 5 mg/kg daily. All children became free of arrhythmias within 5 days of therapy and remained asymptomatic for 5 to 36 months. In 1 patient, successful treatment with amiodarone had to be discontinued because of the appearance of generalized urticaria. When high oral doses of verapamil failed to prevent recurrences of the arrhythmia in this child, amiodarone was reinstituted and completely suppressed the arrhythmia. All 10 children had normal results on thyroid function tests, and no other adverse effects were observed. Shahar and associates recommended the use of amiodarone to control and to prevent sustained supraventricular arrhythmias in pediatric patients with Wolff-Parkinson-White syndrome when traditional antiarrhythmic drugs fail.[25]

Coumel and Fidelle studied the effect of amiodarone in 91 children with atrial tachycardia.[11] In 55 of these patients, the response was favorable; 31 had a fair response, and 7 had a poor response. Among 22 children with junctional tachycardia, a good response was observed in 12 patients and a fair response was noted in 10 patients. Bucknall and co-workers studied 8 children with supraventricular tachycardia and 7 with Wolff-Parkinson-White syndrome, all under 14 years of age.[26] The majority of these patients had no structural cardiac lesions. They were resistant to several other antiarrhythmic agents. The arrhythmia was controlled in almost all these children with doses of amiodarone of 2.7 to 34 mg/kg/day, associated with blood levels of 0.4 to 2.3 mg/L. In several children, amiodarone was given in combination with digoxin or verapamil.

Effects in Atrial Fibrillation

Benaim and Uzan reported that amiodarone converted atrial fibrillation to sinus rhythm or slowed the ventricular response to atrial fibrillation in more than half the patients studied.[27] Santos and colleagues reported that oral amiodarone converted atrial fibrillation to sinus rhythm in 86% of their patients, and sinus rhythm was maintained by amiodarone for at least a year in 72% of their patients.[28] The effect of amiodarone on atrial fibrillation in children was not specifically studied.

Effects in Atrial Flutter

Atrial flutter used to be considered an uncommon cardiac arrhythmia in infancy and childhood. Recently, however, it has become evident that in certain groups of patients, this arrhythmia may be common in infancy and childhood. Included are patients who have undergone Mustard and Blalock-Hanlen procedures for transposition of the great arteries or children with congestive cardiomyopathy or primary endocardial fibroelastosis. Garson and associates reported that 60% of 380 patients who had atrial flutter between 1 and 25 years of age had surgically treated congenital heart disease, most commonly by Mustard and Blalock-Hanlon procedures, and 6% had cardiomyopathy.[29] My colleagues and I have found that 10% of our patients with primary endocardial fibroelastosis develop atrial flutter.

The goal of therapy should be to eliminate all episodes of atrial flutter because the incidence of sudden death is 4 times higher in patients who continue to have episodes of the arrhythmia than in patients who are free of the arrhythmia.[29] Amiodarone may be especially useful in treatment of this arrhythmia in infants and children. Garson and co-workers reported that amiodarone eliminated atrial flutter in 78% of children studied; digitalis with quinidine eliminated the arrhythmia in 53%; digitalis alone was effective in 44%, and digitalis with propranolol was beneficial in 21% of these patients.[29] Bucknall and associates reported that amiodarone was effective in 5 children with atrial flutter.[26]

Effects in Chaotic Atrial Tachycardia

Chaotic atrial tachycardia, uncommon in infants and children, may be difficult to treat. Blieden (personal communication) studied a 4-year-old child with corrected transposition of the great arteries who developed chaotic atrial tachycardia resistant to several Class I and Class II antiarrhythmic drugs and to digitalis. The intravenous administration of amiodarone terminated the arrhythmia, and oral amiodarone prevented its recurrence. I studied a 5-year-old child with the dilated form of primary endocardial fibroelastosis in whom the combination of amiodarone and digitalis controlled chaotic atrial tachycardia.

Effects in Ventricular Arrhythmias

Ventricular tachycardia is an uncommon cardiac arrhythmia in infancy and childhood. When it appears in this age group, it may be difficult to treat. Amiodarone has been effective in several such patients; occasionally, it was the only effective drug. Hesslein and co-workers studied 2 children with ventricular tachycardia and 6 children with ventricular and supraventricular tachycardia.[12] The patients ranged in age from 0.5 to 16.0 years, and most had slow structural heart diseases. Orally administered amiodarone was beneficial in the majority of the children; this group was reported together with children with supraventricular arrhythmias, and the response was not specified.

Paroxysmal idiopathic ventricular tachycardia and premature beats may be aggravated or suppressed by effort. I studied a pair of 14-year-old children who were examined because of constant palpitations, post-exercise dizziness, and syncopal episodes. Physical examinations, electrocardiograms, thoracic roentgenograms, and echocardiograms showed no evidence of underlying structural cardiac disease. One patient had multiple ventricular premature beats with bigeminal and trigeminal rhythm, and the other had paroxysmal ventricular tachycardia. The arrhythmias were completely suppressed during submaximal exercise; however, long runs of paroxysmal ventricular tachycardia started 30 to 120 sec following abrupt cessation of exercise. They were accompanied by a clinical picture of near syncope. Treatment with amiodarone completely abolished the ventricular arrhythmias both at rest and following exercise. An attempt to discontinue the drug was followed by recurrence of the pretreatment arrhythmias. The complaints of palpitations and syncope disappeared during long-term treatment with amiodarone.

Coumel and Fidelle studied the effect of oral amiodarone in 20 children with ventricular arrhythmias.[11] A favorable response was observed in 14 patients, a fair response was seen in 3, and a poor response was noted in 3 patients.

From the experience in adults, it is clear that amiodarone is effective in suppressing various ventricular arrhythmias, either idiopathic or associated with structural heart disease. For example Greene and colleagues studied 54 patients with ventricular arrhythmias who were treated with amiodarone for 6 to 24 months.[30] Only 3 of these patients had ventricular tachycardia, and 4 had ventricular fibrillation during treatment. McKenna and associates reported that oral amiodarone controlled ventricular arrhythmias and increased survival rates in patients with hypertrophic cardiomyopathy.[31]

Pioselli and co-workers studied 46 patients with mitral valve prolapse, almost half of whom had ventricular arrhythmias, including premature ventricular beats, ventricular tachycardia, and ventricular fibrillation.[32] The ages of these patients ranged widely, starting at 7 years of age. Several of these patients were treated with amiodarone, with favorable results. Amiodarone was more effective than other drugs in a 7-year-old child who had more than 190 bouts of ventricular tachycardia daily.

Effects in Sinus Node Dysfunction

Amiodarone depresses the sinus node function and therefore may produce a deleterious effect in patients with sick sinus syndrome. In children, this effect is especially hazardous in those who have had intra-atrial surgical procedures such as Mustard or Blalock-Hanlon operations. Although the majority of patients with sick sinus syndrome tolerate amiodarone well, the drug has produced symptomatic bradycardia and hypotension in such patients.[24, 33, 34] I recommend that amiodarone be given to patients with sick sinus syndrome only in combination with an artificial pacemaker.

Effects in Prolonged QT Syndrome

The prolonged QT syndrome may be congenital, familial, or acquired through the use of several Class I antiarrhythmic drugs. In children, the congenital and familial forms of this syndrome are most important and may be associated with complex arrhythmias. Amiodarone suppressed severely symptomatic arrhythmias in a 17-year-old patient with congenital prolonged QT syndrome.[35]

Intravenous Versus Oral Administration

Unlike the effects of several other antiarrhythmic agents, the electrophysiologic and antiarrhythmic effects of amiodarone administered intravenously on a short-term basis differ from the effects of amiodarone given orally for long periods. Prolonged administration of oral amiodarone produces several effects that are not caused by short-term intravenous administration of the drug. Nademanee and associates reported that oral amiodarone administration lengthened the cycle length of ventricular tachycardia, permanently suppressed premature ventricular beats, and increased the serum levels of reversed T_3, whereas intravenous amiodarone did not alter the tachycardia cycle length or T_3 levels and produced only a transient suppression of premature ventricular beats.[36] Wellens and colleagues reported a similar effect of oral and intravenous amiodarone on the effective refractory period of atrioventricular node.[37] Oral amiodarone prolonged the AH interval and the effective refractory periods of the atria and the ventricles; however, intravenous amiodarone did not alter these parameters. Therefore, oral amiodarone is effective in supraventricular and ventricular arrhythmias, whereas intravenous amiodarone, which only prolongs the atrioventricular nodal refractoriness, is beneficial only in supraventricular arrhythmias. These differences are important, and one should not attempt to shorten the interval of onset of therapeutic effect in ventricular arrhythmias by the intravenous administration of amiodarone.

Comparison with Other Antiarrhythmic Drugs

The efficacy of amiodarone is equal or superior to that of other antiarrhythmic agents. In a study of 74 children resistant to other antiarrhythmic drugs, amiodarone achieved favorable results in 41 children, fair results in 30, and poor results in only 3 children.

Combination with Other Antiarrhythmic Drugs

It is rare to combine amiodarone with other antiarrhythmic drugs, except digitalis, which has a synergistic effect on supraventricular arrhythmias. Many children receiving amiodarone for these arrhythmias have been treated concomitantly with digitalis, usually because of congestive heart failure. Digitalis can also compensate for the slight negative inotropic effect of amiodarone. This feature is especially important in infants and children with primary endocardial fibroelastosis or congestive cardiomyopathy with atrial flutter or other atrial arrhythmias. When a regular dose of amiodarone is ineffective in suppressing an arrhythmia, it may be preferable to add a Class I antiarrhythmic agent rather than to increase the dose of amiodarone.[38] This recommendation is based not only on the higher efficacy of the combination of drugs, but also on the knowledge that several serious adverse effects of amiodarone are dose-dependent.

Electrophysiologic Studies to Predict Effect

Unlike with Class I antiarrhythmic agents, the response to amiodarone cannot be predicted accurately by electrophysiologic studies. A poor response to intravenously administered amiodarone in patients of various ages with Wolff-Parkinson-White syndrome is not necessarily an indicator to a poor response to the long-term administration of oral amiodarone.[39] Even the ability to induce ventricular tachycardia during long-term oral treatment with amiodarone does not preclude a high clinical efficacy of the drug.[40] For example, Waxman and co-workers reported that amiodarone prevented induction of ventricular tachycardia in only 12% of 43 patients who had inducible ventricular tachycardia before treatment, but the drug was clinically effective in 78% of the patients.[8] In another report, these investigators found that the effect of amiodarone on the mode of induction of ventricular arrhythmias could not be used to predict the clinical response to the drug.[41] The cause of the clinical effect is not known. Several investigators have reported a strong correlation between the results of electrophysiologic studies and the drug's clinical effect, however.[42, 43] In patients with supraventricular tachycardia and a concealed bypass tract, prolongation of the effective refractory period of the concealed tract to over 350 msec has been an accurate predictor of a favorable effect of oral amiodarone administration.

Hemodynamic Effects

Like most other antiarrhythmic agents, amiodarone has a slight negative inotropic effect. This effect results, at least in part, from the beta-adrenoreceptor blockade of the drug. The cardiodepressant effect of amiodarone is of a lesser magnitude than that of several other antiarrhythmic agents.

Amiodarone is less deleterious than most other antiarrhythmic agents in patients with congestive heart failure. Moreover, the vasodilatory effect of amiodarone partially compensates for the negative inotropic effect because of afterload reduction. The vasodilatory effect of amiodarone, considered to be its main hemodynamic action, results both from a direct effect on vascular smooth muscle and from an alpha-adrenoreceptor blocking effect.[3,44,45] Because amiodarone decreases myocardial contractility and produces either no change or a decrease in heart rate and peripheral vasodilation, it may reduce blood pressure.

The hemodynamic effect of amiodarone in congestive heart failure has been investigated only in a few patients. In 14 patients with Chagas myocarditis and congestive heart failure, the intravenous administration of amiodarone, 5 mg/kg, decreased heart rate and cardiac index and increased mean right atrial pressure, left ventricular end-diastolic pressure, and pulmonary and systemic vascular resistance. Almost all these parameters returned to control levels within 24 hours of administration of the drug.[46] In another study, 5 of 46 patients treated with amiodarone for 2 weeks to 7 months died of congestive heart failure.[8] In a third study, 9 of 70 patients underwent deterioration of congestive heart failure during treatment with amiodarone. Amiodarone also has a coronary vasodilatory effect.[47] This effect is of little relevance in children, however.

Clinical Pharmacology

Amiodarone may be administered intravenously or orally. The pharmacokinetics and even electrophysiologic properties of these routes of administration are different. Amiodarone has a unique pharmacokinetic profile. It is absorbed from the gastrointestinal tract, with systemic bioavailability of about 50%.[48,49] The drug may be detected in the plasma within 1.5 hours of oral administration, and a peak plasma level is achieved within 4 to 6 hours.[13,50] A steady-state level of 3.84 ± 2.92 µg/ml has been reported. In a study of children under 14 years of age, therapeutic plasma concentrations of amiodarone ranged between 0.4 and 2.3 mg/L, and plasma levels of the metabolite desmethylamiodarone were 0.2 to 2.6 mg/L.[26] Treatment was ineffective in 2 children with amiodarone plasma concentrations of 1.1 and 1.0 mg/L, respectively.

Amiodarone is unique in that its therapeutic effect is evident only after 4 to 5 days of oral administration. Occasionally, the maximal effect may take several weeks or even several months to become evident.[51] Hesslein and associates reported that drug's effect was observable within 2 to 12 days (mean 4 days) of initiation of oral amiodarone treatment in children with ventricular and supraventricular arrhythmias.[12] Coumel and Fidelle reported that, in 91 children treated with oral amiodarone, the delay before response to treatment ranged from 1 to 16 days (mean 4.1 days).[11] In 8 cases of supraventricular tachycardia, an effect was achieved within 5 to 24 hours of administration of a single oral dose. In children, serum amiodarone levels of 0.7 to 1.8 mg/L (mean 1.4) are within the therapeutic range during long-term administration of the drug.[12]

Animal experiments have shown that the concentration of amiodarone in muscle and adipose tissue is 10 to 30 times higher than in the plasma. Determination of plasma concentrations is of little or no value in assessing the efficacy of treatment.

Another unique pharmacokinetic property of amiodarone is its long elimination half-life. In most studies in adults, the elimination half-life has ranged between 6 and 30 days. This long half-life may be, at least partially, explained by the accumulation of the drug in adipose tissue. This hypothesis is supported by the finding of a biphasic elimination of amiodarone after prolonged treatment.[52] Initially, a rapid elimination phase occurs, resulting from elimination of the drug from highly perfused tissues. It is followed by a slow elimination phase, resulting from elimination of the drug from poorly perfused tissues.

The elimination half-life of amiodarone in children is long, but it is shorter than in adults. This difference could be attributed in part to the smaller amount of adipose tissue in children. Because of the drug's long elimination half-life, a considerable delay occurs between termination of treatment and recurrence of the arrhythmias. In adults, the reappearance of arrhythmias may be delayed several months after discontinuance of the drug. In children, the arrhythmias may reappear earlier, because of the more rapid metabolism of the drug. In a group of 31 children, arrhythmias recurred after a mean duration of 3.3 weeks from discontinuance of amiodarone. In 24 of these patients, the arrhythmia recurred within 2 weeks.[11] Age affects the response to the drug, and older children respond similarly to adults.[11]

Side Effects

An important limitation on the use of amiodarone is the high incidence of side effects, some of which are serious. The most important side effects are impairment of thyroid function, sinus bradycardia, corneal microdeposits, skin discoloration, pneumonitis, and neurologic effects. Most of these effects are reversible.

In children, the incidence of side effects of amiodarone is moderate. For example, 7 of 15 children aged 0.5 to 16 years developed side effects that required intervention during oral treatment with amiodarone. Three others had serologic evidence of side effects requiring observation alone. In another study, 3 of 24 children aged 1 week to 14 years required discontinuance of treatment because of side effects.[26] The adverse effects reported in children are usually similar to those observed in adults, but ocular and pulmonary side effects are uncommon in children. A recent study showed the side effects of amiodarone in children are common and are sometimes serious.[26]

Ocular Effects

The most important ocular side effects are corneal microdeposits and the appearance of halos around light sources. The corneal microdeposits are composed of yellow-brown pigmentation consisting of lysosomal inclusion of lipofuscin-like substance. These microdeposits appear mainly in the lower third of the cornea along the line of contact with the inferior eyelid. This location suggests a mechanical factor in the development of the microdeposits. These lesions may be seen only by slit lamp. Corneal microdeposits are common in adults. Harris and co-workers, studying 140 patients treated with amiodarone, stated that corneal microdeposits were found when sought.[53] This adverse effect depends on the dose of amiodarone and on the duration of treatment.

In children, ocular side effects of amiodarone are uncommon, especially when compared with the incidence in adults. Shahar and colleagues, of the Sheba Medical Center in Israel, observed no ocular effects in any of 10 infants and children treated with oral amiodarone.[25] I have seen this effect in 1 of 5 children; amiodarone treatment was initiated in this patient at the age of 7 years, but corneal microdeposits appeared only at the age of 11 years. Coumel and Fidelle found corneal microdeposits in 3 of 135 children treated with amiodarone for a mean duration of 4.2 months.[11] Hesslein and associates did not find ocular side effects in any of 15 children treated with amiodarone for 1 to 19 months (mean 6.1 months).[12] Rosenbaum and co-workers, studying a large series of patients treated with amiodarone, did not find this complication in children under the age of 13 years.[22]

The cause of the rarity of corneal microdeposits in children, as compared with the incidence of this complication in adults, is not known, but a higher degree of tear secretion may be involved in the corneal protection. Although these microdeposits are rare in children every child treated with amiodarone on a long-term basis should undergo ophthalmologic examination at intervals of 6 to 12 months. Such an examination is also recommended before the initiation of amiodarone treatment. Although the microdeposits may interfere with vision, no blindness or permanent visual damage has been observed,[54] and this effect is rarely a reason to discontinue treatment. In 16 patients in whom amiodarone was discontinued for other reasons, corneal microdeposits disappeared within 7 months.[55] The use of artificial tears may prevent this complication.

Bucknall and associates reported that one of 24 children treated with amiodarone developed gritty eyes.[26] Short-term therapy with high doses of amiodarone may cause a transient appearance of halos around lights. Again, no permanent damage occurs.

Discoloration of Skin, Photosensitivity, and Urticaria

Cutaneous side effects appear in up to about half the patients treated with amiodarone,[22] although in large series, the usual incidence of this effect has been about 10%.[56] The main cutaneous side effect is blue discoloration of the skin;[57] it is worsened by exposure to sun, and disappears gradually on discontinuance of the drug or, occasionally, after a reduction in dose. Most physicians discontinue the drug after the appearance of blue discoloration of the skin, however, rather than reducing the dose and waiting the several weeks or even months required for the effect to disappear.

In a group of 135 children treated with amiodarone, photosensitivity developed in 4 children, and bluish skin discoloration occurred in 1 child after 72 hours of treatment. I observed only 1 case of photosensitivity and 1 of bluish skin discoloration in 12 patients treated with amiodarone at the Sheba Medical Center in Israel. Shahar and colleagues observed a sole case of urticaria among 15 children treated with amiodarone.[25] In another group of 24 children, aged 1 week to 14 years and treated with amiodarone at a mean dose of 10.6 mg/kg/day for 2 weeks to 4.6 years, 11 developed photosensitivity, 2 had gray pigmentation, and 1 had a skin rash.[26]

Cardiovascular Effects

Adverse cardiovascular effects associated with amiodarone treatment are uncommon. Although the drug consistently prolongs the spontaneous sinus node cycle length, symptomatic bradycardia is unusual. Complete atrioventricular block and worsening of pre-existing conduction disturbances have been reported during treatment with amiodarone,[22, 58] although these complications are rare in children. One case of complete heart block was found among 24 children treated with amiodarone for a mean period of 1.5 years.[26] Several investigators have not seen any cases of progressive heart block, even in patients with pre-existing conduction disturbances.[27, 56] A transient sinus arrest after electroversion of ventricular fibrillation was reported in 3 patients treated with amiodarone.[59,60] One case of sinus arrest occurred among 24 children treated with amiodarone for a mean period of 1.5 years.[26]

Intravenous administration of amiodarone may cause hypotension. In my experience, intravenous administration of amiodarone to a 60-year-old patient caused bradycardia, hypotension, and sudden death.

Amiodarone may be associated with ventricular fibrillation or polymorphous ventricular tachycardia (torsade de pointes).[61-63] This effect is probably related to prolongation of the QTc interval.

Impairment of Thyroid Function

Impairment of thyroid function is an uncommon but serious complication of treatment with amiodarone. About 200 cases have been reported in the literature or have been observed by me and my co-workers. This complication is especially deleterious in patients with pre-existing coronary artery disease or arrhythmias, which may be worsened by hyperthyroidism. The impairment of thyroid function may appear either as hyperthyroidism or as hypothyroidism. The incidence of thyroid dysfunction varies among reports. Bekaert and associates found an incidence of 3.1% of hyperthyroidism.[64] Rosenbaum and co-workers reported 2 cases of hyperthyroidism and 2 cases of hypothyroidism among 252 patients treated with amiodarone.[22] Thyroid function should be evaluated before initiation of treatment with amiodarone and at regular intervals during treatment.

Although the incidence of impairment of thyroid function in children has usually been considered to be low, a review of the literature shows that the incidence of this complication is not much lower than in adults. For example, in a series of 135 children treated with amiodarone, 1 developed hypothyroidism, and 2 developed hyperthyroidism.[11] In another series of 15 children, 3 developed chemical hypothyroidism, and 2 required hormone replacement.[12] Two of 24 children treated with amiodarone for a mean period of 1.5 years developed an impairment of thyroid function.[26]

Patients with a previous history of thyroid disease are more susceptible to impairment of thyroid function by amiodarone than other patients. These adverse effects, whether manifesting as hyperthyroidism or as hypothyroidism, usually disappear within several weeks or months of discontinuance of the drug. Permanent damage is rare.

The cause of the amiodarone-induced thyroid dysfunction is unknown, but the high content of iodine in the molecule of amiodarone probably plays some role in the development of this side effect.

Neurologic Effects

The incidence of neurologic side effects may be up to 50% in patients treated with amiodarone,[65] although it is usually much lower. These effects include peripheral sensorimotor neuropathy, extrapyramidal symptoms, proximal muscle weakness, tremor, and ataxia. In one study, 4 of 135 children developed nightmares, hallucinations, and personality problems that required cessation of treatment.[11] These signs may have been precursors of hyperthyroidism. In other small series of children treated with amiodarone, no neurologic side effects were reported.

Pulmonary Effects

Prolonged treatment with amiodarone may be associated with pulmonary side effects including pneumonitis and alveolar fibrosis. In one review, the incidence of pulmonary side effects in patients treated with amiodarone was estimated to be 1.4%.[66] Histologic studies showed thickening of the alveolar septa with proliferation of fibroblasts and collagen, fibrosing pneumonitis, accumulation of macrophages in alveolar spaces, and hyperplasia of type-2 pneumocytes, occasionally with bronchiolitis obliterans.

Adverse pulmonary effects usually appear in elderly patients who receive high doses of amiodarone for long periods. These effects appear in younger patients who receive doses as low as 400 mg daily for short periods, however.[67] It is difficult to predict which patients will develop adverse pulmonary effects, although the presence of pre-existing pulmonary disease is a risk factor.[68] Attempts have been made to use the level of the angiotensin-converting enzyme, which is found in the lungs, as an early predictor of pulmonary damage. Patients with pneumonitis and alveolar fibrosis develop dyspnea, cough, pleuritic pain, and hypoxia, complications that may be fatal. In a series of 13 patients with pulmonary complications, 3 patients died and 10 survived after discontinuance of amiodarone and administration of corticosteroids.

Impairment of Hepatic Function

This uncommon complication of amiodarone may occur in children. It was observed in 2 of 24 children treated with a mean dose of 10.6 mg/kg/day for 2 weeks to 14 years.[2, 6]

Drug Interactions

Amiodarone was originally considered to have only minimal interactions with other drugs. Amiodarone does interact with several drugs, however, and some of these interactions may be of special significance in infants and children.

Digoxin

Amiodarone may increase serum digoxin levels in patients or in animals concomitantly treated with digoxin.[69, 70] In 22 patients, treatment with amiodarone for 2 months elevated the serum digoxin level from 1.0 ± 0.4 to 1.9 ± 0.8 ng/ml. This interaction is of special significance in infants and children because many pediatric patients with supraventricular arrhythmias treated with amiodarone are initially given digoxin. Digoxin is the drug of first choice in infants with Wolff-Parkinson-White syndrome. Moreover, many of these infants and children have congestive cardiomyopathy, primary endocardial fibroelastosis, or other causes of congestive heart failure, for which they are treated with digoxin. The addition of amiodarone elevates the serum digoxin levels and may cause toxicity. For example, in a group of 11 children treated with digoxin, the administration of amiodarone increased serum digoxin levels in 6 patients, and changes in digoxin dosage were required in 4 patients.[12] I have studied a child with primary endocardial fibroelastosis and atrial flutter in whom the addition of amiodarone almost doubled the serum level of digoxin.

Koren and associates reported that the addition of amiodarone to digoxin therapy in 9 children caused an increase of 68 to 800% in digoxin plasma concentration in the presence of preserved renal function.[71] The elimination half-life of digoxin was prolonged. These investigators attributed the accumulation of digoxin to the inhibition of tubular secretion of digoxin by amiodarone or to a reduction in the volume of distribution of digoxin. The effect of amiodarone on digoxin may take several weeks to develop because of amiodarone's long half-life. Monitoring of plasma digoxin concentrations is required in all children treated concomitantly with digoxin and amiodarone.

Quinidine

In one report, amiodarone increased the serum levels of quinidine in almost all patients studied.[72] Because children with resistant arrhythmias are likely to receive both drugs, this interaction should be kept in mind.

Procainamide

The administration of amiodarone increased the serum levels of procainamide in the majority of the patients in one study.[72]

Aprindine

Amiodarone may elevate the serum levels of the antiarrhythmic agent aprindine and may exacerbate its side effects.[73] Because aprindine is rarely given to children, however, this interaction is of little relevance to pediatric cardiologists.

Anticoagulant Agents

Amiodarone augments the effect of the anticoagulant agent sodium warfarin by further depressing the coagulation factors that depend on vitamin K.[74, 75] The accurate mechanism of this interaction is not known. One report has suggested that the maintenance dose of warfarin should be reduced by half when amiodarone is added to a therapeutic regimen.[76] This interaction is of special significance in children with arrhythmias after valve replacement.

Effects During Pregnancy and Lactation

Only limited information exists on the effect of amiodarone, administered during pregnancy, on the fetus. Iodine, a major constituent of the amiodarone molecule, does cross the placenta and concentrates in the fetal thyroid gland, however. McKenna and co-workers gave amiodarone to a pregnant woman with atrial fibrillation during the last month of pregnancy.[77] After the child's birth, the levels of amiodarone and its main metabolite in the neonatal plasma were 25% of those in the maternal plasma; the neonate had normal thyroid function. Amiodarone is excreted in breast milk.[77] At present, it is inadvisable to give amiodarone during pregnancy or lactation.

Dosage and Administration

Administration

Amiodarone is given orally in a large loading dose, followed by a smaller maintenance dose. The effect is evident at least 4 days after the initiation of treatment. In adults, a loading dose of 800 to 1600 mg is given for 7 to 10 days, followed by a maintenance dose of 100 to 600 mg daily. The doses prescribed in Europe are usually lower than those used in the United States.

In children, high loading doses of amiodarone are administered, and the maintenance doses are not much lower than in adults. For example, Hesslein and colleagues used loading doses of 200 to 800 mg/day (8.3 to 50 mg/kg, mean 19.1 mg/kg) for 7 to 10 days, followed by maintenance doses of 100 to 300 mg/day (2.2 to 25 mg/kg, mean 7.2 mg/kg), in a group of 15 children with ventricular or supraventricular arrhythmias.[12] Coumel and Fidelle used an initial daily oral dose of 800 mg adjusted according to the child's surface area.[11] This dose was maintained for an average of 2 weeks; it was then reduced by half, and was finally given 5 days a week.

Intravenous Administration

Because of its electrophysiologic properties, intravenously administered amiodarone is effective only in patients with supraventricular tachycardia. In adults, a bolus injection should not exceed 5 mg/kg, injected over 10 min. This dose may be followed by a continuous infusion of 1000 mg over 24 hours. A safe and effective intravenous dose for children has not been determined.

References

1. Gloor, H.O., Urthaler, F., and James, T.N.: The immediate electrophysiologic effects on the canine sinus node and AV junctional region. American College of Cardiology, 1982.
2. Patterson, E., et al.: Depression of cardiac mitochondrial respiratory activity by chronic amiodarone treatment—reversal by T_3. American Heart Association, 1983.
3. Singh, B.N., and Vaughan-Williams, E.M.: The effects of amiodarone, a new antianginal drug, on cardiac muscle. Br. J. Pharmacol., 39:657, 1970.
4. Coutte, R., et al.: Etude electrocardiologique des effects de l'amiodarone sur la conduction intracardiaque chez l'homme. Ann. Cardiol. Angeiol., (Paris), 25:543, 1976.
5. Wellens, H.J.J., et al.: Effect of amiodarone in the Wolff-Parkinson-White syndrome. Am. J. Cardiol., 38:189, 1976.
6. Finerman, W.B., et al.: Electrophysiologic effects of chronic amiodarone therapy in patients with ventricular arrhythmias. Am. Heart J., 104:987, 1982.
7. Nademanee, K., et al.: Refractory life threatening ventricular arrhythmias: control by amiodarone prophylaxis. (Abstract.) Circulation, 62 (Suppl. III):151, 1980.
8. Waxman, H.L., et al.: Amiodarone for control of sustained ventricular tachyarrhythmia: clinical and electrophysiologic effects in 51 patients. Am. J. Cardiol., 50:1066, 1982.
9. Touboul, P., et al.: Bases electrophysiologiques de l'action antiarrythmique de l'amiodarone chez l'homme. Arch. Mal. Coeur, 69:845, 1976.
10. Sicart, M., et al.: Action hémodynamique de l'amiodarone intraveineuse chez l'homme. Arch. Mal. Coeur, 70:219, 1977.
11. Coumel, P., and Fidelle, J.: Amiodarone in the treatment of cardiac arrhythmias in children: one hundred thirty-five cases. Am. Heart J., 100:1063, 1980.
12. Hesslein, P.S., et al.: Oral amiodarone therapy in childhood: early experience. Pediatr. Cardiol., 4:313, 1983.
13. Kannan, R., et al.: Amiodarone kinetics after oral doses. Clin. Pharmacol. Ther., 31:438, 1982.
14. Oreto, G., et al.: Intoxication aigue par l'amiodarone. Arch. Mal. Coeur, 73:857, 1980.
15. Pickoff, A.S., et al.: Dose-dependent electrophysiologic effects of amiodarone in the immature canine heart. Am. J. Cardiol., 52:621, 1983.
17. Charlier, R., et al.: Recherches dans la série des benzofuranes. Cardiologia, 54:83, 1969.
18. Schoenfeld, P.L., and Richard, J.D.: Influence of acute and chronic amiodarone impregnation of spontaneous and induced ventricular dysrhythmias following coronary artery ligation in dogs. J. Am. Coll. Cardiol., 1, 1983.
19. Michat, L., et al.: Effets antiarythmiques de l'amiodarone en injectable en réanimation de chirurgie cardio-vasculaire. Nouv. Presse Med., 5:31, 1976.
20. Rowland, E., and Krikler, D.M.: Electrophysiological assessment of amiodarone in treatment of resistant supraventricular arrhythmias. Br. Heart J., 44:82, 1980.
21. Feld, G. et al.: Oral amiodarone in patients with AV nodal and bypass tract reentrant supraventricular tachycardia: electrophysiology and mechanism of suppression of inducible tachycardia. American College of Cardiology, 1983.
22. Rosenbaum, M.B., et al.: Clinical efficacy of amiodarone as an antiarrhythmic agent. Am. J. Cardiol., 38:934, 1976.
23. Graboys, T.B., Podrid, P.J., and Lown, B.: Efficacy of amiodarone for refractory supraventricular tachyarrhythmias. Am. Heart J. 106:870, 1983.

24. Wheeler, P.J., et al.: Amiodarone in the treatment of refractory supraventricular and ventricular arrhythmias. Postgrad. Med. J., 55:1, 1979.
25. Shahar, E., et al.: Amiodarone in control of sustained tachyarrhythmia in children with WPW syndrome. Pediatrics, 72:813, 1983.
26. Bucknall, C., et al.: Use of amiodarone in children. Proceedings of the British Cardiac Society. Br. Heart J., 51:681, 1984.
27. Benaim, R., and Uzan, C.: The antiarrhythmic effects of amiodarone studied by programmed electrical stimulation of the heart in patients with paroxysmal re-entrant supraventricular tachycardia. J. Electrocardiol., 11:253, 1978.
28. Santos, A.L., et al.: Conversion of atrial fibrillation to sinus rhythm with amiodarone. Acta Med. Port., 1:15, 1979.
29. Garson, A., Jr., et al.: Atrial flutter in the young: a collaborative study of 380 cases. Pediatr. Cardiol., 4:307, 1983.
30. Greene, H.L., et al.: Toxic and therapeutic effects of amiodarone in the treatment of cardiac arrhythmias. J. Am. Coll. Cardiol., 2:1114, 1983.
31. McKenna, W.J., Oakley, C.M., and Goodwin, J.P.: The influence of amiodarone on survival in hyperthropic cardiomyopathy. American Heart Association, 1983.
32. Pioselli, D., et al.: Management of paroxysmal ventricular tachycardia in patients with mitral valve prolapse. In Management of Ventricular Tachycardia. Edited by E. Sandoe et al. Amsterdam, Excerpta Medica, 1978.
33. Grayboys, T.B., Podrid, P., and Lown, B.: Effectiveness of amiodarine for refractory atrial tachyarrhythmias. American College of Cardiology, 1982.
34. Brown, A.K.: Use of amiodarone in bradycardia-tachycardia syndrome. Br. Heart J. 42:573, 1979.
35. Bashour, T., Jokhadar, M., and Cheng, T.: Effective management of the long Q-T syndrome with amiodarone. Chest, 79:704.
36. Nademanee, K., et al.: Does intravenous amiodarone shorten the latency of the onset of antiarrhythmic action of oral amiodarone in ventricular dysrhythmias? J. Am. Coll. Cardiol., 1:630, 1983.
37. Wellens, H.J.J., et al.: A comparison of the electrophysiological effects of intravenous and oral amiodarone. Am. J. Cardiol., 49:1043, 1982.
38. Rotmensch, H.H., Belhassen, B., and Ferguson, R.K.: Amiodarone—benefits and risks in perspective. Am. Heart J., 104:1117, 1982.
39. Frank, R., et al.: Les méthodes provocatives dans l'étude de l'amiodarone per os dans les tachycardies ventricularies et celles du syndrome de Wolff-Parkinson-White. In Colloque sur l'amiodarone. Paris, Documentation Medicale Labaz, 1977, p. 35.
40. Heger, J.J., Rinkenberger, R.L., and Zipes, D.P.: Amiodarone: clinical efficacy and electrophysiology during long-term therapy for recurrent ventricular tachycardia or ventricular fibrillation. N. Engl. J. Med., 305:539, 1981.
41. Waxman, H.L., et al.: Amiodarone for sustained ventricular tachyarrhythmias: electrophysiologic study is not predictive of clinical efficacy. American Heart Association, 1983.
42. McGovern, B., et al.: Predictive accuracy of electrophysiologic testing in the treatment of ventricular arrhythmias with amiodarone. Circulation, 66(Suppl. II):891, 1982.
43. Horowitz, L.N., et al.: Utility of electrophysiologic testing of amiodarone for ventricular tachyarrhythmias. American Heart Association, 1983.
44. Charlier, R.: Cardiac actions in the dog of a new antagonist of adrenergic excitation which does not produce competitive blockade of adrenoceptors. Br. J. Pharmacol., 39:668, 1970.
45. Polster, P., and Broekhuysen, J.: The adrenergic antagonism of amiodarone. Biochem. Pharmacol., 25:131, 1976.
46. Bellotti, G., et al.: Hemodynamic effects of intravenous administration of amiodarone in congestive heart failure from chronic Chagas' disease. Am. J. Cardiol., 52:1046, 1983.
47. Remme, W.J., Hoogenhuyze, D.V., and Kruyssen, D.A.: Acute hemodynamic and anti-ischemic effects of intravenous amiodarone in man. American Heart Association, 1983.

48. Wellens, H.J.J., et al.: A comparison of the electrophysiologic effects of intravenous and oral amiodarone in the same patient. Circulation, 69:120, 1984.
49. Riva, E., et al.: Pharmacokinetics of amiodarone in man. J. Cardiovasc. Pharmacol., 4:264, 1982.
50. Haffajee, C.I., et al.: Clinical pharmacokinetics and efficacy of amiodarone for refractory tachyarrhythmias. Circulation, 67:1349, 1983.
51. Rosenbaum, M.B., et al.: Ten years of experience with amiodarone. Am. Heart J., 106:957, 1983.
52. Holt, D.W., et al.: Amiodarone pharmacokinetics. Am. Heart J., 106:840, 1983.
53. Harris, L., et al.: Side effects of long-term amiodarone therapy. Circulation, 67:145, 1983.
54. Marcus, F.I., et al.: Clinical pharmacology and therapeutic applications of the antiarrhythmic agent, amiodarone. Am. Heart J., 101:480, 1981.
55. Ingram, D.V.: Ocular effects in long-term amiodarone therapy. Am. Heart J 106:902, 1963.
56. Cauchier, J.P., Brochier, M., and Raynaud, R.: Etude clinique des effets antiarythmiques ventriculaires de l'amiodarone (orale et injectable). Ann. Cardiol. Angeiol. (Paris) 22:427, 1973.
57. Heger, J.J., Prystowsky, E.N., and Zipes, D.P.: Relationships between amiodarone dosage, drug concentrations, and adverse side effects. Am. Heart J., 106:931, 1983.
58. Bosc, E., Souchon, H., and Cabasson, J.: Troubles de la conduction intraventriculaire après amiodarone. (Letter.) Nouv. Presse Med., 6:196, 1977.
59. McGovern, B., Garan, H., and Ruskin, J.N.: Sinus arrest during treatment with amiodarone. Br. Med. J., 284:160, 1982.
60. Guanggeng, Cui., and Urthaler, F.: Ventricular flutter during treatment with amiodarone. Brief Reports, 2:609, 1982.
61. McComb, J.M., et al.: Amiodarone induced ventricular fibrillation. Eur. J. Cardiol., 11:381, 1980.
62. Keren, A., et al.: Atypical ventricular tachycardia (torsade de pointes) induced by amiodarone. Chest, 81:384, 1982.
63. Sclarovsky, S., et al.: Amiodarone induced polymorphous ventricular tachycardia. Am. Heart J., 105:1, 1983.
64. Bekaert, J., Solvay, H., and van Schepdael, S.: Etude de l'effet de l'amiodarone sur la fonction thyroidienne. Coeur Med. Interne, 18:241, 1979.
65. Charness, M., et al.: Frequent neurologic toxicity associated with amiodarone therapy. ACC 1983.
66. Sobol, S.M., and Rakita, L.: Pneumonitis and pulmonary fibrosis associated with amiodarone treatment: a possible complication of a new antiarrhythmic drug. Circulation, 65:819, 1982.
67. Dudognon, P., et al.: Neuropathie au chlorhydrate d'amiodarone: étude clinique et histopathologique d'une nouvelle lipidose médicamenteuse. Rev. Neurol. (Paris), 135:527, 1979.
68. Küdenchuk, P.J., et al.: Predicting risk of amiodarone pulmonary toxicity. American Heart Association, 1983.
69. Moysey, J.O., et al.: Amiodarone increases plasma digoxin concentrations. Br. Med. J., 282:272, 1981.
70. Oetgen, W.J., et al.: Amiodarone digoxin interaction: clinical and experimental observations. Circulation, 66(Suppl. II):1529, 1982.
71. Koren, G., et al.: Digoxin toxicity associated with amiodarone therapy in children. J. Pediatr., 104:467, 1984.
72. Saal, A.K., et al.: Interaction of amiodarone with quinidine and procainamide. Circulation, 66(Suppl. II):895, 1982.
73. Southworth, W., Friday, K.J., and Ruffy, R.: Possible amiodarone-aprindine interaction. Am. Heart J., 104:323, 1982.
74. Simpson, W.T.: Amiodarone in cardiac arrhythmias. In International Congress Series No. 16, Royal Society of Medicine. New York, Grune & Stratton, 1979, p. 50.
75. Martinowitz, U., et al.: Interaction between warfarin sodium and amiodarone. (Letter.) N. Engl. J. Med., 304:671, 1981.

76. Hamer, A., et al.: The potentiation of warfarin anticoagulation by amiodarone. American Heart Association, 1982.
77. McKenna, W.J., et al.: Amiodarone therapy during pregnancy. Am. J. Cardiol., 51:1231, 1983.

Chapter 30

Bretylium Tosylate

Bretylium tosylate is an antiarrhythmic drug used mainly for suppression and prevention of recurrent ventricular fibrillation or ventricular tachycardia resistant to conventional Class I antiarrhythmic drugs. The drug has been used for this indication for about 20 years. It has a unique mechanism of action, an effect on postganglionic adrenergic neurons. In children, bretylium tosylate is used mainly in patients with resistant ventricular fibrillation associated with digitalis toxicity.

Pharmacologic Properties

Bretylium tosylate concentrates in sympathetic postganglionic neuron endings and inhibits the release of norepinephrine, which occurs when the neuron is stimulated. Bretylium also inhibits the reuptake of released epinephrine and thereby causes depletion of norepinephrine stores. This effect is responsible for some of the antiarrhythmic actions of this agent, as well as for its antihypertensive effects. Bretylium tosylate also has membrane-stabilizing and weak cholinergic effects.

Electrophysiologic Effects

Bretylium tosylate has a direct antifibrillatory effect. Because it increases refractoriness and the duration of the action potential without altering conduction velocity, bretylium tosylate may be classified as a Class III antiarrhythmic agent. It does not decrease the rate of rise of phase-0 or phase-4 depolarization.[1,2] In at least one study, the drug shortened the duration of the action potential and increased conduction velocity.[3]

Soon after administration, bretylium tosylate may enhance conduction, as a result of the initial release of catecholamines. This characteristic is important in the abolition of re-entrant arrhythmias. This early release also causes a transient acceleration of sinus rhythm in the first 30 min after administration of the drug.[4,5] Bretylium tosylate does not alter electrocardiographic intervals. It increases the fibrillation threshold in damaged myocardium.

Effect in Arrhythmias

The most important use of bretylium tosylate is in the termination of ventricular fibrillation resistant to conventional Class I antiarrhythmic drugs and in the early prevention of recurrences of such arrhythmias. Therapeutic doses of bretylium tosylate have increased the ventricular fibrillation threshold up to 12 times.[6]

In human patients, bretylium tosylate has suppressed ventricular fibrillation associated with acute myocardial infarction or cardiac surgical procedures.[7-9] It is also effective in patients resistant to high doses of lidocaine and D.C. shock. Moreover, the drug increases the efficacy of D.C. shock in patients with ventricular fibrillation.[10] Although the onset of the electrophysiologic effects of bretylium tosylate may be delayed for several hours, the drug is effective in the immediate treatment of ventricular fibrillation.

Bretylium tosylate has also suppressed other ventricular arrhythmias in patients with acute myocardial infarction.[11] It does not prevent the induction of ventricular arrhythmias by programmed electrical stimulation, however.[12]

In children, bretylium tosylate is used rarely, mainly to suppress ventricular fibrillation associated with digitalis toxicity. It is important in such patients to correct hypokalemia not only because of the usual considerations in digitalis toxicity, but also because bretylium tosylate is less effective in the presence of hypokalemia.

Hemodynamic Effects

Bretylium tosylate causes peripheral vasodilation and a reduction in systemic arterial pressure.[8] Soon after administration of the drug, a transient pressor response may occur because of the release of catecholamines.[13] Tolerance to the hypotensive effect usually develops within a few days. The drug has also an early positive inotropic effect.

Clinical Pharmacology

In clinical practice, bretylium tosylate is given only intravenously because oral administration does not provide appropriate and predictable plasma drug levels.[14] The antiarrhythmic effect is evident within 10 to 30 min of injection. The drug concentrates in the myocardium, and its effects are related to the myocardial concentration.[6] Therapeutic plasma levels are 4 to 6 μg/ml.[15] The mean elimination half-life of bretylium tosylate is 9.8 hours, but it varies among patients. Bretylium tosylate is eliminated unchanged in the urine.

Side Effects

Bretylium tosylate is generally well tolerated. The most important side effect is hypotension, which occurs in up to 75% of patients.[16, 17]

An initial hypertensive reaction may also be observed. Other side effects are nausea, vomiting, and pain and swelling of the parotid gland.

Drug Interactions

Class I antiarrhythmic drugs, mainly quinidine, may antagonize the electrophysiologic effects of bretylium tosylate.[18] The antiarrhythmic efficacy of bretylium tosylate is therefore highest when the drug is administered alone.[9]

Dosage and Administration

The initial dose is 5 to 10 mg/kg intravenously. It may be repeated within an hour. The maintenance dose is 5 to 10 mg/kg, 4 times daily, or a continuous infusion at a rate of 1 to 2 mg/min.

References

1. Bigger, J.T., Jr., and Jaffe, C.C.: The effect of bretylium tosylate on the electrophisiologic properties of ventricular muscle and Purkinje fibers. Am. J. Cardiol., 27:82, 1971.
2. Wit, A.C., et al.: Electrophysiologic effects of bretylium tosylate on single fibers of the canine specialized conducting system and ventricle. J. Pharmacol. Exp. Ther., 173:334, 1970.
3. Watanabe, Y., et al.: Electrophysiological mechanisms of bretylium tosylate. (Abstract.) Fed. Proc., 28:269, 1969.
4. Cardinal, R., and Sasyniuk, B.I.: Electrophysiological effects of bretylium tosylate in subendocardial Purkinje fibers from infarcted canine hearts. J. Pharmacol. Exp. Ther., 204:159, 1978.
5. Fujimoto, T., et al.: Electrophysiologic effects of bretylium on canine ventricular muscle during acute ischemia and reperfusion. Am. Heart J., 105:966, 1983.
6. Anderson, J.L., et al.: Kinetics of antifibrillatory effects of bretylium: correlation with myocardial drug concentrations. Am. J. Cardiol., 46:583, 1980.
7. Dhurandhar, R.W., et al.: Bretylium tosylate in the management of refractory ventricular fibrillation. Can. Med. Assoc. J., 105:161, 1971.
8. Holder, D.A., et al.: Experience with bretylium tosylate by a hospital cardiac arrest team. Circulation, 55:541, 1977.
9. Bernstein, J.G., and Koch-Weser, J.: Effectiveness of bretylium tosylate against refractory ventricular arrhythmias. Circulation, 45:1024, 1972.
10. Haynes, R.E., et al.: Comparison of bretylium tosylate and lidocaine in management of out of hospital ventricular fibrillation: a randomized clinical trial. Am. J. Cardiol., 48:353, 1981.
11. Terry, G., et al.: Bretylium tosylate in treatment of refractory ventricular arrhythmias complicating myocardial infarction. Br. Heart J., 32:21, 1970.
12. Bauernfeind, R., et al.: Lack of effectiveness of bretylium in paroxysmal sustained ventricular tachycardia. Am. J. Cardiol., 47:438, 1981.
13. Anderson, J.L., et al.: Serial electrophysiologic effects of bretylium in man. American Heart Association, 198, 1982.
14. Anderson, J.A., et al.: Clinical pharmacokinetics of intravenous and oral bretylium in survivors of ventricular tachycardia or fibrillation. J. Cardiovasc. Pharmacol., 3:485, 1981.
15. Woosley, R.L., et al.: Pharmacologic reversal of hypotensive effect complicating antiarrhythmic therapy with bretylium. Clin. Pharmacol. Ther., 32:313, 1982.
16. Koch-Weser, J.: Drug therapy—bretylium. N. Engl. J. Med., 300:473, 1979.

17. Bauernfeind, R.A., et al.: Electrophysiologic testing of bretylium tosylate in sustained ventricular tachycardia. Am. Heart J., *105*:973, 1983.
18. De Azevedo, I.M., et al.: Electrophysiologic antagonism of quinidine and bretylium tosylate. Am. J. Cardiol., *33*:633, 1974.

Chapter 31

Adenosine and Adenosine Triphosphate

Adenosine and adenosine triphosphate (ATP) are antiarrhythmic agents used to terminate, but not to prevent, re-entrant arrhythmias that incorporate the atrioventricular node in their cycle. Usually, verapamil is considered the drug of choice for this indication, but several investigators have suggested that adenosine and ATP may be the drugs of choice in adults as well as in children.[1,2] These agents are effective in terminating attacks of supraventricular arrhythmia in patients of all age groups, except tiny infants. The most important advantage of adenosine and ATP is their short elimination half-life of less than a minute. This feature allows repeated administration of increasing doses. Moreover, if an adverse hemodynamic effect occurs, it is of short duration. The main disadvantage of these drugs is the high incidence of adverse effects on impulse generation and conduction.

Adenosine or ATP administration is recommended to terminate supraventricular tachycardia when verapamil has failed or when intravenous administration of verapamil is contraindicated, such as in patients with severe impairment of left ventricular function, congestive heart failure due to organic heart disease or prolonged sustained arrhythmia, shock, severe hypotension, or previous administration of beta-adrenoreceptor blocking agents still present in the plasma. Adenosine and ATP are used in Europe, primarily in France.

Pharmacologic Properties

Adenosine and ATP have strong depressant effects on the sinus and atrioventricular nodes.[1,3,4] These direct effects of the drugs result from depression of the slow inward calcium current and increased potassium conductance.[5] These drugs also have a potent vagal effect, but their action in human patients is probably independent of such an effect.[1,4] Adenosine and ATP may have an antiadrenergic effect.[5] These agents are also potent peripheral vasodilators.[3]

Animal studies have shown that the electrophysiologic effects of adenosine are mediated by a specific extracellular receptor that is blocked by methylxanthines, but not by atropine.[1,6] Adenosine may be the active compound, and ATP may act by rapid degradation to adenosine, with release of phosphate.

Electrophysiologic Effects

The electrophysiologic effects of adenosine and ATP have been determined only recently, although these drugs have been used in Europe for many years. In isolated Purkinje fibers, adenosine alone has no effect on the action potential, but it may inhibit the shortening of action potential induced by isoproterenol.[7] In intact animals and in human patients, the main electrophysiologic effects of adenosine and ATP are suppression of the sinus and atrioventricular nodes.[1, 3, 4, 5, 8] In some patients, the drugs affect not only antegrade conduction, but also retrograde conduction in the atrioventricular node.

Administration of ATP during ventricular pacing resulted in transient, complete atrioventricular block or in slight prolongation of ventriculoatrial conduction in 5 of 9 patients with atrioventricular nodal re-entry.[9] In a study of patients with atrioventricular nodal re-entry, termination of re-entrant tachycardia resulted from a block in the antegrade slow pathway.[9] Adenosine released during ischemia may mediate the sinus bradycardia or atrioventricular nodal block seen in this condition.

Endogenous adenosine and ATP have little or no effect on accessory atrioventricular pathways, and termination of supraventricular tachycardia in patients with such pathways results from block in the atrioventricular node.

Effects in Arrhythmias

Adenosine and ATP are used mainly to terminate re-entrant supraventricular tachycardia incorporating the atrioventricular node. Their main advantage is their short elimination half-life. The drug disappears from the plasma in under 2 min. Therefore, repeated injections of increasing doses may be used, and any adverse hemodynamic effect is of short duration.

These drugs terminate 89 to 98% of attacks of paroxysmal supraventricular tachycardia in adults.[9-13] The arrhythmia is terminated within 10 to 40 sec of intravenous administration. Belhassen and Peleg stated that the most rapid effect is achieved by administration into a central vein.[14]

Belhassen and co-workers studied the effect of ATP on atrioventricular re-entrant tachycardia in 18 patients, 15 of them without evidence of organic heart disease.[9] Nine of the patients had atrioventricular nodal re-entrant tachycardia, and the other 9 had atrioventricular re-entrant tachycardia with retrograde conduction in an accessory pathway. ATP was given in a 20-mg intravenous dose. It terminated the tachycardia within 16 sec of administration in 8 of 9 patients with atrioventricular nodal re-entry, by a block in the antegrade slow pathway, and in all 9 patients with an accessory pathway, by an antegrade block in the atrioventricular node. Progressive prolongations of the AH interval were observed before termination of the tachycardia. Although the conversion from tachycardia to sinus rhythm was rapid in this study, it was not smooth. Transient episodes of second-degree or complete atrioventricular block or sinus bradycardia were observed in 8 of the 18 patients. These episodes were of short duration and did not require treatment, however.[9]

Similar findings have also been reported by other investigators. These adverse effects are an important disadvantage of adenosine and ATP over calcium antagonists such as verapamil. Greco and associates reported that ATP was as effective as verapamil and was more effective than digitalis in infants and children with paroxysmal supraventricular tachycardia.[2] Sixty-two children, aged 4 days to 12 years, were selected for the study. Fourteen of them were under a month old. The arrhythmia was terminated in about 90% of the patients treated with ATP or verapamil and in 61 to 71% of the patients treated with digitalis. ATP terminated the tachycardia in less than 1 min, and verapamil was effective within 2 min of intravenous administration. Digitalis, however, terminated the tachycardia only after as long as 2 hours. Therefore, these investigators recommended that ATP or verapamil should be used as drugs of first choice for termination of supraventricular tachycardia in infants and children.

Adenosine does not terminate supraventricular tachycardia due to intra-atrial re-entry or atrial flutter.[1] In animal experiments, adenosine converted induced atrial fibrillation to normal sinus rhythm.[15] Other animal studies, however, showed that atrial fibrillation and flutter can be readily induced by atrial pacing in the presence of adenosine.[15]

The case of a patient in whom atrial fibrillation developed after administration of ATP during both atrial and ventricular pacing has been reported.[16] This phenomenon may be related to shortening of the duration of the atrial action potential. Until this subject is clarified, I advise against using adenosine and ATP in children with atrial fibrillation and/or atrial flutter.

Hemodynamic Effects

Adenosine and ATP are potent peripheral vasodilators.[3] This effect does not usually cause hemodynamic deterioration independent of adverse effects on heart rate. For example, in a study of 17 patients, doses of adenosine sufficient to produce measurable electrophysiologic changes did not alter systemic blood pressure.[1] Despite this finding, one showed monitor blood pressure carefully in all patients treated with adenosine or ATP.

Clinical Pharmacology

Adenosine and ATP are administered only intravenously. The onset of their effect usually occurs within 10 to 50 sec of administration. If a rapid onset of action is desired, the drug should be injected into a central vein. If the effect is not achieved within 2 min, it will probably not occur at all. The elimination half-life of these agents is rapid, less than 1 min, because of a rapid degradation in the plasma and tissues.

Side Effects

Side effects of ATP are common, but they do not usually last long. In this respect, the drug differs from verapamil, which causes side effects only uncommonly, but effects that may be serious or, rarely, lethal. Side effects of adenosine are similar in adults and children. In adults, the important cardiac side effects are sinus arrest, sinus bradycardia, and varying degrees of atrioventricular block, appearing on termination of supraventricular tachycardia.[9, 11, 12] These side effects are usually transient and last no more than a few seconds or a few minutes; they rarely require treatment. Prolonged asystole has required a thoracic blow on rare occasions.[12, 14] None of 26 infants and children treated by Greco and colleagues with ATP developed cardiac arrest or long atrioventricular dissociation, except 1 child with heart failure who had a pause of 780 msec before returning to sinus rhythm.[2] Two of these children developed thoracic discomfort, and 2 developed dyspnea.

Noncardiac adverse effects of adenosine and ATP include flushing (in more than 50% of children), retching (in about 50%), vomiting, cramps, headache, malaise,[2] and, rarely, convulsions and bronchial asthma.[11]

In their review of adenosine and ATP, Belhassen and Pelleg stated that the side effects of these drugs appear to be dose-related.[14] DiMarco and co-workers reported that the use of low doses of 190 ± 88 µg/kg was associated with a low incidence of side effects.[1] It is not known whether adenosine or ATP has a higher incidence of side effects.

Dosage and Administration

Both adenosine and ATP should be given in a rapid intravenous injection lasting less than 5 sec. Slow injection is the most important cause of drug failure with these agents.

Adenosine

Doses of 170 ± 88 µg/kg in a rapid intravenous injection have been used by DiMarco and associates in adults, with high rates of efficacy and safety.[1] Repeated higher doses may be tried within a few minutes.

Adenosine Triphosphate

Doses of 20 mg in a rapid intraveous injection have been used by Belhassen and co-workers in adults.[9] Greco and colleagues used 3 to 5 mg in children younger under a year old and up to 15 mg in older children.[2]

References

1. DiMarco, J.P., et al.: Adenosine: electrophysiologic effects and therapeutic use for terminating paroxysmal supraventricular tachycardia. Circulation, 68:1254, 1983.
2. Greco, R., et al: Treatment of paroxysmal supraventricular tachycardia in infancy with digitalis, adenosine-5'-triphosphate, and verapamil: a comparative study. Circulation, 66:504, 1982.
3. Emelin, N., and Feidberg, W.: Systemic effects of adenosine triphosphate (ATP). Br. J. Pharmacol., 3:273, 1948.
4. Lechat, P., et al.: Mechanism of atrioventricular conduction blockage by adenosine triphosphate. In Recent Advances in Cardiac Arrhythmias. Edited by S. Levy and R. Gerard. London, John Libbey, 1983, p. 39.
5. Belardinelli, L., et al.: Chronotrophic and dromotropic effects of adenosine. In Regulatory Function of Adenosine. Edited by R. M. Berne et al. Boston, Martinus Nijhoff, 1983, p. 377.
6. Belardinelli, L., et al.: Extracellular action of adenosine and the antagonism by aminophylline on the atrioventricular conduction of isolated perfused guinea pig and rat hearts. Circ. Res., 51:569, 1982.
7. Rardon, D.P., and Bailey, J.C.: Attenuation of isoproterenol-induced electrophysiological changes by adenosine in canine cardiac Purkinje fibers. American College of Cardiology, 1983.
8. Leclercq, J.F., and Coumel, P.: Les effets de l'adenosine triphosphate (ATP) sur le noeud sinusal et le noeud auriculoventriculaire chez l'homme: variations selon le lieu d'injection. Coeur Med. Intern. (Paris), 17:541, 1978.
9. Belhassen, B., et al.: Electrophysiologic effects of adenosine-5'-triphosphate on atrioventricular reentrant tachycardia. Circulation, 68:827, 1983.
10. Somlo, E: Adenosine triphosphate in paroxysmal tachycardia. (Letter) Lancet, 268:1125, 1955.
11. Latour, H., et al.: L'utilisation de l-adenosine-5'-triphosphate dans le diagnostic et le traitement des tachycardies paroxystiques nodales. (Abstract.) Arch. Mal. Coeur, 61:239, 1968.
12. Motte, G., et al.: L'adenosine triphosphatique dans les tachycardies paroxystiques: intérêt diagnostique et thérapeutique. Nouv. Presse Med., 1:3057, 1972.
13. Komor, K. and Garas, Z.: Adenosine triphosphate in paroxysmal tachycardia. (Letter) Lancet, 93:269, 1955.
14. Belhassen, B., and Pelleg, A.: Acute management of paroxysmal supraventricular tachycardia: verapamil, adenosine triphosphate or adenosine? Am J Cardiol., 54:225, 1984.
15. Drury, A.N., and Szent-Gyoryi, A.: The physiological action of adenine compounds with especial reference to their action upon the mammalian heart. J. Physiol. (Lond.), 68:213, 1929.
16. Belhassen, B., et al.: Atrial fibrillation induced by adenosine triphosphate. Am. J. Cardiol., 53:1405, 1984.

Section VI
PROSTAGLANDINS AND PROSTAGLANDIN-SYNTHESIS INHIBITORS

The recognition of the effect of prostaglandins and inhibitors of their synthesis on the ductus arteriosus has been one of the most important developments in cardiovascular drug therapy in infants and children. This finding has led to the use of certain prostaglandins for sustaining the patency of the ductus arteriosus in infants with several complex congenital heart diseases, a lifesaving procedure in infants whose circulation depends on the patency of this structure. This development has also led to the use of indomethacin, a prostaglandin-synthesis inhibitor, for pharmacologic closure of patent ductus arteriosus in infants with an otherwise normal heart or in infants whose circulation does not depend on the patency of the ductus arteriosus. This procedure is still controversial. Prostaglandins are also under investigation for use in other cardiovascular diseases in infants and children. At present, prostaglandins and inhibitors of prostaglandin synthesis are vital components of cardiovascular therapy and research in the pediatric age group.

Prostaglandins were identified in the human umbilical cord about 20 years ago.[1] These compounds, which are derivatives of arachidonic acid, underwent various medical investigations, but their role in modulating cardiovascular homeostasis was not recognized until endogenous prostacyclin and thromboxane A_2 were discovered. Although the prostaglandins routinely used in pediatric cardiovascular medicine are of the E group, and prostacyclin (of the I group) is investigational, a general description of all prostaglandins is included here.

Structure and Classification

Prostaglandins are derivatives of arachidonic acid. They are 20-carbon, modified, unsaturated hydroxy fatty acids. They consist of a cyclopentane ring with 2 side chains. The side chains may contain 1 to 3 double bonds, and the prostaglandins are accordingly classified as belonging to group 1, 2, or 3. The compounds of groups 1 and 2 are used clinically in infants, and compounds of group 2 are used in adults.

The prostaglandins are further classified as series E, I, and F (PGE, PGI, PGF). Several other unstable compounds are formed in the processes of synthesis and metabolism of the prostaglandins, but their description is beyond the scope of this text. The prostaglandins are further classified into alpha and beta groups, according to the stereometric position of a hydroxyl group attached to carbon atom number 9 on the side chain. The prostaglandins used in infants are of the E group, with 1 or 2 double bonds. They are referred to by the abbreviations PGE_1 and PGE_2. Prostaglandin I_2 (PGI_2 or prostacyclin) is used in adults and is under investigation for use in children.

General Effects of Prostaglandins and Their Derivatives

In 1938, a report noted the marked sensitivity of placental vessels to an extract of the prostate gland. Not until the specific compounds were isolated and identified 30 years later, however, did it become possible to study their specific effects. The effects of various prostaglandins are often opposing. For example, the PGF compounds cause vasoconstriction of isolated umbilical vessels, whereas PGE_1 and PGE_2 are potent dilators of umbilical vessels. PGI_2 is also a potent vasodilator, but because this agent, which is located in vascular walls, was identified much later than PGE, most of the studies in infants have been conducted with PGE. Because the ductus arteriosus is a fetal vessel, with a structure similar to that of umbilical vessels, the finding that PGE dilates umbilical vessels has stimulated studies of the effect of PGE on the ductus arteriosus. PGI_2 has been investigated for possible use in treatment of angina pectoris and congestive heart failure in adults and treatment of pulmonary hypertension in children.

In the platelets, the predominant prostaglandin is thromboxane A_2 (TxA_2). This unstable compound has a short half-life and potent platelet-aggregating and vasoconstricting properties. It is also produced by phagocytes and, to some extent, by vascular endothelial cells.[3] This compound and agents modulating its metabolism play no role in pediatric cardiovascular therapy.

Thus, it appears that prostaglandins exert various, and occasionally opposing, effects that are important in homeostasis. Most prostaglandins are not circulating hormones, but rather act in the place of their production, namely, vascular walls or platelets. Prostacyclin is unique in several respects, among them the possibility of its being circulating hormone.[4]

References

1. Karim, S.M.M.: The identification of prostaglandins in human umbilical cord. Br. J. Pharmacol. Chemother., 29:230, 1967.

2. Von Euler, U.S.: Action of adrenaline, acetylcholine and other substances on nerve free vessels (human placenta). J. Physiol., 93:129, 1938.
3. Balzman, P.M. et al.: Prostacyclin and thromboxane A_2 synthesis by rabbit pulmonary artery. J. Pharmacol. Exp. Ther., 215:240, 1980.
4. Hwang, D.H., et al.: Species variation in serum levels of prostaglandins (PG's) and their precursor. Fed. Proc., 39:323, 1980.

Chapter 32

Prostaglandin E

Prostaglandin E (PGE_1 and PGE_2) has been used since 1975 to maintain the patency of the ductus arteriosus in infants.[1] This purpose constitutes the primary indication for PGE in cardiovascular medicine. Although prostacyclin also dilates the ductus arteriosus, PGE is still the drug of choice for this indication.[2-6]

Vascular Effects

PGE_1 and PGE_2 are potent vasodilators of fetal and adult vessels, but our understanding of their function is still controversial. For example, studies in adult human patients have shown that PGE_1 is a balanced vasodilator, affecting equally arteries and veins.[7] Animal studies have shown that PGE is mainly an arteriolar dilator; however, PGE also has an inhibiting effect on platelet aggregation, achieved by stimulation of adenyl cyclase in platelets.[8] Although this effect may play some role in the effect of PGE, it appears unlikely because the effect is 30 times less potent than that of prostacyclin. Studies in healthy pregnant women have shown that PGE_2 causes only a moderate peripheral vasodilatation, without altering pulmonary vascular resistance or pressure, and myocardial contractility.[9]

One report suggested that the coronary-vasodilating effect of nitrates may be mediated by PGE.[10] Another study has shown, however, that pretreatment with indomethacin, a prostaglandin-synthesis inhibitor, does not alter the antianginal effect of nitroglycerin.

Effects on the Ductus Arteriosus

Prostaglandins play an important role in maintaining the patency of the ductus arteriosus during embryonal life. This concept is supported by findings of in vitro and in vivo studies. In 1972, Elliott and Starling found that prostaglandins dilated the ductus arteriosus in animals.[11] It was later shown that exogenous PGE_1 and PGE_2 relax isolated strips of ductal tissue in the presence of low oxygen tension in vitro.[2] Inhibitors of prostaglandin synthesis administered to pregnant animals have constricted the ductus arteriosus in the fetuses.[5,6] PGE_2 has dilated indomethacin-constricted ductus arteriosus in animal experiments.[12]

In fetuses the levels of PGE_2 in the plasma are high for the following reasons: (1) PGE_2, like most other prostaglandins, is eliminated mainly by catabolism in the lungs; in the fetus, the circulation by-passes the lungs, and elimination of PGE_2 is limited; and (2) the placenta produces considerable amounts of PGE. The plasma PGE, together with the PGE produced locally in the ductal wall, dilates the ductus arteriosus in the presence of low oxygen tension present in this area during fetal life.[13, 14] After birth, the production of PGE is reduced because of the loss of the placental source, elimination is increased by activation of the pulmonary circulation, and oxygen tension is increased.

These factors contribute to closure of the ductus arteriosus early after birth. Abnormalities of this mechanism or hemodynamic causes may sustain the patency of the ductus arteriosus. This phenomenon can also be produced by the administration of exogenous PGE. Thromboxane A_2, produced in the lungs, may constrict the ductus arteriosus after birth, when pulmonary blood flow increases. For better understanding of the therapeutic capabilities of PGE, one should remember that closure of the ductus arteriosus occurs in two steps: (1) functional closure, caused by constriction of the muscular layer of the ductal wall; the mechanisms described in the previous paragraph are related only to this step; and (2) anatomic closure, including infolding of the endothelium, loss of the normal structure of the subintimal layer, and fibrosis. Once these procedures have occurred, the ductus arteriosus cannot be reopened.

PGE has several hemodynamic effects even in the absence of congenital heart diseases other than patent ductus arteriosus. In animal experiments, in addition to dilation of the ductus arteriosus, PGE_2 increased right ventricular output and decreased cardiac output; therefore, the ratio between right ventricular output and cardiac output became normal.[12] In the foregoing report, pulmonary and systemic vascular resistances were little altered by PGE_2.

Principles of Therapeutic Administration in Children

Infants with several forms of congenital heart diseases are dependent, for maintaining their circulation, on the patency of the ductus arteriosus. These congenital diseases include cyanotic anomalies and aortic arch anomalies. Infants with complete transposition of the great arteries and intact atrial and ventricular septa depend on the patency of the ductus arteriosus for mixing of the systemic and pulmonary circulations, which is essential to life. This mixing through the ductus arteriosus is also important in infants with complete transposition who have a small ventricular or atrial septal defect. In infants with severe, right-sided obstructions, such as pulmonary atresia, severe pulmonic stenosis, or tricuspid atresia with intact ventricular septum, pulmonary supply depends on the ductus arteriosus, and to some extent on the bronchial arteries as well.

In infants with interruption of the aortic arch, blood flow to the inferior part of the body depends on right-to-left shunting through the ductus arteriosus, from the pulmonary artery to the descending aorta distal to the interruption. In infants with severe coarctation of the aorta, patency of the ductus or relaxation of the ductus diverticulum may increase the lumen of the constricting area. In patients with any of these anomalies, maintaining the patency of the ductus arteriosus by administration of PGE is beneficial and may be lifesaving.

Treatment usually begins with an intravenous infusion of PGE_1, which is later replaced by oral administration of the agent. The intervals between oral doses are gradually increased until the infant can be discharged from hospital and managed at home while receiving oral PGE_2.

Effects in Tricuspid Atresia

Freed and co-workers reported 23 infants with tricuspid atresia who received intravenous infusions of PGE_1.[15] Results were favorable in most of these infants, with an increase in arterial oxygen tension, usually evident within 30 min of initiation of the infusion. As with other congenital cardiac anomalies, the best results were obtained in infants less than 4 days old. PGE may be effective in other patients, however. Coe and associates reported the case of an infant with tricuspid atresia and ductus-dependent circulation who responded to orally administered PGE_2.[16] The patient was discharged from the hospital at the age of 46 days with a prescription to receive oral PGE_2 every 4 hours. A repeated cardiac catheterization at the age of 5.5 months showed that the ductus arteriosus had remained patent and the left pulmonary artery had increased in diameter.

Effects in Pulmonary Obstruction

The most common indication for PGE is pulmonary obstruction—either atresia or severe stenosis. Freed and colleagues studied 231 infants with pulmonary atresia and 47 infants with severe pulmonic stenosis who were treated with intravenous or intra-arterial PGE_1 in 56 centers in the United States.[15] A favorable response was observed within 30 min of initiation of the infusion. The mean Pa_{O_2} for the group increased by about 12 mm Hg. Infants over 4 days old had a higher preinfusion Pa_{O_2} and a smaller increase in Pa_{O_2}. Infants weighing more than 4 kg at birth and alkalotic infants had a smaller increase in Pa_{O_2}. No differences in response were observed with respect to mode of administration (whether intra-arterial or intravenous), gender, maternal age, or preinfusion Pa_{CO_2}.[15]

PGE_2 is also effective by oral administration. In 12 children with severe pulmonary obstruction, oral PGE_2 dilated the ductus arteriosus and improved arterial blood oxygenation. The improvement achieved by oral PGE_2 was similar to that seen after intravenous administration of this agent.

The ductus arteriosus remains responsive to the effect of PGE throughout long periods of oral or intravenous therapy.[16, 17] On discontinuance of the drug, the oxygen saturation decreases in the majority of treated infants.

Although PGE_2 maintains the patency of the ductus arteriosus on a long-term basis, its effect on overall survival rates may be limited by pulmonary arterial size, which impairs the effectiveness of systemic-pulmonary shunts, as well as by other factors. Silove and co-workers treated 62 infants, of whom 53 had reduced pulmonary blood flow.[18] Oral PGE_2 was given to 58 of these patients, 26 of whom also received intravenous PGE_1. Fifteen hospital deaths occurred in 46 patients who had undergone operations (33%). Fourteen patients who had not undergone operations died, but not of complications of PGE_2. The influence of oral PGE_2 over long periods on overall survival rates requires further systematic evaluation. Factors determining the response of the ductus arteriosus to PGE are discussed in another section of this chapter, as well as in the literature.[15–30]

Effects in Complete Transposition of the Great Arteries

PGE_1 and PGE_2 dilate the patent ductus arteriosus in infants with complete transposition of the great arteries and ductus-dependent circulation. In infants with complete transposition of the great arteries and intact ventricular and atrial septa, life depends on mixing of the circulations through the ductus arteriosus. In infants with complete transposition of the great arteries and patent foramen ovale or atrial septal defect, the increase in pulmonary blood flow by left-to-right shunting through the ductus arteriosus increases the pulmonary venous return and left atrial pressure and consequently increases interatrial shunting. In such infants, treatment with PGE is effective as initial therapy, even before cardiac catheterization and a balloon atrial septostomy are performed.

Beitzke and Suppan evaluated the efficacy of intravenous administration of PGE_2 in 15 infants with complete transposition of the great arteries and severe hypoxemia.[24] Twelve of the infants had simple transposition, and 3 had small ventricular septal defects. Infusion of

PGE$_2$ resulted in significant increases of Pa$_{O_2}$ from 22 ± 3 to 37 ± 5 mm Hg within 1 to 2 hours of initiation of treatment. Pa$_{O_2}$ remained constantly above 30 mm Hg throughout the infusion. Only 1 of the 15 infants failed to respond to this treatment. When balloon atrial septostomy had been performed, the infusion was stopped. Two patients required reinfusion within 24 hours of the septostomy because of hypoxemia. This approach, of early administration of PGE, appears to be especially suitable when emergency cardiac catheterization is not always possible.

PGE can, of course, be administered after cardiac catheterization. In 1979, Lang and associates reported favorable results of treatment of infants with complete transposition of the great arteries and intact ventricular septum with PGE$_1$.[25] Similar results were reported in 1979 by Benson and colleagues and by Driscoll and co-workers in treating infants with simple transposition of the great arteries who remained severely hypoxic after atrial septostomy.[26, 27] Two years later, Freed and associates reported the results of a multicenter study of the efficacy of PGE$_1$ in congenital heart diseases.[15] Twenty-one infants with complete transposition of the great arteries were included in this study. A significant increase in Pa$_{O_2}$ from 22.9 to 31.8 mm Hg was observed. As in other congenital heart diseases, the responsiveness of the patent ductus arteriosus to PGE is sustained throughout prolonged treatment.[28]

Teixeira and co-workers reported on 7 children with complete transposition of the great arteries and an intact interventricular septum or a small ventricular septal defect.[29] When treated with PGE$_1$, infused intravenously for several weeks, these patients showed an improvement in Pa$_{O_2}$. Heart failure developed in 6 of the patients. The role of shunting through the ductus arteriosus in the development of heart failure in these patients is not clear, but even if it did cause heart failure, patency of the ductus arteriosus is essential for life.

Effects in Aortic Arch Anomalies and Hypoplastic Left Heart Syndrome

PGE is beneficial in infants with interruption of the aortic arch or severe coarctation of the aorta and ductus-dependent circulation. Although blood flow to the descending aorta can be supplied by other collateral arteries in these patients, right-to-left flow through the patent ductus arteriosus plays a major role in maintaining blood supply to the inferior portion of the body. In 1979, Heymann and colleagues first described dilatation of the ductus arteriosus in infants with aortic arch abnormalities.[30]

In 1981, Freed and associates reported on a multicenter study from the United States that evaluated the effect of PGE, infusion on 107 infants with acyanotic congenital heart diseases and ductus-dependent anomalies.[15] Forty-six of these patients had juxtaductal coarctation of the aorta, 34 had complete interruption of the aortic arch, and 8 had miscellaneous lesions. At the onset of infusion, the infants were 1 day to 5 months old (mean age 5 days). Seventy percent of them were under 10 days of age. Clinical improvement occurred in about 80% of the infants with aortic arch anomalies. In the infants with interruption of the aortic arch, blood flow to the descending aorta increased, and the pressure differences across the ductus arteriosus decreased. In infants with coarctation of the aorta, blood pressure in the descending aorta increased and blood pressure in the ascending aorta decreased. Pressure gradient across the coarctation decreased from 45 to 9 mm Hg. The hemodynamic improvement was associated with improved renal function and with the correction of acidosis.

The mean preinfusion Pa_{O_2} for the foregoing group of infants with acyanotic congenital heart diseases was 67 mm Hg. No differences in clinical or arterial pressure response were noted between infants with a low preinfusion Pa_{O_2} and those with a high Pa_{O_2}. As in patients with cyanotic congenital heart diseases, in infants in whom the ductus arteriosus was closed before the infusion, PGE_1 had no beneficial effect.[15]

In the case of a patient with severe coarctation reported by Teixeira and co-workers, PGE_1 decreased blood pressure in the superior limbs, increased blood pressure in the legs, and improved renal function.[29] The infusion was stopped on the thirty-eighth day, when surgical correction was performed. Another infant with coarctation of the aorta and an intact interventricular septum showed hemodynamic deterioration and no control of hypertension; he died suddenly.

PGE_2 is also effective by oral administration. Clinical improvement was observed in two neonates with complete interruption of the aortic arch who were treated with oral PGE_2.

Factors Determining the Response of the Ductus Arteriosus

Several factors may determine the responsiveness of the ductus arteriosus to PGE. The multifactorial regulation accounts for the variability of the response to PGE in infants. Freed and associates reported that the infant's age is an important determinant of such response.[15] Infants under 96 hours of age have responded more favorably than older infants. Treatment initiated even as late as at 3 weeks of age has been effective, however.[16] The responsiveness of the ductus arteriosus is sustained for several months,[19, 20] and discontinuance of treatment after a long period causes deterioration. Thus, age is not an absolute determinant of a patient's response to PGE.

PGE can preserve the patency of a fully patent ductus arteriosus and may dilate a partially constricted ductus arteriosus.[15, 19] An angiocardiographically demonstrated closed ductus arteriosus is considered to be nonresponsive to PGE. Clyman and associates reported that, in fetal lamb, the responsiveness of the ductus arteriosus to PGE was related to the lumen of the ductus.[21] Heymann and co-workers found a similar relationship between the pretreatment luminal cross-sectional area of the ductus arteriosus and the response to PGE_1.[22] The loss of responsiveness after decreased ductal blood flow may result from ischemia of the ductal muscle, caused by decreased flow in the vasa vasorum.

If treatment is initiated soon after functional closure of the ductus arteriosus, a "closed" ductus may reopen. Born and colleagues, studying the ductus arteriosus of fetal lambs, reported that when the ductus was constricted for short periods by infusion of epinephrine or by elevation of arterial oxygen saturation, termination of the infusion or decrease in oxygen saturation produced a rapid dilatation.[23] This phenomenon occurred only when the period of closure was short. In my experience with a week-old infant, PGE reopened a ductus arteriosus that had been closed, as proved by angiocardiographic and oximetric studies.

Administration of PGE does not impair the ability of the ductus arteriosus to close spontaneously when PGE is discontinued. For example, in 10 of 11 infants with complete transposition of the great arteries who underwent total correction and who received early infusions of PGE_2, the initially large ducti have spontaneously closed.[24]

Comparative Effects in Cyanotic and Acyanotic Congenital Heart Diseases

Because the therapeutic goals in infants with cyanotic and acyanotic congenital heart diseases differ, the criteria for a favorable clinical response to PGE are also different: improved oxygenation in cyanotic congenital heart disease and improved blood flow in the descending aorta and decreased pressure gradients across aortic coarctation in infants with acyanotic lesions. In addition to these obvious differences, Freed and associates found two other important factors: (1) age of the patient; and (2) time to onset of effect.[15]

In the infants with cyanotic congenital heart diseases studied by Freed and co-workers, the response depended on age; the best responders were under 4 days old.[15] In infants with acyanotic congenital heart diseases, age was not so critical for a positive response. One infant responded favorably at 36 days of age. This difference is only relative, however. For example, Coe and colleagues reported on an infant with tricuspid atresia who responded favorably to PGE initiated at the age of 3 weeks.[16]

The time to onset of effect is longer in infants with acyanotic than cyanotic congenital heart diseases. Freed and co-workers reported that in cyanotic infants, the maximal Pa_{O_2} response usually occurred within 30 min of initiation of the infusion.[15] In contrast, in infants with interruption of the aortic arch, the maximal response was observed in 1.5 hours (range 15 min to 4 hours). In infants with coarctation of the aorta, the maximal response was observed within 3 hours (range 15 min to 11 hours) of the initiation of treatment.[15] I treated an infant with interruption of the aortic arch in whom maximal effect was observed 20 hours after initiation of the infusion. Therefore, in infants with acyanotic cardiac anomalies, infusion of PGE should be continued for longer periods, until its maximal efficacy is determined.

Effects in Persistent Fetal Circulation with Pulmonary Hypertension

Prolonged administration of PGE has decreased the amount of pulmonary arterial musculature.[31] This subject is further discussed in the section of this chapter on side effects of PGE. In infants with congenital heart disease, abnormally thick pulmonary vascular walls, and pulmonary hypertension, or in infants with persistent fetal circulation and pulmonary hypertension, such an effect may be beneficial. No clinical studies of the efficacy of PGE in these conditions have been performed. In the presence of a patent and partially constricted ductus arteriosus, however, the administration of PGE may dilate the ductus and may aggravate pulmonary hypertension and congestive heart failure, despite the favorable effects of PGE in patients with congestive heart failure not associated with a patent ductus arteriosus.[32]

Effects in Congestive Heart Failure

In adults with congestive heart failure, endogenous PGE may play an important role in modulating circulatory homeostasis.[32] The exogenous administration of PGE has produced hemodynamic improvement in patients with congestive heart failure. This improvement probably resulted from the peripheral vasodilatory effect of PGE, although not all researchers agree on whether the arterial or the venous vasodilatory effects predominate in modulating the hemodynamic improvement.

Awan and colleagues reported that, in 9 patients with severe chronic congestive heart failure due to coronary artery disease, PGE_1 reduced mean systemic arterial pressure from 85 ± 6 to 76 ± 5 mm Hg and left ventricular filling pressure from 19 ± 3 to 15 ± 2 mm Hg.[33] Heart rate was not altered, whereas cardiac index increased from 1.9 ± 0.2

to 2.5 ± 0.2 L/min/m^2, and stroke volume index increased from 28 ± 2.4 to 35 ± 2.9 ml/beat/m^2. Systemic vascular resistance was reduced.[33] Popat and Pitt reported that, in 5 patients with acute myocardial infarction and congestive heart failure, PGE$_1$ decreased systemic vascular resistance, mean systemic arterial pressure, pulmonary capillary wedge pressure, and pulmonary vascular resistance and increased cardiac index.[7] No studies have been performed, however, on the effect of exogenous PGE on the hemodynamic condition of children with congestive heart failure not associated with a patent ductus arteriosus.

Initiation of Treatment

In management of critically ill infants suspected of having ductus-dependent congenital heart diseases, treatment is often delayed until diagnosis is confirmed by cardiac catheterization. It is common practice to initiate PGE infusion once such a diagnosis is confirmed. The several hours required for establishing the diagnosis may be critical, however. Heymann suggested that treatment should be initiated in critically ill infants suspected to have a ductus-dependent congenital cardiac anomaly even before confirmation of diagnosis.[13] This suggestion is based on the excellent results achieved in clinical studies and on the relative safety of PGE.

The foregoing approach has several problems, however. First is the risk of deterioration of congestive heart failure in certain infants. Second, the influence of PGE treatment on overall mortality rates has not yet been determined, even in infants in whom the diagnosis of a ductus-dependent congenital cardiac anomaly has already been confirmed. I believe that, at present, no unequivocal answer exists to the question whether PGE treatment should be initiated before cardiac catheterization in infants with cyanotic congenital heart diseases.

A similar problem is seen in infants with acyanotic congenital heart diseases and ductus-dependent circulation. Because PGE can improve the clinical and hemodynamic condition of infants with aortic arch anomalies amenable to surgical correction, PGE infusion can be started in critically ill infants in whom this diagnosis is suspected, even before confirmation of the diagnosis by cardiac catheterization. PGE can produce transient hemodynamic and clinical improvement even in infants with hypoplastic left heart syndrome that is not amenable to surgical correction, however.

Echocardiographic studies do not always differentiate between aortic arch anomalies and hypoplastic left heart syndrome. Therefore, it is not possible to rely on the results of echocardiography when deciding whether to start PGE infusion. It is a common practice in many centers to administer PGE whenever a diagnosis of aortic arch anomaly is suspected, even before confirmation; if cardiac catheterization later shows a hypoplastic left heart not amenable to surgical correction, the infusion may be discontinued.

Monitoring of Treatment

Prostaglandins may produce a variety of adverse effects, which are discussed later in this chapter. Therefore, one must monitor heart rate, systemic arterial blood pressure, rate of respiration, signs of central nervous system involvement, body temperature, and electrocardiogram carefully during infusion of PGE. Careful ambulatory monitoring is required in infants treated at home with oral PGE_2 for several months.

Side Effects

PGE is usually well tolerated by infants, especially when the agent is given for short periods and at low doses. Side effects occasionally occur, however. They include cardiovascular disorders, effects related to the central nervous system, respiratory depression, and alteration of the pulmonary arterial musculature. Infants treated with high oral doses of PGE can develop gastrointestinal side effects.

Lewis and associates reported on the incidence and types of side effects in 492 infants with congenital cardiac anomalies (385 with cyanotic congenital heart diseases and 107 with aortic arch anomalies) who were treated with PGE_1 administered intravenously, in a multicenter study in the United States.[34] These workers reported that 43% of the infants developed at least one adverse effect, but in only about half these patients were the effects attributed to treatment with PGE. The most common adverse effects were cardiovascular, seen in 18% of the patients. Effects on the central nervous system developed in 16% of the patients, and respiratory depression occurred in 12%. It is impossible to evaluate the incidence and extent of impairment of pulmonary vascular musculature in this series. No death was directly attributed to administration of PGE_1 in the report of Lewis and co-workers.[34] These investigators noted that some of the adverse effects could be eliminated by lowering the dose of PGE_1.[34] In another study, Silove and colleagues found that low doses of PGE_2, administered intravenously, produced adverse effects in only 7 of 30 patients.[18] This incidence is lower than that observed by Lewis and associates with intravenous PGE_1.[34] In only 3 of these 7 infants did major complications occur.[18]

The incidence and types of adverse effects are different in infants treated with oral PGE_2. Silove and co-workers reported that 25 of 58 infants developed complications during oral therapy.[18] These complications included apnea and/or necrotizing enterocolitis in 4 and diarrhea in 13 infants.

Cardiovascular Effects

Cardiovascular side effects are the most common complications of intravenous and intra-aortic administration of PGE. They include bradycardia or tachycardia, arrhythmias, hypotension, and cutaneous vasodilation and edema. These adverse effects are more common in infants who weigh less than 2.0 kg and in those who receive PGE_1 infusion for more than 48 hours. These effects are reported to be rare in infants treated for longer periods with oral PGE_2,[18] although bradycardia may be a significant adverse effect of PGE_2.[35] In the study reported by Lewis and colleagues, infants with cyanotic lesions had more adverse cardiovascular effects than infants with aortic arch anomalies.[34] This difference could be attributed to the more common use of intra-aortic catheters for infusion of PGE_1 in cyanotic infants. This route of administration, which produces much more cutaneous vasodilation than intravenous infusion, could have been the cause of the circulatory impairment reported in this study.

In infants with various congenital heart diseases, heart failure may develop or may worsen during PGE therapy.[29] In infants with transposition of the great arteries or ductus-dependent pulmonary blood flow, heart failure has been easily managed by conventional treatment or by a decrease in the rate of PGE_1 infusion. In infants with coarctation of the aorta, however, an improvement in heart failure has been observed only on discontinuing the infusion.

Effects Related to the Central Nervous System

Side effects related to the central nervous system have been observed mainly with intravenous or intra-aortic administration of PGE_1 and PGE_2 and less frequently with oral administration of PGE_2. Lewis and associates reported that the incidence of effects on the central nervous system was 16%.[34] This incidence was not influenced by the type of cardiac anomaly, whether cyanotic or acyanotic, by the birth weight of the patient, or by the patient's preinfusion Pa_{O_2} level. The incidence of those effects was the same in patients who received PGE_1 intravenously as in those who were given the agent intra-arterially.

The adverse effects reported by Lewis and colleagues included seizure-like activity, elevation of body temperature, irritability, and lethargy. Of these effects, seizure-like activity was the most common with intravenous administration and elevation of body temperature was the most common with intra-arterial administration.[34] These effects were more frequent in infants with a preinfusion pH of less than 7.15 and in those treated for long periods. These adverse effects required discontinuance of treatment in only a few infants. In the majority of infants, effects were abolished by a reduction in the infusion rate.

Respiratory Depression

Respiratory depression, a common side effect in infants treated with intravenous or intra-aortic PGE,[34] may also occur in infants treated with oral PGE_2.[18] It is more common among infants with cyanotic congenital heart diseases and among infants weighing less than 2.0 kg at birth. Respiratory depression has been reported less frequently in infants with a pH of less than 7.15, perhaps because more infants in this group undergo mechanical ventilation. The incidence of this adverse effect is not influenced by the route of administration, by the preinfusion arterial blood Pa_{O_2}, or by the duration of the infusion.

Structural Changes in the Pulmonary Circulation

PGE may produce structural changes in the pulmonary circulation. Haworth and Silove studied at autopsy the pulmonary circulation of eight infants with pulmonary atresia who received PGE_1 infusions.[36] These investigators found profound changes in the musculature of the pulmonary arteries. The relative thickness of the pulmonary arterial media was reduced; the muscular layer was terminated more proximally in the pulmonary arterial tree of the treated infants than in the arterial tree of normal infants or infants with pulmonary artresia who did not receive PGE and who died at the same age. Local aneurysmal dilatations were observed in the arterial walls. The intra-acinar arteries were abnormally small, whereas the preacinar arteries were dilated. These changes were directly correlated with the duration of the infusion.[31]

The long-term effect of these changes on mortality and morbidity rates is not known. It is also not known whether prolonged oral administration of PGE_2 can produce similar changes. Two infants treated with PGE_2 did not develop the pulmonary arterial changes described with PGE_1.[36] Further studies are required to clarify this point, but if PGE_2 does not affect the pulmonary vasculature, one should use this agent for prolonged therapy. At present, however, treatment with PGE should be given for as short a time as possible, to prevent such changes. It is not known whether the changes in the musculature of the pulmonary arteries will disappear on termination of treatment.

Structural Changes in the Ductus Arteriosus

Prolonged treatment with PGE has weakened the walls of the ductus arteriosus.[37] Cole and associates reported that, in an infant treated with

PGE_1 for several weeks, the ductus arteriosus showed disruption of the internal elastic membrane, localized increase in elastic tissue in the media, destruction of the normal medial structure, fragmentation of the elastic fibers in the media, and edema, thickening, and infiltration of the adventitia.[38] In two other studies, however, no histologic difference has been found between the ducti of infants who received PGE_1 and those of untreated infants.[29,39] The histologic changes in the ductus arteriosus were attributed by Teixeira and co-workers to the normal process of ductal closure.[29] These changes do not prevent the normal functional and anatomic closure of the ductus arteriosus when treatment is discontinued.[24,40]

Park and co-workers found that prolonged administration of PGE_1 may delay the normal closing process or maturation of the ductus arteriosus, but it does not have any significant deleterious or clinical effect, nor does it prevent the normal closure of the ductus arteriosus when PGE_1 therapy is discontinued.[41] Angiocardiograms performed up to 33 months after PGE_1 treatment in 28 infants showed no abnormality of the ductus arteriosus.

Cutaneous Effects

Cutaneous side effects have resulted mainly from cutaneous vasodilation and edema. These effects may be localized, by inadvertent positioning of the catheter tip in a brachiocephalic or intercostal artery. Such local cutaneous effects have responded to repositioning of the catheter tip.[34] This problem has caused a greater incidence of cutaneous abnormalities in infants when PGE was infused into the aorta than when it was infused intravenously.

Gastrointestinal Effects

Gastrointestinal side effects were observed in about 30% of patients treated with oral PGE_2 and in 2% of patients treated with intravenous or intra-aortic PGE_1.[18,34] The major gastrointestinal adverse effect is necrotizing enterocolitis, which developed in only a few of a study of 492 infants treated with PGE_1, but in about 5% of those treated with oral PGE_2; diarrhea developed in 9 of the 492 infants treated with PGE_1 intravenously or intra-arterially.[34] In another study, diarrhea occurred in 13 of 58 infants treated with PGE_2 orally.[18] In a more recent study, refractory diarrhea was reported in 1 of 17 infants treated for several weeks with PGE_1 intravenously.[29] Diarrhea, which often limits the tolerance of infants to therapeutic doses of oral PGE_2, may be partially controlled by reducing the dose. Hyperbilirubinemia has been uncommon.[34]

Metabolic Effects

Metabolic side effects, including hypocalcemia and hypoglycemia, were seen in about 1% of the patients in a study.[34]

Hematologic Effects

Hematologic side effects, including hemorrhage, disseminated intravascular coagulation, and thrombocytopenia, were observed in under than 4% of the patients treated with PGE_1 reported by Lewis and associates.[34] It is not known whether these effects were directly attributable to treatment. Disseminated intravascular coagulation was much more common in acyanotic infants than in cyanotic infants in the foregoing study.

Renal Failure

Lewis and colleagues reported that renal failure occurred in 4% of infants with acyanotic lesions and 1% of infants with cyanotic lesions treated with PGE_1.[34]

Cortical Hyperostosis

Symmetric laminar cortical hyperostosis of long bones of the limbs was first described in Japan, in infants treated on a long-term basis with a low-dose infusion of PGE_1.[42, 43] These changes resemble those of Caffey's disease, but the symmetry of the lesions, the absence, or limited presence, of clavicular involvement, and the absence of mandibular changes differentiate between the cortical hyperostosis associated with PGE_1 and Caffey's disease. Cortical hyperostosis of the long bones was reported in three of seven infants with complete transposition of the great arteries and in three of 8 infants with ductus-dependent, right-sided cardiac obstruction who were treated for several weeks with an infusion of PGE_1 in Canada.[29] The cause of this adverse effect is not known. Certain concentrations of prostaglandins can stimulate bone formation, but the reason for the distribution of this effect and for its predominance in the long bones of the limbs is unknown.

Dosage and Administration

Intravenous Administration

One should start an infusion of PGE_1 at a rate of 0.05 µg/kg/min.[13] After 30 min of infusion, one should attempt to reduce the rate of infusion because the beneficial effect may be maintained at lower infusion rates, and the incidence and severity of adverse effects may be reduced.

An infusion of PGE_2 should be started at a rate of 0.002 to 0.006 µg/kg/min.[19] The dose may be increased up to about 0.06 µg/kg/

min. If the patient responds favorably to a high dose, one should try to reduce the dose gradually. If required, initial infusion rates of 0.1 µg/kg/min may be used.[24] Because the clinical response to oral and intravenous PGE_2 is similar, the intravenous route is recommended mainly for infants who, during oral therapy, develop diarrhea that does not respond to a reduction in the oral dose.

Intra-arterial Administration

PGE can be given intra-arterially, and attempts have been made to administer the agent into the aorta, as close as possible to the aortic origin of the ductus arteriosus; however, intra-arterial administration has no advantage over other routes of administration.

Oral Administration

PGE_2 can be given orally, and Silove and associates recommend it as the route of choice.[19] They suggest initiating an oral regimen of 30 to 45 µg/kg/hour, given at intervals of 1 hour. If no response is observed within 2 hours, the dose can be increased gradually to a maximum of 65 µg/kg/hour. Occasionally, doses as high as 90 µg/kg/hour are used, but they are poorly tolerated. Most patients require 30 to 45 µg/kg given every hour for first 2 weeks.

It is, of course, desirable to reduce the frequency of oral PGE administration, especially in infants who are to be discharged from hospital. Although this goal is rarely achieved in infants under 3 weeks old,[19] wider dosage intervals are available to older patients. The case of 7-week-old infant who was discharged from hospital and received oral PGE_2 every 4 hours has been reported.[16]

References

1. Elliott, R.B., et al.: Medical manipulation of the ductus arteriosus. Lancet, *1*:140, 1975.
2. Coceani, F., and Olley, P.M.: The response of the ductus arteriosus to prostaglandins. Can. J. Physiol. Pharmacol., *51*:220, 1973.
3. Pace-Asciak, C.R., and Rengaraj, G.: The 6-ketoprostaglandin $F_{1-alpha}$ pathway in the lamb ductus arteriosus. Biochim. Biophys. Acta, *486*:583, 1977.
4. Clyman, R.I., et al.: Formation of prostacyclin (PGI_2) by the ductus arteriosus of fetal lambs at different stages of gestation. Prostaglandins, *16*:633, 1978.
5. Coceani, F., and Olley, P.M.: Role of prostaglandins, prostacyclin, and thromboxanes in the control of prenatal patency and postnatal closure of the ductus arteriosus. Semin. Perinatol., *4*:109, 1980.
6. Clyman, R.I.: Ontogeny of the ductus arteriosus response to postaglandins and inhibitors of their synthesis. Semin. Perinatol., *4*:115, 1980.
7. Popat, K.D., and Pitt, B.: Hemodynamic effects of prostaglandin E infusion in patients with acute myocardial infarction and left ventricular failure.
8. Vane, J.R.: Inhibition of prostaglandin synthesis as a mechanism of action of aspirin-like drugs. Nature (New Biol.), *231*:232, 1971.
9. Thayssen, P., et al.: Systolic time intervals and haemodynamic changes during intravenous infusion of prostaglandins F_{2a} and E_2. Br. Heart J., *45*:447, 1981.

10. Morcillio, E.: Myocardial prostaglandin E release by nitroglycerin and modification by indomethacin. Am. J. Cardiol., *45*:5, 1980.
11. Elliott, R.B., and Starling, M.D.: The effects of prostaglandin F_2 in the closure of the ductus arteriosus. Prostaglandins, *5*:339, 1972.
12. Sideris, E.B., et al.: Effects of indomethacin and prostaglandins E_2, I_2, and D_2 on the fetal circulation. Adv. Prostaglandin Thromboxane Leukotriene Res., *12*:477, 1983.
13. Heymann, M.A.: Pharmacologic use of prostaglandin E_1 in infants with congenital heart disease. Am. Heart J., *101*:837, 1981.
14. Challis, J.R.G., et al.: Prostaglandin in the circulation of the fetal lamb. Prostaglandins, *11*:1041, 1976.
15. Freed, M.D., et al.: Prostaglandin E_1 in infants with ductus arteriosus-dependent congenital heart disease. Circulation, *64*:899, 1981.
16. Coe, J.Y., et al.: Management of tricuspid atresia with orally administered prostaglandin E_2. J. Pediatr., *100*:496, 1982.
17. Von Euler, U.S.: Action of adrenaline, acetylcholine and other substances on nerve free vessels (human placenta). J. Physiol., *93*:129, 1938.
18. Silove, E.D., et al.: Long-term oral prostaglandin E_2 therapy in ductus dependent circulation. American Heart Association, 1983.
19. Silove, E.D., et al.: Oral prostaglandin E_1 in ductus dependent pulmonary circulation. Circulation, *63*:682, 1981.
20. Lewis, A.B., et al.: Administration of prostaglandin E_1 in neonates with critical congenital cardiac defects. J. Pediatr., *93*:481, 1978.
21. Clyman, R.I., et al.: Factors determining the loss of ductus arteriosus responsiveness to prostaglandin E. Circulation, *68*:433, 1983.
22. Heymann, M.A., and Rudolph, A.M.: Ductus arteriosus dilatation by prostaglandin E_1 in infants with pulmonary atresia. Pediatrics, *53*:325, 1977.
23. Born, G.V.R., et al.: The constriction of the ductus arteriosus caused by oxygen and by asphyxia in newborn lambs. J. Physiol., *132*:304, 1956.
24. Beitzke, A., and Suppan, C.H.: Use of prostaglandin E_2 in management of transposition of great arteries balloon atrial septostomy. Br. Heart J., *49*:341, 1983.
25. Lang, P., et al.: Use of prostaglandin E_1 in infants with d-transposition of the great arteries and intact ventricular septum. Am. J. Cardiol., *44*:76, 1979.
26. Benson, L.N., et al.: Role of prostaglandin E_1 infusion in the management of transposition of the great arteries. Am. J. Cardiol., *44*:691, 1979.
27. Driscoll, D.J., et al.: The use of prostaglandin E_1 in a critically ill infant with transposition of the great arteries. J. Pediatr., *95*:259, 1979.
28. Levy, H.H., et al.: Prolonged use of prostaglandin E_1 to maintain patency of the ductus arteriosus in congenital heart disease. (Abstract.) Pediatr. Res., *12*:384, 1978.
29. Teixeira, O.H.P., et al.: Long-term prostaglandin E_1 therapy in congenital heart defects. J. Am. Coll. Cardiol., *3*:838, 1984.
30. Heymann, M.A., et al.: Dilation of the ductus arteriosus by prostaglandin E_1 in aortic arch abnormalities. Circulation, *59*:169, 1979.
31. Haworth, S.G., et al.: Effect of prostaglandin E_1 on pulmonary circulation in pulmonary artesia. Br. Heart J., *43*:306, 1980.
32. Dzau, V.J., et al.: Prostaglandins in severe congestive heart failure. N. Engl. J. Med., *310*:347, 1984.
33. Awan, N.A., et al.: Cardiocirculatory and myocardial energetic effects of prostaglandin E_1 in severe left ventricular failure due to chronic coronary heart disease. Am. Heart J., *102*:703, 1981.
34. Lewis, A.B., et al.: Side effects of therapy with prostaglandin E_1 in infants with critical congenital heart disease. Circulation, *64*:893, 1981.
35. Silove, E.D.: Administration of E-type prostaglandins in ductus-dependent congenital heart disease. Pediatr. Cardiol., *2*:303, 1982.
36. Haworth, S.G., and Silove, E.D.: Pulmonary arterial structure in pulmonary atresia following prostaglandin E_2 administration. Br. Heart J., *45*:311, 1981.
37. Gittenberger-de Croot, A.C., et al.: Histopathology of the ductus arteriosus after prostaglandin E_1 administration in ductus dependent cardiac anomalies. Br. Heart J., *40*:215, 1978.

38. Cole, R.B., et al.: Prolonged prostaglandin E_1 infusion: histologic effects on the patent ductus arteriosus. Pediatrics, 67:816, 1981.
39. Silver, M.S., et al.: The morphology of the human newborn ductus arteriosus: a reappraisal of its structure and closure with special reference to prostaglandin E_1 therapy. Hum. Pathol., 12:1123, 1981.
40. Lewuis, A.B., and Lurie, P.R.: Prolonged PGE_1 infusion in an infant with cyanotic congenital heart disease. Pediatrics, 61:534, 1978.
41. Park, I.S., et al.: Morphologic features of the ductus arteriosus after prostaglandin E_1 administration for ductus-dependent congenital heart defects. J. Am. Coll. Cardiol., 1:471, 1983.
42. Sone, K., et al.: Long-term low-dose prostaglandin E_1 administration. J. Pediatr., 97:866, 1980.
43. Ueda, K., et al.: Cortical hyperostosis following long-term administration of prostaglandin E_1 in infants with cyanotic congenital heart disease. J. Pediatr., 97:834, 1980.

Chapter 33

Prostacyclin

Prostacyclin (PGI_2) is a potent vasodilatory prostaglandin that is formed in walls of blood vessels, mainly in the intima.[1-3] It participates in regulation of the circulation and is considered to be the most important prostaglandin producing coronary vasodilation.[4] PGI_2 is formed in various organs, but it is not clear whether it acts as a circulating hormone as well as locally. It is released by the lungs to the blood.[5-8]

Since 1976, when it was synthesized, PGI_2 has been extensively evaluated in various aspects of cardiovascular therapy in adults and children. In adults, PGI_2 has been studied mainly with respect to treatment of angina pectoris, coronary spasm, systemic hypertension, and congestive heart failure. In children, it has been evaluated primarily for its role in maintaining the patency of the ductus arteriosus and treatment of primary pulmonary hypertension.

Pharmacologic Properties

The most important pharmacologic properties of PGI_2 are vasodilation and inhibition of platelet aggregation. PGI_2 thereby opposes the effects of thromboxane A_2.[1,9,10]

Hemodynamic Effects

PGI_2 produces peripheral vasodilation, mainly arterial, without any significant effect on myocardial contractility. These effects decrease peripheral resistance, systemic arterial pressure, and left ventricular filling pressure and increase cardiac output. Like many other vasodilators, PGI_2, in high doses, increases heart rate. Pulmonary vascular resistance is reduced. These hemodynamic effects have been observed in animal experiments, in healthy human subjects, and in patients with various cardiovascular diseases, although not all changes have occurred in all groups. For example, in a group of persons without evidence of heart disease, an infusion of PGI_2 reduced systemic vascular resistance by 30% and pulmonary vascular resistance by 22%; heart rate was increased. Cardiac output, stroke volume, left ventricular filling pressure, and right atrial pressure were not altered, however. In a group of 20 patients with unstable angina pectoris, PGI_2 increased heart rate in 40% of the patients and decreased blood pressure in 50%.[11]

Effects in the Fetus

In contrast to studies of PGI_1, most hemodynamic studies of PGI_2 have been conducted in adults. Nonetheless, it has been important to determine the hemodynamic effects of PGI_2 in early stages of life. Sideris and colleagues studied the hemodynamic effects of PGI_2 in 19 fetal lambs.[12] At infusion rate of 0.1 µg/kg/min, PGI_2 increased the pressure gradient across the ductus arteriosus between the main pulmonary artery and the aorta. Infusion rates of 0.05 µg/kg/min or higher caused redistribution of right ventricular output, by decreasing ductal blood flow and by increasing pulmonary flow. The total cardiac output was not altered.

Effects in Patent Ductus Arteriosus

Because PGI_2 is a potent vasodilator, one might have expected that it would be beneficial in dilating and maintaining the patency of the ductus arteriosus. Several studies have shown, however, that PGI_2 is not effective for this indication. In animal experiments, that PGI_2 failed to dilate the ductus arteriosus sufficiently to abolish the pressure gradient across it; PGI_2 even increased the pressure gradient. It increased pulmonary arterial flow, decreased pulmonary vascular resistance, and did not alter systemic vascular resistance.[12a] Another animal study showed that, whereas PGE_2 had more effect on the ductus arteriosus than on the pulmonary circulation, PGI_2 had no effect on the ductus arteriosus but was an effective pulmonary vasodilator.[12]

Effects in Primary Pulmonary Hypertension

Theoretically, PGI_2 should be beneficial to patients with primary pulmonary hypertension. In animal studies, the agent has produced a dose-dependent decreased in pulmonary vascular resistance. Studies in fetal lambs have shown that PGI_2 has a potent pulmonary vasodilatory effect, without affecting the ductus arteriosus.[12] PGI_2 also reversed pulmonary hypertension induced in piglets by hypoxia.[13] In healthy men, PGI_2 produced a decrease of about 20% in pulmonary vascular resistance. Human patients may be more sensitive than animals to the effect of PGI_2 on the pulmonary vascular bed.[14-16]

In several studies of patients with primary pulmonary hypertension, short-term administration of PGI_2 produced a beneficial effect.[17-19] Four patients with primary pulmonary hypertension showed an increase in cardiac output and decreases in pulmonary and systemic vascular resistances and pressures during an infusion of PGI_2.[20]

In another study, the effect of PGI_2, at infusion rates of 2 to 12 ng/kg/min, was evaluated in 7 patients with primary pulmonary hypertension.[19] The drug increased heart rate from 83 ± 13 to 94 ± 11

beats/min and cardiac output from 4.22 ± 1.64 to 6.57 ± 2.04 L/min and reduced total pulmonary vascular resistance from 17.1 ± 8.7 to 9.7 ± 5.9 U and pulmonary arterial pressure from 65 ± 15 to 55 ± 16 mm Hg. In 3 of these patients, the reduction in pulmonary vascular resistance was maintained for up to 48 hours of infusion, when measurements were stopped. Systemic arterial pressure and resistance were also reduced.

PGI_2 may play a beneficial role in the short-term management of children with primary, and perhaps secondary, pulmonary hypertension. The long-term response to this agent has yet to be determined.

Effects in Persistent Fetal Circulation

Persistence of the fetal circulation is an important cause of pulmonary hypertension in the neonate. One report cites the case of a neonate with this condition in whom pulmonary vasoconstriction was completely reversed by PGI_2.[21]

Effects in Congestive Heart Failure

Endogenous PGI_2 plays an important role in regulating circulatory homeostasis in patients with congestive heart failure,[22] especially in hyponatremic patients. In a study of patients with refractory congestive heart failure, the intravenous administration of PGI_2 produced a significant hemodynamic improvement, as seen by reductions in pulmonary and systemic vascular resistances and pressures and by increases in cardiac output and stroke volume.[23] The effect of PGI_2 on congestive heart failure in infants and children has not been studied.

Effects in Systemic Hypertension

In adults with systemic hypertension, PGI_2 has produced hemodynamic improvement, by means of the arterial vasodilatory effect.[24] The effect of PGI_2 on hypertension in young age groups has not been studied.

Clinical Pharmacology

PGI_2 may be administered intravenously, intra-arterially, or by inhalation. Steady-state plasma levels can be achieved within 15 min of the initiation of the infusion. Although PGI_2 is metabolized mainly in the liver and kidney, it may be metabolized in the lungs, but to a much lesser extent than the other prostaglandins. PGI_2 is converted to an active metabolite, 6-keto PGE_1, as well as to several inactive metabolites. The forms of conversion are enzymatic and nonenzymatic.[25-28] The elimination half-life of PGI_2 in vivo is about 3 min.[29]

Side Effects

Intravenous administration of PGI$_2$ is associated with a high incidence of side effects, usually at infusion rates exceeding 4ng/kg/min and often requiring discontinuance of the infusion. In patients with primary pulmonary hypertension, the most significant adverse effect of prostacyclin is systemic arterial hypotension; it rapidly disappears with a reduction in the infusion rate. Other adverse effects are nausea, vomiting, restlessness, and anxiety. Flushing and headache may develop from to the agent's vasodilatory effect. Widening of the QRS complex and bradycardia are uncommon.[20]

Dosage and Administration

Intravenous and intra-arterial infusion rates of 2 to 15 ng/kg/min are used.

References

1. Moncada, S., and Vane, J.R.: Pharmacology and endogenous roles of prostaglandin endoperoxides, thromboxane A$_2$, and prostacyclin. Pharmacol. Rev., 30:293, 1979.
2. Goehlert, U.G., et al.: Biosynthesis of prostacyclin in rat cerebral microvessels and the choroid plexus. J. Neurochem., 36:1192, 1981.
3. Vane, J.R.: Prostaglandins and the cardiovascular system. Br. Heart J., 49:405, 1983.
4. Raz, A., et al.: Characterization of a novel metabolic pathway of arachidonate in coronary arteries which generates a potent endogenous coronary vasodilator. J. Biol. Chem., 252:1123, 1977.
5. Moncada, S., et al.: An enzyme isolated from arteries transforms prostaglandin endoperoxides to an unstable substance that inhibits platelet aggregation. Nature, 263:663, 1976.
6. Moncada, S., et al.: Human arterial and venous tissues generate prostacyclin (prostaglandin X), a potent inhibitor of platelet aggregation. Lancet, 1:18, 1977.
7. Gryglewski, R.J., et al.: Generation of prostacyclin by lungs in vivo and its release into the arterial circulation. Nature, 273:765, 1978.
8. Moncada, S., et al.: Prostacyclin is a circulating hormone. Nature, 273:767, 1978.
9. Szczeklik, K., et al.: Circulatory and antiplatelet effects of intravenous prostacyclin in healthy men. Pharmacol. Res., 10:545, 1978.
10. Szozeklik, A., et al.: Successful therapy of advanced arteriosclerosis obliterans with prostacyclin. Lancet, 1:1111, 1979.
11. Lichstein, E., et al.: Prostacyclin in unstable angina. American Heart Association, 1983.
12. Sideris, E.B., et al.: Effects of indomethacin, prostacyclin and prostaglandin E$_2$ on the fetal cardiac output and its distribution. American Heart Association, 1983.
12a. Sideris, E.B., et al.: Effects of indomethacin and prostaglandins E$_2$, I$_2$, and D$_2$ on the fetal circulation. Adv. Prostaglandin Thromboxane Leukotriene Res., 12:477, 1983.
13. Starling, M.B., et al.: Treatment of elevated pulmonary vascular resistance in neonatal animals. N.Z. Med. J., 91:363, 1980.
14. Szczeklik, J., et al.: Haemodynamic changes induced by prostacyclin in man. Br. Heart J., 44:254, 1980.
15. Leffler, C.W., and Hessler, J.R.: Pulmonary and systemic vascular effects of exogenous prostaglandin I$_2$ in fetal lambs. Eur. J. Pharmacol., 54:37, 1979.
16. Spannhake E.W., et al.: Pulmonary and systemic vasodilator effects of prostacyclin. (Abstract.) Fed. Proc. 37:731, 1978.
17. Watkins, W.D., et al.: Prostacyclin and prostaglandin E$_1$ for severe idiopathic pulmonary artery hypertension. (Letter.) Lancet, 1:1083, 1980.

18. Szczeklik, J., et al.: Prostacyclin for pulmonary hypertension. (Letter.) Lancet, 2:1076, 1980.
19. Rubin, L.J., et al.: Prostacyclin-induced acute pulmonary vasodilation in primary pulmonary hypertension. Circulation, 66:334, 1982.
20. Guadagni, D.N., et al.: Haemodynamic effects of prostacyclin (PGI$_2$) in pulmonary hypertension. Br. Heart J., 45:385, 1981.
21. Lock, J.E., et al.: Use of prostacyclin in persistent fetal circulation. (Letter.) Lancet, 1:1343, 1979.
22. Dzan, V.J., et al.: Prostaglandins in severe congestive heart failure. N. Engl. J. Med., 310:347, 1984.
23. Yui, Y., et al.: Prostacyclin therapy in patients with congestive heart failure. Am. J. Cardiol., 50:320, 1982.
24. Chaignon, M., et al.: Prostacyclin infusion in hypertension: acute hemodynamic and hormonal effects. (Letter.) N. Engl. J. Med., 307:559, 1983.
25. Wong, P.Y.K., et al.: Metabolism of prostacyclin by 9-hydroxyprostaglandin dehydrogenase in human platelets. J. Biol. Chem., 255:9021, 1980.
26. Sun, F.F., et al.: Metabolism of prostacyclin (PGI$_2$). (Abstract.) Prostaglandins, 15:724, 1978.
27. Wong, P.Y.K., et al.: Hepatic metabolism of prostacyclin (PGI$_2$) in the rabbit: formation of a potent novel inhibitor of platelet aggregation. Biochem. Biophys. Res. Commun., 93:486, 1980.
28. Rosenkranz, B., et al.: Prostacyclin metabolites in human plasma. Clin. Pharmacol. Ther., 29:420, 1981.
29. Lucas, F.V., et al.: Pharmacokinetics of prostacyclin. American Heart Association, 1983.

Chapter 34
Indomethacin

Several nonsteroidal anti-inflammatory drugs, including indomethacin, aspirin, and ibuprofen, constrict the patent ductus arteriosus in infants and even in fetuses when the drugs are administered to pregnant women. The mechanism responsible for this effect is believed to be inhibition of the synthesis of prostaglandins. Chapter 32 discusses the role of these agents in maintaining the patency of the ductus arteriosus during fetal life and in contributing, by a reduction in level, to the postnatal constriction of this structure.

The main use of prostaglandin-synthesis inhibitors, which are usually nonsteroidal anti-inflammatory drugs, in pediatric cardiovascular medicine is in pharmacologic closure of the patent ductus arteriosus in infants. The drug most widely used for this purpose is indomethacin. In the following chapter, the pharmacology, efficacy and adverse effects of indomethacin are discussed. The question whether pharmacologic or surgical closure is preferable for infants with a patent ductus arteriosus is mentioned only briefly because it is beyond the scope of this book.

Indomethacin is a nonsteroidal anti-inflammatory agent used in pediatric cardiovascular medicine for pharmacologic closure of patent ductus arteriosus. This end is achieved by inhibition of the enzyme cyclo-oxygenase, which participates in the synthesis of prostaglandins.

Structure

Indomethacin is a derivate of indoleacetic acid.

Pharmacologic Properties

Indomethacin is an acidic anti-inflammatory drug. In 1971, Vane found that this drug inhibited the enzyme cyclo-oxygenase. Many of the effects of indomethacin are attributed to this mechanism.[1]

Closure of Patent Ductus Arteriosus

Treatment with indomethacin promotes closure of patent ductus arteriosus and improves survival rates in infants with this anomaly. Indomethacin is effective in the majority of patients. It has been in use since the mid-1970s, when trials with aspirin did not have favorable results.

Heymann and co-workers studied the efficacy of indomethacin in infants with a patent ductus arteriosus, aged 4 to 21 days (mean age 10 days).[2] A dose of 0.1 mg/kg promoted closure of the ductus in 8 of 10 infants, and a dose of 0.3 mg/kg was effective in all 5 infants studied. The effect was evident within 30 hours of administration of indomethacin. Friedman and associates reported that a single dose of indomethacin promoted closure of patent ductus arteriosus in 6 infants with respiratory distress syndrome.[3] All infants in this series weighed more than 1000 g at birth. Yanagi and colleagues studied 39 infants with hemodynamically significant patent ductus arteriosus and symptoms of congestive heart failure or respiratory distress.[4] Closure of the ductus arteriosus occurred in 85% of the infants receiving indomethacin, as compared with 11% of those receiving placebo. Birth weight of the infants treated with indomethacin in this study was 1.5 ± 0.2 kg. Animal experiments have shown that indomethacin-induced constriction of the ductus arteriosus is associated with decreased right ventricular output and increased left ventricular output, although total cardiac output remains unchanged.[5]

As more experience was gained with the use of indomethacin, the drug was also given to preterm low-birth-weight infants with symptomatic patent ductus arteriosus. The results of these studies were less favorable. For example, indomethacin produced an improvement in only 2 of 7 preterm low-birth-weight infants with patent ductus arteriosus, congestive heart failure, and respiratory disturbances resistant to conventional treatment.[6] Even in these 2 infants, the ductus arteriosus remained open, and the improvement was only partial. The patients who responded weighed more at birth the other patients in this study. In another group of 6 infants weighing under 1000 g at birth, indomethacin produced only partial improvement, without complete closure of the ductus arteriosus.[7]

The poor response in these studies could have resulted from the late age at which indomethacin was given (between 7 and 30 days of age). PGE is more effective when given at an early age; therefore, the response to indomethacin may also be better if the drug is given early. Another cause of failure of the drug when given at later ages is the large left-to-right shunt that has developed, with associated hemodynamic impairment.

Nadas, in summarizing the subject in 1981, stated that until 1978, pharmacologic closure of the ductus arteriosus had been achieved in 18 to 100% of patients in several studies, and the issue was far from settled. Nadas reported the preliminary results of a multicenter study in the United States including 342 infants with a hemodynamically significant patent ductus arteriosus. Indomethacin was effective in closing the ductus arteriosus in more than two-thirds of these patients.[20]

Merritt and co-workers summarized the results of several studies using intravenous indomethacin in infants with patent ductus arteriosus and found a response rate of 79 to 91% in preterm infants treated during the first 2 weeks of life.[8] These findings were based on 10 studies reported between 1978 and 1982. The mean postnatal age of the infants in these studies ranged from 2.3 to 9.8 days.

The optimal timing for administration of indomethacin has not been determined. Current practice is to treat only those infants with hemodynamic deterioration due to a hemodynamically significant left-to-right shunt through the patent ductus arteriosus and in whom conventional therapy has been unsuccessful. In the critically ill preterm infant, however, the pulmonary edema resulting from patent ductus arteriosus, with its surfactant-inhibitory effect, imposes an additional burden on the premature lungs, with pulmonary congestion and acidosis.[8] Several studies have shown reduced responsiveness with late treatment.[9-17]

In a study by Mahony and associates, infants were treated as soon as a patent ductus arteriosus was diagnosed, but before signs of a significant shunt became noticeable.[18] The mean age at which indomethacin was administered was 2.9 days. Among infants weighing under 1000 g at birth, administration of indomethacin was associated with a significant decrease in morbidity, despite the absence of clinical or echocardiographic signs of a hemodynamically significant shunt before or during treatment. Mahony and colleagues stated that infants weighing under 1000 g at birth are at a high risk for developing a potentially deleterious shunt through a patent ductus arteriosus.[18] These workers suggested that early treatment of such infants with indomethacin may prevent this development and may decrease morbidity.

Merritt and co-workers studied 11 preterm infants who had received indomethacin as soon as signs of left-to-right shunting through a patent ductus were detected, at a mean age of 48.8 hours, and compared their clinical course with 12 infants treated initially by conventional therapy and only later, at a mean age of 167.4 hours, with indomethacin.[19] Only 2 of the 11 infants treated early developed chronic lung disease, as compared with 8 of the 12 infants treated later.

Halliday and associates reported that, in 36 preterm infants weighing under 1500 g, indomethacin produced a better response in those aged 8 to 14 days than in those older than 14 days, irrespective of birth weight or gestational age.[12] Nadas reported no statistically significant difference in hospital mortality rates whether indomethacin was given concurrently with conventional therapy, immediately on diagnosis of patent ductus arteriosus, or only when evidence of a patent ductus arteriosus persisted after 48 hours of conventional therapy, however.[20]

Preterm infants of low birth weight appear to be more resistant to indomethacin than those of higher birth weight. Because indomethacin probably acts by blocking prostaglandin synthesis in the ductal wall, among other sites, it may be assumed that the underdevelopment of the muscular layer of the ductal wall in these infants is the cause of the resistance. Indomethacin not only closes the patent ductus arteriosus, but is also associated with improved survival in infants with this anomaly.[2, 3, 21]

In summary, indomethacin appears to be effective in closing patent ductus arteriosus in infants. The question whether to select surgical ligation or pharmacologic closure with indomethacin depends, however, on the side effects of the drug and on other practical considerations. The time for initiation of treatment is controversial.

Gestational Age and Response

The question whether gestational age effects the response to indomethacin is controversial. McCarthy and associates reported that infants with gestational age of under 33 weeks showed a maximal response to indomethacin.[22] In contrast, Yeh and co-workers reported that all their 10 patients of more than 37 weeks' gestation responded to the drug.[21] Halliday and co-workers reported that gestational age did not affect the response to indomethacin.[12] In vitro studies have shown that gestational age affects the response of isolated strips of the ductus arteriosus from lambs to indomethacin.[23] At present, the question of a possible relationship between gestational age and response to indomethacin remains open.

Morphology of the Ductus Arteriosus and Response

The morphologic features of the patent ductus arteriosus may affect the response to indomethacin. Four stages of morphologic, and probably also a corresponding functional, maturation of the ductus arteriosus have been described[24]: In stage 1, the ductus arteriosus resembles in structure a small artery, consisting of a thin intima and an internal elastic membrane. In stage 2, intimal cushions that may protrude into the lumen are formed. In stage 3, the ductus is functionally closed with intimal cushions protruding into the lumen or occluding it, cytolytic necrosis, and mucoid lakes. Stage 3a resembles stage 3, but with a subendothelial elastic lamina around the ductal lumen. Stage 4 consists of complete occlusion with fusion of the intimal cushions. No strict relationship exists between gestational age and stage of ductal maturation. Infants with a ductus arteriosus at stages 1 or 3a may not respond completely to indomethacin.

Clyman and associates suggested that the maturation of the ductus arteriosus may be influenced by glucocorticoids.[25, 26] They also suggested that glucocorticoids can alter the sensitivity of lamb ductus arteriosus to PGE_2. These findings may indicate a potential direction for prenatal prophylaxis.

Drug Levels and Ductal Response

As stated earlier, indomethacin is effective in about 80 to 90% of patients. Inadequate plasma levels of the drug or rapid excretion may be responsible for some failures.

Pharmacologic Versus Surgical Closure of Patent Ductus Arteriosus

The decision whether to attempt pharmacologic closure of a patent ductus arteriosus or to ligate the ductus surgically depends on several factors. Most important is the mortality rate in infants undergoing these procedures. In a multicenter study in the United States, the mortality rate was the same in infants treated surgically without ever having received indomethacin and in those treated with indomethacin.[20] Merritt and colleagues summarized the results of 10 studies using intravenous indomethacin for closure of a patent ductus arteriosus and found a mortality rate of 3 to 23%.[8] This rate was comparable to the mortality rate of 7 to 24% reported in several surgical series since 1981.[27-29] The selection of therapy depends on other factors as well, however, such as availability of surgical facilities, the general condition of the patient, and the presence of a contraindication to indomethacin administration. In the large study in the United States, for example, 44% of infants with a patent ductus could not be randomized because of contraindications. I believe that the decision should be made individually in each case.

Based on the results of the United States co-operative study, Ellison and Nadas suggested that the preferable strategy for the management of small premature infants with patent ductus arteriosus is an initial trial of conventional medical therapy, with indomethacin given only if this regimen is not effective.[30] Surgical ligation should be performed if indomethacin is ineffective.

Contraindications

In the co-operative multicenter study in the United States, the presence of one of the following factors was considered to be a contraindication to administration of indomethacin[20]: (1) blood urea nitrogen levels of 30 mg/dl or more; (2) serum creatinine levels of 1.8 mg/dl or more; (3) total urine output of 0.5 ml/kg/hour or less over the past 8 hours; (4) a platelet count of under 60,000; (5) a positive stool blood test; (6) evidence of bleeding diathesis; (7) evidence or suspicion of necrotizing entercolitis; and (8) evidence of intracranial hemorrhage, either suspected within 24 hours or confirmed (unless it occurred at least a week before; the infant would then be considered to be completely recovered).

Clinical Pharmacology

Indomethacin may be given orally, rectally, or intravenously. The response is usually evident within 24 to 48 hours. The drug is rapidly and almost completely absorbed from the gastrointestinal tract after oral administration. Peak plasma levels are usually reached within 3 hours of oral administration. Food may delay the absorption of indomethacin.

In patients who do not respond, the drug may not reach adequate levels at the ductus arteriosus. Alpert and co-workers reported that plasma levels were the same in responders as in nonresponders, however.[31]

About 90% of the drug in the plasma is bound to plasma proteins. It penetrates various tissues, including the ductus arteriosus and, to some extent, the central nervous system. The penetration of the drug into the central nervous system is greater in premature neonates than in adults. Indomethacin is eliminated by hepatic metabolism, converting it to inactive metabolites. The main pathways of metabolism are O-demethylation and N-deacetylation.[32] The free and conjugated metabolites are excreted in the urine and bile and possibly also by the intestinal walls. The highest efficacy of ductal constriction has been achieved with a peak plasma level of 1.0 μg/ml after a loading dose and 0.5 μg/ml during maintenance therapy.[33]

Side Effects

Although side effects of indomethacin in infants are uncommon, some of these effects may be severe. In contrast, long-term indomethacin use in adults is associated with a high incidence of side effects.

Cardiovascular Effects

The inhibition of prostaglandin synthesis may be deleterious. In adult patients with coronary artery disease and congestive heart failure, indomethacin may produce hemodynamic deterioration. In one study, indomethacin caused hemodynamic deterioration, as seen by increases in systemic vascular resistance and pulmonary capillary wedge pressure and by a decrease in cardiac output.[34] This effect occurred in patients who had also hyponatremia, whereas patients with congestive heart failure and normal sodium levels had no significant hemodynamic changes. It is not known whether indomethacin produces hemodynamic deterioration in infants with patent ductus arteriosus and congestive heart failure. Animal experiments have shown, however, that indomethacin may increase the fetal pulmonary blood flow even if it partially constricts the ductus arteriosus.[5] The potential of hemodynamic deterioration should be weighed against the marked improvement achieved by closure of the ductus arteriosus.

Renal Effects

Renal failure may be produced in infants receiving high doses of indomethacin. An increase in serum creatinine and decreases in serum sodium levels and urinary volume have been observed.[12-14, 16, 35] These effects may occur in addition to pre-existing impairment of renal function or general hemodynamic impairment in preterm low-birth-weight infants with patent ductus arteriosus. The indomethacin-induced renal failure may be life-threatening, although it usually responds to discontinuance of the drug.[2, 3, 6] Merritt and colleagues reported a 30% reduction or more in urine formation in the 12 hours after indomethacin administration in 55% of their patients.[8] In most of these patients, urine formation returned to pretreatment levels within 24 hours. In 25 of the 67 patients, not necessarily those with decreased urine formation, transient elevations of serum or creatinine by more than 30% were observed.[13] The transient impairment in renal function appears to be independent of plasma levels of indomethacin and duration of therapy.[33]

Gastrointestinal Effects

Like other acidic nonsteroidal anti-inflammatory agents, indomethacin may cause gastrointestinal side effects. Gastrointestinal bleeding may result from indomethacin-induced inhibition of platelet aggregation.[36] Yanagi and associates reported that 23% of infants in their study who were treated with indomethacin developed mild and transient gastrointestinal bleeding that disappeared spontaneously within 24 hours.[4] A few cases of necrotizing enterocolitis and focal intestinal performation have been reported. Nagaraj and co-workers reported that 13 of 82 infants treated with indomethacin developed necrotizing enterocolitis, and 8 of 82 had focal gastrointestinal perforation.[37] Other studies have not reported a higher incidence of these effects in infants treated with indomethacin than in infants who undergo surgical ligation of the patent ductus arteriosus.[11, 15, 16, 38, 39]

Increased Bleeding Time

Indomethacin prolongs bleeding time, probably by inhibiting thromboxane A_2 in platelets. This effect does not increase the incidence of spontaneous bleeding, however.

Hyponatremia

Hyponatremia was reported in several neonates treated with indomethacin.[12] For example, 8 of 67 infants treated by Merritt and associates experienced a transient reduction in serum sodium levels.[8] Fourteen of 48 infants studied by Bhat and colleagues had serum sodium levels lower than 130 meq/L.[9] The effect of indomethacin in potentiating antidiuretic hormone may be the cause of this adverse effect. In patients with congestive heart failure and hyponatremia, prostaglandins play an especially important role in regulating the circulation.[34] By inhibiting the synthesis of prostaglandins and by producing hyponatremia in infants who already have congestive heart failure, indomethacin may be potentially deleterious.

Hyperkalemia

Halliday and co-workers found a rise in serum potassium levels to more than 6.0 meq/L in 25% of infants treated with indomethacin.[12] The mechanism of this effect is not clear, but it may be related to impaired renal function.

Retrolental Fibroplasia

Patent ductus arteriosus is a risk factor for the development of retrolental fibroplasia. Treatment with indomethacin does not increase this risk.[39]

Drug Interactions

Indomethacin interacts with several drugs. The mechanism of most interactions is inhibition of prostaglandin synthesis by indomethacin; the effect of the interacting drugs depends, at least partially, on normal synthesis of prostaglandins. The interactions relevant to the pediatric age group are with furosemide, hydralazine, digoxin, and possibly with methylxanthines.

Furosemide

Furosemide is a potent diuretic and natriuretic agent that also has some vasodilatory properties. Some of these effects may be partially mediated by prostaglandins. Several investigators have reported an interaction between indomethacin and furosemide. Patak and co-workers reported that administration of furosemide after pretreatment with indomethacin decreased the effect of furosemide in normal persons and in hypertensive patients.[40] Chennovasin and colleagues reported that indomethacin decreased the natriuretic effect of furosemide.[41] Other investigators, however, did not find such an interaction.[42]

Nies and associates reported that the most important mechanism of the interaction between indomethacin and furosemide is the effect of indomethacin in blocking the renal vasodilation produced by furosemide.[43] Indomethacin blocks the proximal tubular effect of furosemide and thus decreases the delivery of electrolytes to the loop of Henle. Other possible mechanisms are blockade of furosemide-induced inhibition of chloride transport in the loop of Henle or competition for the acid transport system in the proximal tubule. Indomethacin is usually given to infants with large left-to-right shunts. If these patients are treated for congestive heart failure, the interaction between furosemide and indomethacin may be significant.

Hydralazine

Inhibition of prostaglandin synthesis by indomethacin may reduce the effect of hydralazine.[44]

Digoxin

Wikerson and colleagues reported a significant elevation of serum digoxin levels in anesthetized dogs following the administration of indomethacin.[45] In human infants, digoxin and quinidine interactions with indomethacin, even leading to digitalis intoxication, have been reported;[46, 47] these interactions may be partially attributed to the reduced renal function in the neonates that decreased the renal clearance of digoxin.

Interactions of combined quinidine and digoxin with indomethacin may be significant in infants with patent ductus arteriosus, congestive heart failure, and arrhythmias who are receiving conventional anticongestive therapy. In a study of six healthy volunteers, indomethacin did not alter the elimination half-life, systemic clearance, or distribution of digoxin, however.[48]

Methylxanthines

No interaction between methylxanthines and indomethacin has been reported, although in vitro studies showed that methylxanthines can relax the ductus arteriosus.[49] In infants with patent ductus arteriosus and respiratory distress syndrome, treatment with methylxanthines such as aminosphylline possibly may inhibit the effect of indomethacin. This potential interaction has not been studied.

Other Drugs

Indomethacin has been reported to reduce the effect of nitroglycerin.[50] This interaction is controversial and is not relevant to infants. Indomethacin has also reduced the effect of propranolol and pindolol.[51]

Dosage and Administration

Intravenous Administration

In adults, doses of 0.5 mg/kg were used in clinical studies.[34] In infants of low birth weight, under 1000 g, an intravenous dose of 0.2 mg/kg was given, followed by 0.1 mg/kg in 12 hours and an additional 0.1 mg/kg in 36 hours.

Oral and Rectal Administration

Friedman and associates used oral doses of 2.5 mg/kg and rectal doses of 5 mg/kg with success.[3] Heymann and co-workers used lower oral doses of 0.1 to 0.3 mg/kg, repeated up to 3 times, with success.[2] Yanagi and colleagues administered 3 doses of 0.2 mg/kg each, at 8 hour intervals, through an orogastric tube.[4]

Administration to Pregnant Women

Experimentally, several nonsteroidal anti-inflammatory drugs have constricted the fetal ductus arteriosus when administered to pregnant women. Among these agents are indomethacin, aspirin, ibuprofen, and flurbiprofen.[52-54] The reason for this effect is that these agents cross the placenta and inhibit prostaglandin synthesis in the fetus. Intrauterine constriction of the fetal ductus arteriosus may cause pulmonary hypertension in the neonate or congestive heart failure in the fetus.[55] Therefore, one should not give nonsteroidal anti-inflammatory drugs to pregnant women. A recent study has shown, however, that acidic and basic nonsteroidal anti-inflammatory drugs are different; every acidic drug tested had some constrictive effect on the fetal ductus arteriosus. In contrast, six basic nonsteroidal anti-inflammatory drugs showed no significant constriction of the fetal ductus arteriosus even at doses up to a hundred fold higher than regular therapeutic doses. Among these basic drugs are benzydamine, MK-447, and ONO-3144, which do not inhibit cyclo-oxygenase or prostaglandin synthetase.[52] If future studies confirm these findings, certain basic nonsteroidal antiflammatory drugs might be used with safety in pregnant women.

References

1. Vane, J.R.: Inhibition of prostaglandin synthesis as a mechanism of action of aspirin-like drugs. Nature (New Biol.), 231:232, 1971.
2. Heymann, M.A., et al.: Closure of the ductus arteriosus in premature infants by inhibition of prostaglandin synthesis. N. Engl. J. Med., 295:530, 1976.

3. Friedman, W.F., et al.: Pharmacologic closure of patent ductus arteriosus in the premature infant. N. Engl. J. Med., 295:526, 1976.
4. Yanagi, R.M., et al.: Indomethacin treatment for symptomatic patent ductus arteriosus: a double-blind controlled study. Pediatrics, 67:647, 1981.
5. Sideris, E.B., et al.: Effects of indomethacin and prostaglandins E_2, I_2, and D_2 on the fetal circulation. Adv. Prostaglandin Thromboxane Leukotriene Res., 12:477, 1983.
6. Cooke, R.W.I. and Pickering, D.: Poor response to oral indomethacin therapy for persistent ductus arteriosus in very low birthweight infants. Br. Heart J., 41:301, 1979.
7. Ivey, H.H., et al.: Failure of indomethacin to close persistent ductus arteriosus in infants weighing under 1000 grams. Br. Heart J., 41:304, 1979.
8. Merritt, T.A., et al.: Clinical trials of intravenous indomethacin for closure of the patent ductus arteriosus. Pediatr. Cardiol., 4(Suppl. II):71, 1983.
9. Bhat, R., et al.: Patent ductus arteriosus: recent advances in diagnosis and management. Pediatr. Clin. North Am., 29:1117, 1982.
10. Firth, J., and Pickering, D.: Timing of indomethacin therapy in persistent ductus. Lancet, 2:144, 1980.
11. Gersony, W., et al.: Effects of indomethacin in premature infants with patent ductus arteriosus: results of a national collaborative study. J. Pediatr., 102:895, 1983.
12. Halliday, H., et al.: Indomethacin therapy for large patent ductus arteriosus in the very low birth weight infant: results and complications. Pediatrics, 64:154, 1979.
13. Harris, J., et al.: Parenteral indomethacin for closure of the patent ductus arteriosus. Am. J. Dis. Child., 136:1005, 1982.
14. McCarthy, J., et al.: Age-dependent closure of the patent ductus arteriosus by indomethacian. Pediatrics, 62:706, 1978.
15. Yeh, T., et al.: Intravenous indomethacin therapy in premature infants with patent ductus arteriosus. Am. J. Dis. Child., 136:803, 1982.
16. Merritt, T.A.: Closure of the patent ductus arteriosus with ligation and indomethacin: a consecutive experience. J. Pediatr., 93:639, 1978.
17. Vert, P., et al.: Effectiveness and pharmacokinetics of indomethacin in premature newborns with patent ductus arteriosus. Eur. J. Clin. Pharmacol., 18:83, 1980.
18. Mahony, L., et al.: When to treat the patent ductus arteriosus with indomethacin in very-low-birth-weight infants. Adv. Prostaglandin Thromboxane Leukotriene Res., 12:1983.
19. Merritt, T.A., et al.: Early closure of the patent ductus arteriosus in very low birth weight infants: a controlled trial. J. Pediatr., 99:281, 1981.
20. Nadas, A.S.: Mannheimer lecture. Pediatr. Cardiol., 3:71, 1982.
21. Yeh, T.F., et al.: Intravenous indomethacin therapy in premature infants with persistent ductus arteriosus—a double-blind controlled study. J. Pediatr., 98:137, 1981.
22. McCarthy, I.S., et al.: Age dependent closure of patent ductus arteriosus by indomethacin. Pediatrics, 62:706, 1978.
23. Clyman, R.I., et al.: Age dependent sensitivity of the ductus arteriosus to indomethacin and prostaglandins. J. Pediatr., 96:94, 1980.
24. Gittenberger de Groot, A.C., et al.: The ductus arteriosus in the preterm infant: histologic and clinical observations. J. Pediatr., 96:88, 1980.
25. Clyman, R.I., et al.: Prenatal administration of betamethasone for prevention of patent ductus arteriosus. J. Pediatr., 97:123, 1981.
26. Clyman, R.I., et al.: Glucocorticoids alter the sensitivity of the lamb ductus arteriosus to prostaglandin E_2. J. Pediatr., 98:126, 1981.
27. Eggert, L., et al.: Surgical treatment of the patent ductus arteriosus in preterm infants. Pediatr. Cardiol., 2:15, 1982.
28. Mikhail, M., et al.: Surgical and medical experience with 734 premature infants with patent ductus arteriosus. J. Thorac. Cardiovasc. Surg., 83:349, 1982.
29. Nagle, M., et al.: Ligation of patent ductus arteriosus in very low birth weight infants. Am. J. Surg., 142:681, 1981.
30. Ellison, R.C., and Nadas, A.S.: Indomethacin and patent ductus arteriosus in premature infants: report from a collaborative study in the United States. Pediatr. Cardiol., 4(Suppl. II):93, 1983.

31. Alpert, B.S., et al.: Plasma indomethacin levels in preterm newborn infants with symptomatic patent ductus arteriosus: clinical and echocardiographic assessments of response. J. Pediatr., *95*:578, 1979.
32. Duggan, D.E., et al.: The metabolism of indomethacin in man. J. Pharmacol. Exp. Ther., *181*:563, 1972.
33. Seyberth, H.W., et al.: Indomethacin in preterm infants with patent ductus arteriosus: disposition, benefit and side effects. Pediatr. Cardiol, *4(Suppl. II)*:81, 1983.
34. Dzau, V.J., et al.: Prostaglandins in severe congestive heart failure. N. Engl. J. Med., *310*:347, 1984.
35. Friedman, W., et al.: The inhibition of prostaglandin and prostacyclin synthesis in the clinical management of patent ductus arteriosus. Semin. Perinatol., *4*:125, 1980.
36. Friedman, Z., et al.: Indomethacin disposition and indomethacin-induced platelet dysfunction in premature infants. J. Clin. Pharmacol., *18*:272, 1978.
37. Nagaraj, H., et al.: Gastrointestinal perforation following indomethacin therapy in very low birth weight infants. J. Pediatr. Surg., *16*:1003, 1981.
38. Merritt, T.A., et al.: Patent ductus arteriosus treated with ligation or indomethacin: a follow-up study. J. Pediatr., *95*:588, 1979.
39. Merritt, T.A., et al.: Preschool assessment of infants with a patent ductus arteriosus. Am. J. Dis. Child., *136*:507, 1982.
40. Patak, R.V., et al.: Antagonism of the effects of furosemide by indomethacin in normal and hypertensive man. Prostaglandins, *10*:649, 1975.
41. Chennovasin, P., et al.: J. Pharmacol. Exp. Ther. *215*:77, 1980.
42. Weber, P., et al.: Increase of free arachidonic acid by furosemide in man as the cause of prostaglandin and renin release. Eur. J. Pharmacol., *41*:329, 1977.
43. Nies, A.S., et al.: Indomethacin-furosemide interaction: the importance of renal blood flow. Adv. Prostaglandin Thromboxane Leukotriene Res., *11*:1983.
44. Slack, B.L., et al.: The effect of prostaglandin synthetase inhibition on the action of hydralazine. (abstract.) Circulation, *58(Suppl. II)*:II-21, 1978.
45. Wilkerson, R.D., et al.: Effects of selected drugs on serum digoxin concentrations in dogs. Am. J. Cardiol., *45*:1201, 1980.
46. Mayes, L.C., and Boerth, R.C.: Digoxin-indomethacin interaction. Pediatr. Res., *14*:263, 1980.
47. Schimmel, M.S.: Toxic digitalis levels associated with indomethacin therapy in a neonate. Clin. Pediatr (Phila.), p. 768, 1980.
48. Finch, M.B., et al.: Pharmacokinetics of digoxin alone and in the presence of indomethacin therapy. Br. J. Clin. Pharmacol., *17*:353, 1984.
49. Kreil, E., et al.: Effects of cyclic AMP on isolated ductus arteriosus. Pediatr. Res., *7*:300, 1973.
50. Morcillio, E.: Myocardial prostaglandin E release by nitroglycerin and modification by indomethacin. Am. J. Cardiol., *45*:5, 1980.
51. Durao, V., and Rico, J.M.G.T.: Modification by indomethacin of the blood pressure lowering effect of pindolol and propranolol in conscious rabbits. Eur. J. Pharmacol., *43*:377, 1977.
52. Momma, K., and Takeuchi, H.: Constriction of fetal ductus arteriosus by nonsteroidal antiinflammatory drugs. Adv. Prostaglandin Thromboxane Leukotriene Res., *12*:1983.
53. Heymann, M.A., and Rudolph, A.M.: Circ. Res., *38*:418, 1976.
54. Olley, P.M., et al.: Eur. J. Pharmacol., *34*:247, 1975.
55. Levin, D.L.: *In* Prostaglandins in the Perinatal Period. Edited by M.A. Heymann. New York, Grune & Stratton, 1980, p. 35.

Section VII
CENTRALLY ACTING ANTIHYPERTENSIVE AGENTS

Regulation of blood pressure is a complex mechanism in which the central nervous system plays an important role. It is possible to affect the peripheral vascular resistance, and thus also the systemic arterial pressure, by altering the sympathetic discharge from the central nervous system. Most conventional antihypertensive agents act on the end organs in the regulation of blood pressure, namely, the peripheral arteries and arterioles, the heart, and the kidneys. Several centrally acting antihypertensive agents have been used for many years as conventional therapy, however. They include agents such as methyldopa, clonidine, Guanabenz, and guanfacine. Some experience with these agents, mainly methyldopa and clonidine, has also been gained in young age groups.

These agents have in common a central mechanism of action. Methyldopa exerts its effect when it has been metabolized to the active form of the drug, which acts as a central false transmitter. Clonidine acts by direct stimulation of postsynaptic alpha-2-adrenoreceptors in the central nervous system. In both cases, the result is a decrease in sympathetic discharge and in vascular resistance, without an increase in cardiac output, leading to a reduction in blood pressure. The centrally acting antihypertensive agents are discussed in Chapters 35 and 36.

Chapter 35

Clonidine

Clonidine, an antihypertensive agent with a central mechanism of action, reduces sympathetic discharge and thereby causes vasodilation and a hypotensive effect. The drug is effective alone or in combination with other antihypertensive drugs in controlling essential and renovascular hypertension. Clonidine may be useful in certain patients with congestive heart failure, but the specific hemodynamic profile of this drug may be disadvantageous in children with congestive heart failure because clonidine may reduce cardiac output.

The bulk of experience with clonidine has been in treatment of hypertension in adults. Several children and adolescents with essential hypertension have been treated with clonidine, however. Clonidine may produce side effects, including severe bradycardia, which is uncommon, drowsiness, and dry mouth.

I advise against giving clonidine to infants and young children. In older children and in adolescents with hypertension, the drug may be given if all forms of oral conventional treatment have failed. The long-term effects of prolonged clonidine treatment in children have not been studied.

Mechanism of Action

Clonidine is an antihypertensive agent acting mainly by a central mechanism. Its primary effect is stimulation of alpha-adrenoreceptors in the central nervous system. These receptors are most probably postsynaptic alpha-2-adrenoreceptors.[1-5] The effect of clonidine can be inhibited by alpha-adrenoreceptor blocking agents. The question whether the central mechanism of the antihypertensive effect of clonidine is mediated by opiate receptors is controversial. In hypertensive rats, the antihypertensive effect of clonidine has been antagonized by central administration of antiserum to beta-endorphin[6,7] or by the opiate antagonists naloxone and noltrexone.[6, 8-10] These findings may indicate an involvement of opiate receptors in regulation of blood pressure by clonidine. Because other investigators have reported that opiate antagonists do not inhibit the effect of clonidine,[11] however, the role of opiate receptors in this mechanism is not clear.

The stimulation of central alpha-adrenoreceptors results in a reduction in sympathetic discharge and in the levels of plasma catecholamines and plasma renin activity. These effects, in turn, decrease peripheral resistance and blood pressure by reducing the sympathetic tone and the pressor effects of plasma catecholamines and the renin-angiotensin system. The peripheral vasodilation is not associated with an increase in cardiac output because heart rate is reduced and myocardial contractility is not enhanced.

Cardiovascular, Renal, and Humoral Effects

Clonidine decreases peripheral resistance, arterial pressure, and heart rate. It does not usually alter myocardial contractility. In hypertensive patients, clonidine has not altered cardiac output,[12] but in patients with congestive heart failure, a decrease in cardiac output has been observed.[13] Clonidine inhibits, but does not prevent, the normal responses of heart rate and blood pressure to exercise.[14] Renal hemodynamics are not altered or are even improved by clonidine. In a group of patients with renovascular hypertension, clonidine reduced the renal vascular resistance.[15] In a group of patients with essential hypertension, clonidine did not alter renal blood flow or glomerular filtration rate.[12] Clonidine lowers the levels of plasma catecholamines and plasma renin activity,[15–17] although in a study of several patients with low-renin hypertension, clonidine elevated plasma renin activity.[18] Clonidine may have a suppressant effect on aldosterone, an effect independent of the renin-suppressant action of the drug.[19]

Effects in Hypertension

Clonidine has effectively controlled hypertension in numerous clinical studies. It lowers both elevated systolic and diastolic blood pressures, at rest and during exercise, in patients with essential hypertension as well as in those with renovascular hypertension. Clonidine may be used either as the sole antihypertensive agent or in combination with other antihypertensive drugs, preferably excluding alpha-adrenoreceptor blocking agents. Its effect in monotherapy is comparable to that of hydrochlorothiazide.[20–26]

Effects in Young Hypertensive Patients

The pharmacologic profile of clonidine makes it suitable for treatment of hypertension in young age groups. The drug has the following advantages: (1) it can be used alone; (2) short- and long-term control of blood pressure may be achieved with the same dose of the drug; (3) clonidine does not cause fluid and sodium retention; (4) cardiac output, renal blood flow, and glomerular filtration rate are not altered;

(5) plasma catecholamine levels decline; and (6) no overt changes in blood chemistry occur.[26] On the other hand, adverse effects such as sexual dysfunction and sedation may be troublesome in various young age groups.

Falkner and co-workers studied the efficacy and tolerance of clonidine in a group of 14 adolescents treated with hydrochlorothiazide.[20] The group treated with clonidine included 12 males and 2 females; 10 were blacks. The mean age of the group was 16 years. Systolic blood pressure was 146 ± 15.8, and diastolic blood pressure was 96 ± 6.2 mm Hg. Heart rate was 85 ± 9.3 beats/min. After a placebo phase, therapy was initiated with a low oral dose of clonidine, 0.1 mg twice daily, for 12 weeks. This regimen resulted in decreases in systolic blood pressure of about 10 mm Hg, in diastolic blood pressure of about 8 mm Hg, and in heart rate of about 10 beats/min. Ten of the patients continued treatment with clonidine, 0.2 mg twice daily, and had a greater reduction of blood pressure with this dose. In comparison, the adolescents treated with 25 mg hydrochlorothiazide twice daily showed a decrease in systolic pressure only. Some of these patients developed reductions in serum potassium levels. Falkner and associates stated that clonidine effectively controlled blood pressure in 85% of the patients in the group studied, and hydrochlorothiazide was effective in only 40% of these patients.

Only a few cases of clonidine treatment in children with severe hypertension have been reported. In my experience, clonidine was ineffective in a child whose condition was resistant to multiple conventional and investigational agents. Pennisi and associates reported on 2 patients, aged 18 and 17 years, respectively, who received clonidine as part of multiple drug therapy for severe hypertension.[27] In both patients, this regimen failed to control the elevated blood pressure, and frequent intravenous administration of diazoxide was required. Control of blood pressure with oral therapy was achieved only when minoxidil was added.[27]

In the report of the Task Force on Blood Pressure Control in Children, clonidine was not evaluated, and clinical data were not available.

Effects in Congestive Heart Failure

In patients with congestive heart failure, clonidine has an interesting and unique hemodynamic profile. It produces vasodilation without enhancing myocardial function. This hemodynamic profile has only recently been recognized.[13] Clonidine may be beneficial to adult patients with congestive heart failure and active coronary artery disease. In such patients, the lack of increase in myocardial contractility is important because myocardial oxygen demand is not heightened. This feature is not usually of benefit in children, and it may even be deleterious, by limiting the hemodynamic improvement produced by vasodilation. The hemodynamic features of clonidine in patients with congestive heart failure were evaluated by Hermiller and colleagues.[13] In a group of 14 patients, clonidine, at doses of 0.2 and 0.4 mg orally, had no effect on myocardial contractility. The 0.4-mg dose increased stroke volume by 15%, whereas the 0.2-mg dose did not alter this parameter. The 0.2-mg dose decreased heart rate by 11%, mean pulmonary arterial pressure by 20%, pulmonary capillary wedge pressure by 27%, and mean systemic arterial pressure by 15%. The calculated pulmonary and systemic vascular resistances were also decreased, but to a lesser extent than the corresponding pressures because cardiac output was also reduced.[13] The hemodynamic effects of clonidine result from a decrease in central sympathetic discharge that leads not only to vasodilation, but also to depression of heart rate. The reflex increase in myocardial contractility, seen with conventional vasodilators, does not occur with clonidine because of the decrease in sympathetic discharge.

Effects in Bronchospasm

The effect of clonidine on pulmonary function has not been evaluated in pediatric patients with bronchial asthma, but in a study of adults with hypertension and bronchospasm, the drug did not produce any adverse effect on pulmonary function.[28]

Drug Discontinuance

Clonidine withdrawal syndrome is a significant problem in some patients who abruptly discontinue treatment with this drug. It is difficult to evaluate the incidence of this syndrome, but a well-controlled study showed that none of 20 patients with essential hypertension developed this syndrome after abrupt cessation of treatment.[29] The symptoms of abrupt clonidine withdrawal include tachycardia, arrhythmias, palpitations, rebound hypertension, flushing, nausea, and vomiting.[30–34] The syndrome probably results from increases in sympathetic discharge, plasma catecholamine levels, and plasma renin activity on discontinuance of the drug. Opioid receptors may play a role in the development of symptoms.

Clinical Pharmacology

Clonidine may be given intravenously or orally. It is well and rapidly absorbed from the gastrointestinal tract after oral administration.[35–37] A strong correlation exists between plasma levels of the drug and its antihypertensive effect; therapeutic plasma levels range between 0.8 and 2.0 ng/ml in patients with normal renal function. At least one study has indicated that the therapeutic effect of clonidine is maximal within a narrow range of plasma concentration and does not increase when plasma levels are higher than the upper limit of this range.[38]

The half-life of clonidine is about 8 hours. The drug is eliminated mainly by the kidneys, and about 60% of the dose is eliminated unchanged in the urine.[39, 40] In patients with renal failure, the drug accumulates, and high plasma levels are reached.

Side Effects

The most serious side effect of clonidine is severe bradycardia, which may be produced by high doses; it responds to atropine. The most common side effects are drowsiness and dry mouth. They may be dose-related and may appear only when the dose is increased, as in 1 of 14 adolescents treated with clonidine in a study.[20]

Dosage and Administration

Oral doses of 0.1 to 0.2 mg daily are administered to older children and to adolescents.

References

1. Schmitt, H.: The pharmacology of clonidine and related compounds. Handbook Exp. Pharmacol., *39*:299, 1977.
2. U'Prichard, D.C., et al.: Multiple apparent alpha-noradrenergic receptor binding sites in rat brain: effect of 6-hydroxydopamine. Mol. Pharmacol., *16*:47, 1979.
3. Rouot, B.M., et al.: Multiple α_2-noradrenergic receptor sites in rat brain: selective regulation of high affinity [^{3}H] clonidine binding by guanyl nucleotides and divalent cations. J. Neurochem., *34*:374, 1980.
4. Summers, R.J., et al.: Selectivity of a series of clonidine-like drugs for α_1 and α_2 adrenoreceptors in rat brain. Neurosci. Lett., *20*:347, 1980.
5. Holman, R.B., et al.: Simultaneous determination of indole and catecholamines in small brain regions in the rat using a weak cation exchange resin. Neuroscience, *1*:147, 1976.
6. Ramirez-Gonzalez, M.D., et al.: Beta-endorphin acting on the brainstem is involved in the antihypertensive action of clonidine and α-methyldopa in rats. Circ. Res., *53*:150, 1983.
7. Petty, M.A., and de Jong, W.: Does β-endorphin contribute to the central antihypertensive action of α-methyldopa? Clin. Sci. *63*:293, 1982.
8. Farsang, C., and Kunos, G.: Naloxone reverses the antihypertensive effect of clonidine. Br. J. Pharmacol., *67*:161, 1979.
9. Farsang, C., et al.: Possible role of an endogenous opiate in the cardiovascular effects of central α-adrenoceptor stimulation in spontaneously hypertensive rats. J. Pharmacol. Exp. Ther., *214*:253, 1980.
10. Farsang, C., et al.: Reversal by naloxone of the antihypertensive action of clonidine: involvement of the sympathetic nervous system. Circulation, *69*:461, 1984.
11. Rogers, J.F., and Cubeddu, L.X.: Naloxone does not antagonize the antihypertensive effect of clonidine in essential hypertension. Clin. Pharmacol. Ther., *34*:68, 1983.
12. Thananopavarn, C., et al.: Clonidine, a centrally acting sympathetic inhibitor, as monotherapy for mild to moderate hypertension. Am. J. Cardiol., *49*:153, 1982.
13. Hermiller, J.B., et al.: Clonidine in congestive heart failure: a vasodilator with negative inotropic effects. Am. J. Cardiol., *51*:791, 1983.

14. Lowenthal, D.T., et al.: Dynamic and biochemical responses to single and repeated doses of clonidine during dynamic physical activity. Clin. Pharmacol. Ther., *32*:18, 1982.
15. Cohen, I.M., et al.: Reduced renovascular resistance by clonidine. Clin. Pharmacol. Ther., *26*:572, 1979.
16. Manhem, P., et al.: Plasma clonidine in relation to blood pressure, catecholamines, and renin activity during long-term treatment of hypertension. Clin. Pharmacol. Ther., *31*:445, 1982.
17. Hokfelt, B., et al.: The effect of clonidine and penbutolol respectively on catecholamines in blood and urine, plasma renin activity and urinary aldosterone in hypertensive patients. Arch. Int. Pharmacodyn. Ther., *213*:307, 1975.
18. Colub, M.S., et al.: Hormonal and hemodynamic effects of short- and long-term clonidine therapy in patients with mild-to-moderate hypertension. Chest, *83*:377, 1983.
19. Weber, M.A., et al.: Effects on the renin-angiotensin system of agents acting at central and peripheral adrenergic receptors. Chest, *83*:374, 1983.
20. Falkner, B., et al.: Effectiveness of centrally acting drugs and diuretics in adolescent hypertension. Clin. Pharmacol. Ther., *32*:577, 1982.
21. Bravo, E.L.: Effects of clonidine on sympathetic function. Chest, *83*:369, 1983.
22. Kokubu, T., et al.: Effect of clonidine on blood pressure in chronic one-kidney, one-clip and two-kidney, one-clip hypertensive rats. Chest, *83*:359, 1983.
23. Mathias, C.J., et al.: Clonidine lowers blood pressure independently of renin suppression in patients with unilateral renal artery stenosis. Chest, *83*:357, 1983.
24. Lilja, M., et al.: Clonidine twice daily in hypertension. Acta Med. Scand., *214*:111, 1983.
25. Thananopavarn, C., et al.: Clonidine in the elderly hypertensive. Chest, *83*:410, 1983.
26. Sambhi, M.P.: Clonidine monotherapy in mild hypertension. Chest, *83*:427, 1983.
27. Pennisi, A.J., et al.: Minoxidil therapy in children with severe hypertension. J. Pediatr., *90*:813, 1977.
28. Ziment, I.: Management of hypertension in the asthmatic patient. Chest, *83*:392, 1983.
29. Whitsett, T.L.: Abrupt cessation of treatment with centrally acting antihypertensive agents: a review. Chest, *83*:400, 1983.
30. Brenner, W.I., and Lieberman, A.N.: Acute clonidine withdrawal following open heart operation. Ann. Thorac. Surg., *24*:80, 1977.
31. Bruce, D.L., et al.: Preoperative clonidine withdrawal syndrome. Anesthesiology, *51*:90, 1979.
32. Geyskes, G.G., et al.: Clonidine withdrawal: mechanism and frequently of rebound hypertension. Br. J. Clin. Pharmacol., *7*:55, 1979.
33. Weber, M.A.: Discontinuation syndrome following cessation of treatment with clonidine and other antihypertensive agents. J. Cardiovasc. Pharmacol., *20(Suppl. 1)*:573, 1980.
34. Whitsett, T.L., et al.: Abrupt cessation of clonidine administration: a prospective study. Am. J. Cardiol., *41*:1285, 1978.
35. Frisk-Holmberg, M., et al.: Pharmacokinetics of clonidine and its relation to the hypotensive effect in patients. Br. J. Clin. Pharmacol., *6*:227, 1978.
36. Velasco, M., et al.: A sliding dose schedule for clonidine in hypertensive patients. Clin. Pharmacol. Ther., *20*:31, 1976.
37. Velasquez, M.T., et al.: Plasma clonidine levels in hypertension. Clin. Pharmacol. Ther., *34*:341, 1983.
38. Frisk-Holmberg, M.: Clinical pharmacology of clonidine. Chest, *83*:395, 1983.
39. Thurau, K.W., et al.: Activation of renin in the single juxtaglomerular apparatus by sodium chloride in the tubular fluid at the macula densa. Circ. Res., *31(Suppl. 2)*:183, 1972.
40. Morgan, T., and Gillies, A.: Factors controlling the release of renin: a micropuncture study in the cat. Pflugers Arch., *368*:13, 1977.

Chapter 36

Methyldopa

Methyldopa is a widely used antihypertensive agent with a central mechanism of action. In adults, it is effective mainly in short- and long-term treatment of essential hypertension. In children and adolescents, methyldopa is effective in essential hypertension as well as in hypertension resulting from renal artery stenosis, renal parenchymal diseases, and coarctation of the aorta. Methyldopa is used alone more often than most antihypertensive agents other than diuretics. Its efficacy may be increased, especially during long-term therapy, when it is combined with diuretics or beta-adrenoreceptor blocking agents. A specific adverse effect of methyldopa is hemolytic anemia.

Structure

Methyldopa is alpha-methyl-3,4-dihydroxyphenylalanine.

Effect in Hypertension

Methyldopa is a potent antihypertensive agent, effective in patients with almost all forms of hypertension. The drug reduces elevated systolic and diastolic hypertension at rest as well as during exercise.[1] Standing blood pressure is reduced to a greater degree by methyldopa than supine blood pressure.[2] Methyldopa is effective in mild as well as in severe and malignant hypertension. The antihypertensive effect is sustained throughout long periods of treatment.

Methyldopa is also beneficial in childhood hypertension of various causes. The number of studied cases is small, however, and only a few short series have been reported in the literature. Several cases of hypertensive children resistant to methyldopa, but responsive to modern antihypertensive agents, have been reported.

I treated 4 patients with essential hypertension, aged 15 to 18 years, with methyldopa for 3 months to 2 years, and blood pressure became normal in these patients. No other medications were used. It appears that, at these young ages, monotherapy with methyldopa may be especially effective.

Sinaiko and Mirkin treated a child with systolic hypertension and 8 children with systolic and diastolic hypertension.[3] These patients ranged in age from 1 month to 16 years. Two of them had essential hypertension, 1 had hemolytic uremic syndrome, 1 had renal artery stenosis, and the others had various renal parenchymal diseases. The mean blood pressure was 148/98 ± 8/4 mm Hg during administration of hydrochlorothiazide alone and 142/88 ± 8/4 mm Hg following the addition of methyldopa to the regimen. Propranolol added to hydrochlorothiazide had a similar effect. Triple therapy with minoxidil, propranolol, and hydrochlorothiazide was more effective than the previous therapeutic regimens.

Monotherapy with intravenously administered methyldopa was effective in a study of infants and children with severe malignant hypertension resulting from renal artery stenosis.[4]

Methyldopa is often used for treatment of renovascular hypertension until surgical correction can be performed. Foster and colleagues reported on the case of a child with renal artery stenosis and hypertension adequately controlled by methyldopa, in whom the drug was discontinued preoperatively.[4] In this child, blood pressure rose, and cardiac arrest developed after induction of anesthesia. Since that report, it has been common practice to continue methyldopa administration until surgical correction of renal artery stenosis has been performed. Methyldopa is effective in hypertensive patients with low, normal, or high plasma renin activity.[5,6] In hypertensive patients, left ventricular myocardial mass is reduced by methyldopa. Echocardiographic studies have shown significant regression of myocardial hypertrophy,[7] regression unrelated to the antihypertensive effect and therefore perhaps resulting from an independent mechanism.

Treatment with methyldopa may be associated with fluid retention, which may be reversed by addition of a diuretic agent. Renal function is not impaired during treatment with methyldopa.

Hemodynamic Effects

Methyldopa reduces blood pressure by decreasing peripheral vascular resistance.[8,9] Heart rate is not much increased, probably because the drug inhibits the compensatory increase in sympathetic stimulation. Heart rate may also decrease, especially if it is high during the control period. Methyldopa decreases heart rate during exercise. Myocardial contractility, ejection fraction, and cardiac output are increased, probably because of the decrease in peripheral vascular resistance.[10] Cardiac output may also be reduced by methyldopa, perhaps from venodilation.[11,12] A reduction in cardiac output may contribute to the antihypertensive effect of the drug.

Effect on the Renin-Angiotensin System

Methyldopa usually reduces plasma renin activity and aldosterone excretion.[5,13] No correlation exists between this effect and the antihypertensive action of the drug.

Mechanism of Action

Several mechanisms have been suggested to account for the antihypertensive effect of methyldopa. The main site of action is probably the central nervous system. Small doses of methyldopa injected directly into the vertebral artery of animals have a potent antihypertensive effect.[14] The inhibition of metabolic transformation of methyldopa in the central nervous system prevents the antihypertensive effect.[15,16] The effect of methyldopa is thought to be exerted by its metabolite, alpha-methyl-norepinephrine, which acts by stimulation of alpha-adrenoreceptors in the central nervous system.[17]

Another suggested mechanism involves the theory of peripheral false transmitters. According to this theory, metabolites of methyldopa replace natural catecholamines in peripheral nerve endings. When the nerves are stimulated, these metabolites are released as false transmitters and thereby attenuate the pressor response to sympathetic stimulation.[18,19]

Clinical Pharmacology

Methyldopa may be given intravenously or orally. The drug is rapidly absorbed from the gastrointestinal tract. The peak plasma concentration is reached within 1 to 4 hours of oral administration. Absorption is incomplete, and the drug undergoes significant first-pass hepatic metabolism, resulting in systemic bioavailability of 20 to 60%.[20,21] Therapeutic plasma levels range between 1.0 and 3.0 $\mu g/ml$.[22] Protein binding is 15% only; the total volume of distribution is 0.6 L/kg. Methyldopa is eliminated by metabolic transformation and by renal excretion of the metabolites. The elimination half-life is about 2 hours.

Side Effects

The incidence of side effects of methyldopa is high. Such effects include drowsiness, fatigue, dryness of mouth, postural hypotension, depression, and impotence. Up to 30% of patients treated with methyldopa for more than 6 months have a positive Coombs' test; up to 3% of these patients develop hemolytic anemia.

Dosage and Administration

Although methyldopa may be given intravenously as well as orally, only oral administration is widely used in clinical practice. The pediatric dose is 10 to 60 mg/kg daily, in 4 divided doses. The daily dose should not exceed 1750 mg in older children.

References

1. Mallion, J.M., et al.: Study of the action of methyldopa on 20 hypertensive subjects during rest and effort. *In* Methyldopa in Hypertension. Edited by A. Zanchetti. Rahway, NJ, Merck Sharp and Dohme International, 1978, p. 70.

2. Mancia, G., et al.: Methyldopa and neural control of circulation in essential hypertension. Am. J. Cardiol., 45:1237, 1980.
3. Sinaiko, A.R., and Mirkin, B.L.: Management of severe childhood hypertension with minoxidil: a controlled clinical study. J. Pediatr., 91:138, 1977.
4. Foster, J.H., et al.: Malignant hypertension secondary to renal artery stenosis in children. Ann. Surg., 164:700, 1966.
5. Weidmann, P., et al.: Plasma renin and blood pressure during treatment with methyldopa. Am. J. Cardiol., 34:671, 1974.
6. Leonetti, G., et al.: Relationship between the hypotensive and renin-suppressing activities of alpha-methyldopa in hypertensive patients. Am. J. Cardiol., 40:762, 1977.
7. Fouad, F.M., et al.: Reversal of left ventricular hypertrophy in hypertensive patients treated with methyldopa. Am. J. Cardiol., 49:795, 1982.
8. Sannerstedt, R., et al.: Hemodynamic effects of methyldopa (Aldomet®) at rest and during exercise in patients with arterial hypertension. Acta Med. Scand., 171:75, 1962.
9. Weil, M.H., et al.: Alpha-methyldopa for the treatment of hypertension. Circulation, 28:165, 1963.
10. Alcocer, L., and Aspe, J.: Hemodynamic, metabolic, and ventricular function effects of methyldopa in the treatment of hypertension. In Methyldopa in Hypertension. Edited by A. Zanchetti. Rahway, NJ, Merck Sharp and Dohme International, 1978, p. 33.
11. Lund-Johansen, P.: Hemodynamic changes in long-term alpha methyldopa therapy of essential hypertension. Acta Med. Scand., 192:221, 1972.
12. Wilson, W.R., et al.: The acute hemodynamic effects of alpha-methyldopa in man. J. Chronic Dis., 15:907, 1961.
13. Mancia, C., et al.: Effect of treatment with methyldopa on hemodynamics and on neural circulatory control. In Methyldopa in Hypertension. Edited by A. Zanchetti. Rahway, NJ, Merck Sharp and Dohme International, 1978, p. 50.
14. Henning, M., and Van Zwieten, R.A.: Central hypotensive effect of α-methyldopa. J. Pharm. Pharmacol., 20:409, 1968.
15. Henning M., and Rubenson, A.: Evidence that the hypotensive action of methyldopa is mediated by central actions of methylnoradrenaline. J. Pharm. Pharmacol., 23:40, 1971.
16. Henning M.: Studies on the mode of action of α-methyldopa. Acta Physiol. Scand., 322(Suppl.):1, 1969.
17. Heise, A., and Kroneberg, G.: Central nervous α-adrenergic receptors and the mode of action of α-methyldopa. Naunyn Schmiedebergs Arch Pharmacol., 279:285, 1973.
18. Day, M.D., and Rand, M.J.: A hypothesis for the mode of action of α-methyldopa in relieving hypertension. J. Pharm. Pharmacol., 15:221, 1963.
19. Day, M.D., and Rand, M.J.: Some observations on the pharmacology of α-methyldopa. Br. J. Pharmacol., 22:72, 1964.
20. Kwan, K.F., et al.: Pharmacokinetics of methyldopa in man. J. Pharmacol. Exp. Ther., 198:264, 1976.
21. Stenbaek, O., et al.: Pharmacokinetics of methyldopa in normal man. Clin. Pharmacol. Ther., 12:117, 1977.
22. Barnett, A.J., et al.: Pharmacokinetics of methyldopa plasma levels following single intravenous, oral and multiple oral dosage in normotensive and hypertensive subjects. Clin. Exp. Pharmacol. Physiol., 4:331, 1977.

Index

Accessory atrioventricular pathways, digitalis glycoside effects on, 10-11
  diltiazem effect on, 96
  mexiletine effect on, 277
  phenytoin effect on, 267
  procainamide effect on, 247
  propafenone effect on, 289
  propranolol effect on, 199-200
  verapamil effect on, 65
Action potential, digitalis glycoside effects on, 9
  procainamide effect on, 246
  propafenone effect on, 288
Acute myocardial infarction, nitroprusside effects on, 127-128
Adenosine and adenosine triphosphate, 331-335
  clinical pharmacology of, 334
  compared with verapamil, 68-69
  dosage and administration of, 334-335
  effects in arrhythmias, 332-333
  electrophysiologic effects of, 332
  hemodynamic effects of, 333
  pharmacologic properties of, 331
  side effects of, 334
Agents affecting renin-angiotensin system, 159-180
  captopril, 161-178
  introduction to, 159
  saralasin, 179-180
  See also specific agents
Agranulocytosis, hydralazine and, 118
  procainamide and, 251
Alpha-adrenoreceptor blocking agents, 149-158
  prazosin, 149-155
  tolazoline, 157-158
  See also specific agents
Amiodarone, 305-325
  administration of, intravenous vs oral, 312
  clinical pharmacology of, 314-315
  combined with other antiarrhythmic drugs, 313
  compared with other antiarrhythmic drugs, 312
  dosage and administration of, 321-322
  drug interactions of, 319-321
    with anticoagulant agents, 321
    with aprindine, 320
    with digitalis glycosides, 26-27
    with digoxin, 319-320
    with procainamide, 320
    with propafenone, 296
    with quinidine, 320
  effects during pregancy and lactation, 321
  effects in arrhythmias, 308-311
    experimentally induced, 308
    in atrial fibrillation, 309
    in atrial flutter, 309-310
    in chaotic atrial tachycardia, 310
    in supraventricular tachycardia, 308-309
    in ventricular arrhythmias, 310-311
  effects in prolonged QT syndrome, 312
  effects in sinus node dysfunction, 311-312
  electrophysiologic effects of, 306-308
  electrophysiologic studies to predict effect of, 313
  hemodynamic effects of, 313-314
  pharmacologic properties of, 305-306
  side effects of, 315-319
    cardiovascular, 317-318
    impaired hepatic function, 319
    impaired thyroid function, 318
    neurologic, 318-319
    ocular, 316-317
    photosensitivity, 317
    pulmonary, 319
    skin discoloration, 317
    urticaria, 317
  structure of, 305
Amrinone, 55-59
  clinical pharmacology of, 57
  dosage and administration of, 58
  effect on pulmonary hypertension, 57
  electrophysiologic effects of, 57
  hemodynamic effects of, 55-56
    in young age groups, 56
  side effects of, 57-58
  structure of, 55
Angina pectoris, nifedipine effect on, 87
  propranolol effect on, 198
  verapamil effect on, 75
Antacids, drug interaction of, with digitalis glycosides, 28
Anterior pituitary hormone(s), propranolol effect on, 206

Index

Antiarrhythmic agents, 233-335
  adenosine, 331-335
  adenosine triphosphate, 331-335
  amiodarone, 305-325
  bretylium, 327-330
  class I agents, 234
  class II agents, 234
  class IV agents, 234-235
  digitalis glycosides, 235
  disopyramide, 255-260
  ethmozin, 301-303
  flecainide, 285-286
  introduction to, 233-235
  lidocaine, 261-264
  mexiletine, 275-283
  phenytoin, 265-273
  procainamide, 245-254
  propafenone, 287-299
  quinidine, 237-244
  See also specific agents
Antibiotics, drug interaction of, with digitalis glycosides, 27-28
Anticoagulant agent(s), drug interaction of, with amiodarone, 321
Aortic arch, anomalies of, prostaglandin E effects on, 345-346
Aortic insufficiency, hydralazine effects on, 114
Aortic stenosis, hydralazine effects on, 113
Aprindine, drug interaction of, with amiodarone, 320
Arterial hypertension, nitroprusside effects on, 124-125
Aspirin, drug interaction of, with digitalis glycosides, 27
Atenolol, 219-223
  clinical pharmacology of, 222
  compared with methyldopa, 222
  compared with propranolol, 221-222
  dosage and administration of, 223
  effect in hypertension, 221
  effect on plasma lipid(s), 222
  hemodynamic effects of, 219-220
  pharmacologic properties of, 219
  side effects of, 222-223
  structure of, 219
  treatment during pregnancy with, 220-221
Atrial fibrillation, amiodarone effect on, 309
  digitalis glycosides for, 15
  diltiazem effects on, 98
  propranolol effect on, 202-203
  quinidine effect of, 238
  verapamil effect on, 67
Atrial flutter, amiodarone effect on, 309-310
  digitalis glycosides for, 14-15
  diltiazem effects on, 98
  propranolol effect on, 201-202
  quinidine effect of, 238
  verapamil effect on, 68
Atrial tachycardia, chaotic, amiodarone effect on, 310
Atrioventricular node, digitalis glycoside effects on, 10
  diltiazem effect on, 96
  mexiletine effect on, 276-277
  phenytoin effect on, 266-267
  procainamide effect on, 246-247
  propafenone effect on, 289
  propranolol effect on, 199
  verapamil effect on, 64-65
Atrioventricular pathways, accessory. *See* Accessory atrioventriuclar pathways
Atrium(ia), digitalis glycoside effects on, 10
  diltiazem effect on, 96
  mexiletine effect on, 276
  minoxidil effects on, 142
  phenytoin effect on, 266
  procainamide effect on, 246
  propafenone effect on, 288-289
  verapamil effect on, 64

Beta-adrenoreceptor blocking agents, atenolol, 219-223
  bucindolol, 223-225
  classification of, 182-184
  diltiazem effect with, 99-100
  drug discontinuance effects, 186
  effect on peripheral circulation, 185
  hemodynamic effects of, 185
  intrinsic sympathomimetic activity of, 183-184
  introduction to, 181-187
  labetalol, 226-227
  membrane-stabilizing activity of, 184
  metoprolol, 225-226
  oxyhemoglobin dissociation and, effect on, 184
  pharmacokinetic differences of, 185
  pindolol, 226
  potency of, 182
  propranolol, 189-218
  pulmonary effects of, 185
  selectivity of, 182
  side effects of, 186
  sotalol, 228
  structure of, 182
  therapeutic indications for, 186
  timolol, 227-228
  vasodilatory activity of, 184
  verapamil and, 73-74
  See also specific agents

Index

Bipyridine derivatives, 55-59. *See also* Amrinone
Bleeding time, indomethacin effects on, 372
Bradycardia, propranolol and, 209
Bretylium tosylate, 327-330
   clinical pharmacology of, 328
   dosage and administration of, 329
   drug interactions of, 329
   effect in arrhythmias, 328
   electrophysiologic effects of, 327
   hemodynamic effects of, 328
   pharmacologic properties of, 327
   side effects of, 328-329
Bronchospasm, clonidine effects on, 382
   propranolol effects on, 210
Bucindolol, 223-225
   clinical pharmacolocy of, 224-225
   dosage and administration of, 225
   electrophysiologic effects of, 224
   hemodynamic effects of, 2245
   pharmacologic properties of, 223-224
   side effects of, 225
   structure of, 223

Calcium antagonists, 61-103
   diltiazem, 95-103
   introduction to, 61
   nifedipine, 85-94
   verapamil, 63-83
   See also specific agents
Captopril, 161-178
   clinical pharmacology of, 172-173
   discontinuance of, 172
   dosage and administration of, 175
   drug interactions of, 175
   hemodynamic effects of, 162-172
      in coarctation of the aorta, 169-170
      in congestive heart failure, 167-169
      in pulmonary hypertension, 167
      in systemic hypertension, 162-167
      in Takayasu's disease, 170-171
      in ventricular septal defect, 171-172
      on coronary circulation and myocardial energetics, 171
      on renal function, 171
   pharmacologic effects of, 161-162
   side effects of, 173-175
      cardiovascular, 173-174
      dysgeusia and, 174
      hematopoietic depression and, 174
      hyperkalemia and, 174
      renal damage and, 174
   structure of, 161
Cardiac surgical procedures, nitroprusside effects on, 126-127
Cardiovascular system, amiodarone effect on, 317-318

captopril effect on, 173-174
   clonidine effects on, 380
   indomethacin effects on, 370-371
   prostaglandin E effects on, 351
Central nervous system, propranolol effects on, 210
Centrally acting antihypertensive agents, 377-388
   clonidine, 379-384
   introduction to, 377
   methyldopa, 385-388
   See also specific agents
Cimetidine, drug interaction of, with propranolol, 211
Clonidine, 379-384
   cardiovascular effects of, 380
   clinical pharmacology of, 382-383
   discontinuance of drug, 382
   dosage and administration of, 383
   effects in bronchospasm, 382
   effects in congestive heart failure, 381-382
   effects in hypertension, 380-381
   humoral effects of, 380
   mechanism of action of, 379-380
   renal effects of, 380
   side effects of, 383
Coarctation of the aorta, captopril effect on, 169-170
Complete atrioventricular block, propranolol and, 209
Congenital heart disease(s), cyanotic vs acyanotic, prostaglandin E effects in, 347-348
Congestive heart failure, captopril effects on, 167-169
   clonidine effects on, 381-382
   diazoxide effects on, 146-147
   digitalis glycoside effects on, 7-8
   hydralazine effects on, 108-111
   minoxidil effects on, 138-140
   nifedipine and, 91
   nitroprusside effects on, 122-123
   prazosin effects on, 150-151
   propranolol and, 210
   prostacyclin effects on, 361
   prostaglandin E effects on, 348-349
Constipation, verapamil and, 78
Coronary arteries, nifedipine effect on, 86
Coronary circulation, captopril effect on, 171

Diazoxide, 145-148
   clinical pharmacology of, 147
   dosage and administration of, 147
   hemodynamic effects of, 145-147
      on congestive heart failure, 146-147

Diazoxide, hemodynamic effects of *(continued)*
  on pulmonary hypertension, 146
  on systemic hypertension, 145-146
  pharmacologic properties of, 145
  side effects of, 147
  structure of, 145
Digitalis glycosides, 3-33
  clinical pharmacology of, 16-18
    digitoxin, 18
    digoxin, 16-18
  dosage and administration of, 28
  drug interactions of, 26-28
    with amiodarone, 26-27
    with antacids, 28
    with antibiotic agents, 27
    with aspirin, 27
    with indomethacin, 27
    with quinidine, 26
    with vasodilators, 27
    with verapamil, 26
  electrophysiologic effects of, 8-11
    accessory atrioventricular pathways and, 10-11
    action potential and, 9
    atria and, 10
    atrioventricular node and, 10
    sinoatrial node and, 9-10
    ventricles and, 11
  for arrhythmias, 12-16
    atrial fibrillation, 15
    atrial flutter, 14-15
    supraventricular tachycardia, 12-14
    ventricular, 15-16
  hemodynamic effects of, 4-8
    age and, 5
    in endocardial fibroelastosis, 5-7
    in left-to-right shunt and congestive heart failure, 7-8
    in obstructive cardiac lesions, 8
    renal function and, 5
  in myocardial infarction, 11-12
  mechanism of action of, 3
  toxicity of, 19-26. *See also* Digitalis toxicity
    clinical manifestations of, 20-21
    plasma levels in, 21-22
    treatment of, 22-26
  treatment during pregnancy with, 19
  See also Digitoxin; Digoxin
Digitalis toxicity, 19-26
  cardiac effects of, 20-21
  clinical manifestations of, 20-21
  extracardiac effects of, 21
  incidence of, 19-20
  plasma levels in, determination of, 21-22
    prevention of further elevations in, 22
    reducing, 24
  treatment of, 22-26
    arrhythmias and, 24-25
    conduction disturbances and, 24
    digoxin-specific antibody, 22-24
    electrolytic disturbances and, 25-26
    hyperkalemia and, 25-26
    hypokalemia and, 25
    plasma level reduction of, 22, 24
Digitoxin, clinical pharmacology of, 18
  dosage and administration of, 28
  See also Digitalis glycosides
Digoxin, clinical pharmacology of, 18
  combined with dopamine, 40
  diltiazem interaction with, 101
  dosage and administration of, 28
  drug interactions of, with amiodarone, 319-320
    with indomethacin, 373
    with quinidine, 240-241
  See also Digitalis glycosides
Diltiazem, 95-103
  clinical pharmacology of, 100
  dosage and administration of, 101
  drug interactions of, 101
  effects in lactation, 101
  effects on arrhythmias, 97-98
  electrophysiologic effects of, 95-97
  hemodynamic effects of, 98-100
  mechanism of action of, 95
  side effects of, 101
  structure of, 95
Diphenylhydantoin. *See* Phenytoin
Direct-acting vasodilators, 107-148
  diazoxide, 145-148
  hydralazine, 107-120
  minoxidil, 137-144
  nitroglycerin, 133-136
  nitroprusside, 121-131
  See also specific agents
Disopyramide, 255-260
  clinical pharmacology of, 258
  compared with other antiarrhythmic agents, 257
  compared with propafenone, 294
  contraindications to use of, 258
  dosage and administration of, 258
  effects on arrhythmias, 256-257
  electrophysiologic effects of, 255-256
  hemodynamic effects of, 257-258
  pharmacologic properties of, 255
  side effects of, 258
  structure of, 255
Dizziness, prazosin and, 153
Dobutamine, 43-49
  clinical pharmacology of, 48
  combined with other drugs, 47-48
  comparison with other positive inotropic agents, 46-47

dosage and administration of, 48
hemodynamic effects of, 43-46
  in young age groups, 44-46
mechanism of action of, 46
side effects of, 48
structure of, 43
Dopamine, 35-42
adverse effects of, 41
clinical pharmacology of, 40
combined with dobutamine, 47
combined with other drugs, 39-40
  digoxin, 40
  dobutamine, 39
  nitrates, 40
  phenoxybenzamine, 39-40
compared with dobutamine, 46
dosage and administration of, 41
hemodynamic effects of, 35-37
maturity and drug response to, 39
neonatal uses of, 38-39
pediatric use of, 37-38
pharmacologic properties of, 35
structure of, 35
Ductus arteriosus, indomethacin response of, 365-368
  drug levels and, 369
  gestational age and, 368
  morphology and, 368-369
  pharmacologic vs surgical closure of, 369
  prostacyclin effects in, 360
  prostaglandin E effects on, 341-342
    factors determining, 346-347
    structural changes and, 352-353
Dysgeusia, captopril and, 174

Edema, peripheral, nifedipine and, 92
Electrocardiograph, changes in, minoxidil effects on, 142
Endocardial fibroelastosis, digitalis glycoside effects on, 5-7
Ethmozin, 301-303
Eye(s), amiodarone effects on, 316-317

Fetal circulation, persistent, prostacyclin effects in, 361
Flecainide, 285-286
  compared with propafenone, 293
Flushing, hydralazine and, 118
  nifedipine and, 92
  verapamil and, 78
Furosemide, drug interactions of, with indomethacin, 372-373

Gastrointestinal system, indomethacin effects on, 371
  prostaglandin E effects on, 353

Gingival hyperplasia, nifedipine and, 92
  phenytoin effect on, 270
Glucose metabolism, propranolol effect on, 206
Growth, propranolol effects on, 211

Headache, hydralazine and, 118
Heart rate, hydralazine and, 117
  nifedipine effect on, 91
Heat sensation, nifedipine and, 92
Hematopoietic depression, captopril and, 174
Hydralazine, 107-120
  clinical pharmacology of, 116-117
  compared with minoxidil, 139-140
  compared with nitroprusside, 116
  compared with prazosin, 151
  dosage and administration of, 118
  drug interactions of, with indomethacin, 373
    with propranolol, 118
  effects during pregnancy and lactation, 118
  hemodynamic effects of, 108-116
    on aortic insufficiency, 114
    on aortic stenosis, 113
    on congestive heart failure, 108-111
    on mitral insufficiency, 114
    on pulmonary vascular diseases, 114-115
    on systemic hypertension, 115-116
    on ventricular septal defect, 111-113
    postoperative use and, 115
  pharmacologic properties of, 107-108
  side effects of, 117-118
  structure of, 107
Hyperkalemia, captopril and, 174
  indomethacin effects and, 372
Hyperostosis, prostaglandin E effects on, 354
Hypertension. *See* Pulmonary hypertension; Systemic hypertension
Hypertrichosis, minoxidil and, 142
Hypertrophic cardiomyopathy, verapamil effect on, 69-73
  hemodynamic effects, 69-70
  mechanism of action, 72-73
  relief of symptoms, 70-72
  selection of patients, 72
  diltiazem effect on, 98-99
  disopyramide effect on, 257-258
  nifedipine effect on, 90
Hypertrophic obstructive cardiomyopathy, propranolol effect on, 193-195
Hyponatremia, indomethacin effects and, 372
Hypoplastic left heart syndrome, prostaglandin E effects on, 345-346

Ibuprofen, captopril interaction with, 175
Indomethacin, 365-376
　captopril interaction with, 175
　clinical pharmacology and, 370
　closure of patent ductus arteriosus and, 365-368
　　drug levels and response, 369
　　gestational age and response, 368
　　morphology of ductus and response, 368-369
　　surgical closure vs, 369
　contraindications to use, 369-370
　dosage and administration of, 374
　drug interactions of, 372-374
　　with digitalis glycosides, 27
　　with digoxin, 373
　　with furosemide, 372-373
　　with hydralazine, 373
　　with methylxanthines, 373
　pharmacologic properties of, 365
　pregnancy and, administration during, 374
　side effects of, 370-372
　　cardiovascular, 370-371
　　gastrointestinal, 371
　　hyperkalemia and, 372
　　hyponatremia and, 372
　　increased bleeding time and, 372
　　renal, 371
　　retrolental fibroplasia and, 372
　structure of, 365
Inotropic agents. See Positive inotropic agents
Isoprenaline. See Isoproterenol
Isoproterenol, 51-53
　clinical pharmacology of, 52
　compared with dobutamine, 47
　hemodynamic effects of, 51-52
　phamacologic properties of, 51
　pulmonary function and, 52
　pulmonary hypertension and, 52
　side effects of, 52
　structure of, 51

Kidney(s), captopril and, 171, 174
　clonidine effects on, 380
　digitalis glycoside effects on, 5
　indomethacin effects on, 371
　minoxidil and, 140
　prostaglandin E effects on, 354

Labetalol, 226-227
Lactation, amiodarone effect on, 321
　hydralazine effect on, 118
Left to right shunt, digitalis glycoside effects on, 7-8
Lidocaine, 261-264
　clinical pharmacology of, 262-263
　compared with propafenone, 293-294
　dosage and administration of, 263
　drug interactions of, with propranolol, 211
　effect on ventricular arrhythmias, 262
　electrophysiologic effects of, 261-262
　pharmacologic properties of, 261
　side effects of, 263
　structure of, 261
Liver, amiodarone effect on, 319
Lung(s), amiodarone effect on, 319
Lupus erythematosus, procainamide effect on, 251

Methyldopa, 385-388
　clinical pharmacology of, 387
　compared with atenolol, 222
　dosage and administration of, 387
　effects in hypertension, 385-386
　effects on renin-angiotensin system, 386
　hemodynamic effects of, 386
　mechanism of action, 387
　side effects of, 387
　structure of, 385
Methylxanthines, drug interactions of, with indomethacin, 373
Metoprolol, 225-226
Mexiletine, 275-283
　clinical pharmacology of, 280
　compared with propafenone, 293
　dosage and administration of, 281
　drug interactions of, 281
　effects in arrhythmias, 277-279
　electrophysiologic effects of, 275-277
　hemodynamic effects of, 279-280
　pharmacologic properties, 275
　side effects of, 280-281
　structure of, 275
Minoxidil, 137-144
　adverse effects of, 141-142
　clinical pharmacology of, 141
　dosage and administration of, 142-143
　effects in congestive heart failure, 138-140
　　compared with hydralazine, 139-140
　　compared with nitroprusside, 140
　effects in hypertension, 137-138
　　compared with prazosin, 138
　neurohumal effect of, 140-141
　pharmacologic properties of, 137
　renal effects of, 140
　structure of, 137
Mitral insufficiency, hydralazine effects on, 114
Myocardial energetics, captopril effect on, 171
Myocardial infarction, digitalis glycoside effects on, 11

N-acetylprocainamide, 252
NAPA, 252
Neonatal hypoxemia, tolazoline effect on, 157
Nervous system, amiodarone effect on, 318-319
Neurohumoral effect(s), of minoxidil, 140-141
Nifedipine, 85-94
  clinical pharmacology of, 91
  dosage and administration of, 92
  hemodynamic effects of, 85-91
    in neonates, 86-87
    on angina pectoris, 87
    on coronary arteries, 86
    on hypertrophic cardiomyopathy, 90
    on pulmonary hypertension, 87-90
    on systemic hypertension, 90-91
  side effects of, 91-92
  structure of, 85
Nitrates, combined with dobutamine, 48
  combined with dopamine, 40
Nitroglycerin, 133-136
  clinical pharmacology of, 135
  dosage and administration of, 135
  for ischemic heart disease, 134-135
  hemodynamic effects of, 133-135
  pharmacologic properties of, 133
  side effects of, 135
Nitroprusside, 121-131
  adverse effects of, 128-129
  clinical pharmacology of, 128
  combined with dobutamine, 48
  compared with hydralazine, 116
  compared with minoxidil, 140
  dosage and administration of, 129
  hemodynamic effects of, 121-128
    after cardiac surgical procedures, 126-127
    in acute myocardial infarction, 127-128
    in arterial hypertension, 124-125
    in ventricular septal defect, 125-126
    regional, 123-124
    with congestive heart failure, 122-123
    without congestive heart failure, 122
  pharmacologic properties of, 121
  toxicity of, 128

Obstructive cardiac lesions, digitalis glycoside effects on, 8
Ocular effect(s), of amiodarone, 316-317
Osteomalacia, phenytoin effect on, 271
Oxygenation, impairment of, with nitroprusside, 128-129
Oxyhemoglobin dissociation, propranolol effect on, 197

Palpitations, hydralazine and, 118
Patent ductus arteriosus. *See* Ductus arteriosus
Pericardial effusion, minoxidil and, 141
Pericarditis, minoxidil and, 141
Peripheral vascular resistance, propranolol and, 210
Persistent fetal circulation, prostaglandin E effects in, 348
Phenoxybenzamine, combined with dopamine, 39-40
Phenytoin, 265-273
  clinical pharmacology of, 269-270
  dosage and administration of, 271
  effects on arrhythmias, 267-269
  electrophysiologic effects of, 265-267
  hemodynamic effects of, 269
  pharmacologic properties of, 265
  side effects of, 270-271
  structure of, 265
Photosensitivity, amiodarone and, 317
Pindolol, 226
  drug interactions of, with indomethacin, 374
Plasma lipid(s), atenolol effect on, 222
  prazosin effect on, 152-153
  propranolol effect on, 205-206
Platelet function, propranolol effect on, 197
Positive inotropic agents, 1-59
  bipyridine derivatives, 55-59
  digitalis glycosides, 3-33
  dobutamine, 43-49
  dopamine, 35-42
  introduction to, 1-2
  isoproterenol, 51-53
  See also specific agents
Prazosin, 149-155
  clinical pharmacology of, 153
  compared with minoxidil, 138
  dosage and administration of, 154
  effect on plasma lipid levels, 152-153
  effect on pulmonary function, 152
  hemodynamic effects of, 149-152
    in valvar diseases, 151
    on congestive heart failure, 150-151
    on hypertension, 152
    on normal circulation, 149-150
  pharmacologic properties of, 149
  side effects of, 153
  structure of, 149
Pregnancy, amiodarone effect on, 321
  hydralazine effect on, 118
  indomethacin administration and, 374
Prenalterol, compared with dobutamine, 47
Procainamide, 245-254
  clinical pharmacology of, 249-251
  compared with propafenone, 294

Procainamide *(continued)*
  dosage and administration of, 252
  drug interaction of, with amiodarone, 320
  effect on arrhythmias, 248-249
  electrophysiologic effects of, 246-248
  hemodynamic effects of, 249
  pharmacologic properties of, 246
  side effects of, 251-252
  structure of, 245
Propafenone, 287-299
  clinical pharmacology of, 294-295
  compared with other drugs, 293-294
  dosage and administration of, 297
  drug interactions with, 296
  effects on arrhythmias, 290-293
    experimentally induced, 290
    supraventricular tachyarrhythmias, 290-292
    ventricular, 292-293
  electrophysiologic effects of, 288-290
    on accessory atrioventricular pathways, 289
    on action potential, 288
    on atria, 288-289
    on atrioventricular node, 289
    on sinoatrial node, 288
    on ventricles, 289-290
  pharmacologic properties of, 287
  side effects of, 295-296
  structure of, 287
Propranolol, 189-218
  clinical pharmacology of, 207-209
  compared with atenolol, 221-222
  dosage and administration of, 211-212
  drug discontinuance effects, 206-207
  drug interactions of, 211
    with diltiazem, 101
    with hydralazine, 118
    with indomethacin, 374
    with propafenone, 296
  effect in angina pectoris, 198
  effect on anterior pituitary hormones, 206
  effect on arrhythmias, 200-204
    in atrial fibrillation, 202-203
    in atrial flutter, 201-202
    in supraventricular tachycardia, 200-201
    in ventricular arrhythmias, 203-204
  effect on glucose metabolism, 206
  effect on oxyhemoglobin dissociation, 197-198
  effect on plasma lipids, 205-206
  effect on platelet function, 197
  effect on pulmonary function, 197
  effect on sex hormones, 206
  effect on thyrotoxicosis, 204205
  electrophysiologic effects of, 198-200
    on accessory atrioventricular pathways, 199-200
    on atrioventricular node, 199
    on sinus node, 198-199
    on ventricles, 200
  hemodynamic effects of, 189-197
    in hypertrophic obstructive cardiomyopathy, 193-195
    in systemic hypertension, 191-193
    in tetralogy of Fallot, 195-197
  pharmacologic properties of, 189
  side effects of, 209-211
    arrhythmogenic, 210-211
    bradycardia, 209
    complete atrioventricular block, 209
    congestive heart failure, 210
    growth retardation, 211
    on central nervous system, 210
    peripheral vascular effects, 210
    pulmonary, 210
Prostacyclin, 359-363
  clinical pharmacology of, 361
  dosage and administration of, 362
  effects in congestive heart failure, 361
  effects in patent ductus arteriosus, 360
  effects in persistent fetal circulation, 361
  effects in primary pulmonary hypertension, 360-361
  effects in systemic hypertension, 361
  hemodynamic effects of, 359-360
  pharmacologic properties of, 359
  side effects of, 362
Prostaglandin E, 341-357
  comparative effects of, in cyanotic and acyanotic congenital heart diseases, 347-348
  dosage and administration of, 354-355
  effects in aortic arch anomalies, 345-346
  effects in complete transposition of great arteries, 344-345
  effects in congestive heart failure, 348-349
  effects in ductus arteriosus, 341-342
    factors determining, 346-347
  effects in hypoplastic left heart syndrome, 345-346
  effects in persistent fetal circulation with pulmonary hypertension, 348
  effects in pulmonary obstruction, 343-344
  effects in tricuspid atresia, 343
  side effects of, 350-354
    cardiovascular, 351
    cortical hyperostosis, 354
    cutaneous, 353

gastrointestinal, 353
hematologic, 354
metabolic, 354
related to central nervous system, 351-352
renal failure, 354
respiratory depression, 352
structural change in ductus arteriosus, 352-353
structural change in pulmonary circulation, 352
therapeutic administration in children, initiation of, 349-350
monitoring of, 350
principles of, 342-343
vascular effects of, 341
Prostaglandins and prostaglandin-synthesis inhibitors, 337-376
general effects of, 338
indomethacin, 365-376
introduction to, 337-339
prostacyclin, 359-363
prostaglandin E, 341-357
structure and classification of, 337-338
See also specific agents
Pulmonary circulation, prostaglandin E effects on, 352
Pulmonary function, prazosin effect on, 152
propranolol effect on, 197
Pulmonary hypertension, captopril effect on, 167
diazoxide effect on, 146
diltiazem effect on, 100
nifedipine effect on, 87-90
prostacyclin effects in, 360-361
prostaglandin E effects in, 348
verapamil effect on, 74-75
Pulmonary obstruction, prostaglandin E effects on, 343-344
Pulmonary vascular disease(s), hydralazine effects on, 114-115

QT syndrome, prolonged, amiodarone effect on, 312
Quinidine, 237-244
clinical pharmacology, 240
compared with propafenone, 294
dosage and administration of, 242
drug interactions of, 240-241
with amiodarone, 320
with digitalis glycosides, 26
with propranolol, 211
effects on arrhythmias, 238-239
electrophysiologic effects of, 237-238
hemodynamic effects of, 239-240
pharmacologic properties of, 237

side effects of, 242
structure of, 237

Respiratory depression, prostaglandin E effects on, 352
Retrolental fibroplasia, indomethacin effects and, 372

Salbutamol, compared with dobutamine, 47
Saralasin, 179-180
Sex hormones(s), propranolol effect on, 206
Sinoatrial node, digitalis glycoside effects on, 9-10
diltiazem effect on, 96
phenytoin effect on, 266
propafenone effect on, 288
verapamil effect on, 64
Sinus node, dysfunction of, amiodarone effect on, 311-312
mexiletine effect on, 276
procainamide effect on, 246
propranolol effect on, 198-199
Sinus tachycardia, verapamil effect on, 65
Skin, amiodarone effect on, 317
phenytoin effect on, 270
prostaglandin E effects on, 353
Sotalol, 228
Supraventricular arrhythmia(s), mexiletine effect on, 279
phenytoin effect on, 268-269
Supraventricular tachycardia, amiodarone effect on, 308-309
digitalis glycosides for, 12-14
diltiazem effects on, 97-98
propafenone effect on, 290-292
propranolol effect on, 200-201
quinidine effect on, 239
verapamil effect on, 65-67
Systemic hypertension, captopril effect on, 162-167
combined with other drugs, 164
in children, 164-165
in chronic renal failure and renal transplantation, 167
in neonates, 165-167
mechanisms of, 163
clonidine effects on, 380
diazoxide effects on, 145-146
diltiazem effects on, 100
hemodynamic effects of, 386
hydralazine effects on, 115-116
methyldopa effects on, 385-386
minoxidil effects on, 137-138
nifedipine effects on, 90-91
nitroprusside effects on, 124-125

Systemic hypertension *(continued)*
  prazosin effects on, 152
  propranolol effects on, 191-193
  prostacyclin effects in, 361
  saralasin effects on, 179
  verapamil effects on, 74
Systemic lupus erythematosus, hydralazine and, 117

Takayasu's disease, captopril effect on, 170-171
Tetralogy of Fallot, propranolol effect on, 195-197
Thrombocytopenia, hydralazine and, 117
Thyroid, amiodarone effect on, 318
Thyrotoxicosis, propranolol effect on, 204-205
Timolol, 227-228
Tolazoline, 157-158
Transposition of great arteries, prostaglandin E effects on, 344-345
Tricuspid atresia, prostaglandin E effects on, 343

Urticaria, amiodarone and, 317

Valvar disease(s), prazosin effects on, 151
Vasodilators, 105-180
  agents affecting renin-angiotensin system, 159-180
    introduction to, 159
  alpha-adrenoreceptor blocking agents, 149-158
  direct-acting, 107-148
  drug interaction of, with digitalis glycosides, 27
  introduction to, 105-106
  See also specific agents
Ventricle(s), digitalis glycoside effects on, 11
  diltiazem effect on, 97
  mexiletine effect on, 277
  phenytoin effect on, 267
  procainamide effect on, 247-248
  propafenone effect on, 289-290
  propranolol effect on, 200
  verapamil effect on, 65
Ventricular arrhythmia(s), amiodarone effect on, 310-311
  digitalis glycosides for, 15-16
  mexiletine effect on, 278-279
  phenytoin effect on, 267-268
  propafenone effect on, 292-293
  propranolol effect on, 203-204
  quinidine effect on, 239
Ventricular septal defect, captopril effect on, 171-172
  hydralazine effects on, 111-113
  nitroprusside effects on, 125-126
Verapamil, clinical pharmacology of, 75-76
  compared with other antiarrhythmic drugs, 68-69
  determination of plasma levels in, 80
  dosage and administration of, 79-80
  drug interaction of, with digitalis glycosides, 26
  effects on arrhythmias and, 65-69
    atrial fibrillation and flutter, 67-68
    sinus tachycardia, 65
    supraventricular tachycardia, 65-67
    ventricular arrhythmias, 68
  effects on hypertrophic cardiomyopathy, 69-73
    hemodynamic effects and, 69-70
    mechanism of action and, 72-73
    relief of symptoms and, 70-72
    selection of patients and, 72
  electrophysiologic effects of, 63-65
    accessory atrioventricular pathways and, 65
    atria and, 64
    atrioventricular node and, 64-65
    sinoatrial node and, 64
    ventricles and, 65
  electroversion after administration of, 68
  hemodynamic effects of, 73-75
    angina pectoris and, 75
    in presence of beta-adrenergic blockade, 73-74
    pulmonary hypertension and, 74-75
    systemic hypertension and, 74
  mechanism of action of, 63
  overdose of, 78-79
  side effects of, 77-78
  structure of, 63

Warfarin, drug interaction of, with propafenone, 296

**NO LONGER THE PROPERTY
OF THE
UNIVERSITY OF R. I. LIBRARY**